D1544859

WITHDRAWN

UNDERSTANDING NICOTINE AND TOBACCO ADDICTION

Novartis Foundation Symposium 275

UNDERSTANDING NICOTINE AND TOBACCO ADDICTION

2006

John Wiley & Sons, Ltd

Contents

Participants

David Balfour Section of Psychiatry, Division of Pathology & Neuroscience, Ninewells Hospital & Medical School, Dundee DD1 9SY, UK

Daniel Bertrand Department of Neurosciences, Faculty of Medicine, University of Geneva, CH-1211 Geneva 4, Switzerland

Arthur L. Brody UCLA Department of Psychiatry, 300 UCLA Medical Plaza, Ste 2200, Los Angeles, CA 90095, USA

Lisiane Bizarro *(Novartis Foundation Bursar)* Instituto de Psicologia, Universidade Federal do Rio Grande do Sul, Rua Ramiro Barcelos 2600, RS-90035-003, Brazil

Anthony Caggiula Department of Psychology, University of Pittsburgh, 3131 Sennott Square, 210 Bouquet Street, Pittsburgh, PA 15260, USA

Jean-Pierre Changeux Receptors and Cognition Laboratory, Institut Pasteur, 25 Rue du Dr Roux, F-75724 Paris 15, France

Cristiano Chiamulera Section in Pharmacology, Department of Medicine and Public Health, University of Verona, P.le L. Scuro, 10, I-37100 Verona, Italy

Paul B. S. Clarke Department of Pharmacology and Therapeutics, McGill University, 3655 Promenade Sir-William-Osler, Room 1325, Montreal, QC H3G 1Y6, Canada

William A. Corrigall *(Chair)* Corrigall Consulting, 48 Highland Park Blvd., Thornhill, ON L3T 1B3, Canada, and Minneapolis Medical Research Foundation, 914 South Eighth Street Minneapolis, MN 55404, USA

Fabrizio Gasparini Neuroscience Research, Novartis Institute for BioMedical Research Basel, WSJ-386.715, Postfach, CH-4002 Basel, Switzerland

Peter Hajek Tobacco Dependence Research Centre, Barts and The London, Queen Mary's School of Medicine and Dentistry, Turner Street, Whitechapel, London E1 2AD, UK

Christian Heidbreder   Centre of Excellence for Drug Discovery in Psychiatry, GlaxoSmithKline Pharmaceuticals, I-37135 Verona, Italy

Martin J. Jarvis   Department of Epidemiology and Public Health, University College London, Gower Street, London WC1E 6BT, UK

Caryn Lerman   Transdisciplinary Tobacco Use Research Center, University of Pennsylvania, 3535 Market Street, Suite 4100, Philadelphia, PA 19104, USA

Athina Markou   Molecular and Integrative Neurosciences Department, SP2400 The Scripps Research Institute, 10550 North Torrey Pines Road, La Jolla, CA 92037, USA

Kenneth Perkins   WPIC University of Pittsburgh, 3811 O'Hara St, Pittsburgh, PA 15213, USA

Richard Peto   Clinical Trial Service Unit and Epidemiological Studies Unit, Radcliffe Infirmary, Oxford OX2 6HE, UK

Marina R. Picciotto   Yale University, Department of Psychiatry, 34 Park Street, CMHC 3 Fl, New Haven, CT 06520, USA

Jane Powell   Room 309 Whitehead Building, Psychology Department, Goldsmiths College, University of London, New Cross, SE14 6NW

Saul Shiffman   Department of Psychology, University of Pittsburgh, Sennott Square, 3rd Floor, 210 S. Bouquet Street (corner of Forbes), Pittsburgh, PA 15260, USA

Ian Stolerman   Section of Behavioural Pharmacology, Institute of Psychiatry PO49, King's College London, De Crespigny Park, London SE5 8AF, UK

Rachel F. Tyndale   Centre for Addiction and Mental Health, Department of Pharmacology, Room 4326, Medical Sciences Building, 1 King's College Circle, University of Toronto, Toronto, Ontario M5S 1A8, Canada

Gino Van Heeke   Novartis Institute for Biochemical Research, Wimblehurst Road, Horsham, West Sussex RH12 5AB, UK

Robert Walton   Department of Clinical Pharmacology, University of Oxford, Radcliffe Infirmary, Woodstock Road, Oxford, OX2 6HE, UK

Robert West   Cancer Research UK Health Behaviour Unit, Department of Epidemiology and Public Health, University College London, Brook House, 2–16 Torrington Place, London WC1E 6BT, UK

Chair's introduction

William A. Corrigall

Corrigall Consulting, 48 Highland Park Blvd., Thornhill, ON L3T 1B3, Canada

The presentations at this meeting break down into five areas. The first is the characterization and definition of nicotine and tobacco addiction. The second deals with nicotinic receptors. The third involves brain pathways and neurotransmitters involved in nicotine and tobacco addiction. Genetic susceptibility is a fourth issue, and the fifth is medications for nicotine and tobacco addiction.

In terms of characterizing nicotine and tobacco addiction, there are some immediate issues that need discussion. How do we define nicotine and tobacco addiction? In my opinion, resolution of this is something that should be high on our list of priorities. If we look across the range of current definitions, there are disparate elements, factors and dimensions being used.

How do we reduce tobacco and nicotine addiction to studiable elements? Is there a single concept or definition for the disease but various sub-dimensions, the study of which is logical to advance the field and to advance medication development? What cellular or animal models can we use to achieve such advances in basic biology? How can we deconstruct the disease into logical models for human experimental research? And what are appropriate components of the disease in clinical trials?

We need to turn our attention to the full set of nicotinic receptors that could be involved in nicotine addiction. An extensive focus on the mid-brain dopamine system has guided some of the focus on the nicotinic receptor subtypes involved in addictive processes. This is only sensible. As the span of neurochemical targets is broadening, however, we should look at how other nicotinic receptors might be involved. Where is this full set of receptors located in the CNS? How do they influence local CNS function, both at the individual cell level and at the local circuitry level? What are the response dynamics of these receptors when ligand binding occurs?

At the last of these meetings on this topic, 16 years ago (Ciba Foundation 1990), there was clearly a focus on the midbrain dopamine system. This focus has remained, as indeed it has with drug abuse in general. The present meeting affords a good opportunity for us to review where we have been and where we might go with this concept, while at the same time broadening our focus to other neurochemical targets.

1

What are the new approaches that exist by which we might make progress in understanding neurochemical pathways involved in nicotine addiction?

With regard to genetic susceptibility, the obvious issue is the question of what underlies the high heritability of nicotine addiction. What are the phenotypes of interest? What are the polymorphisms of interest? These relate to the neurochemical substrates that have been discovered. However, we have not yet accounted for all of the variance, and there must be other key elements.

Finally, we come to medications for nicotine and tobacco addiction. Here we need to examine the mechanisms of the various nicotine-replacement therapies that account for their effectiveness. Also, what is their effectiveness? What are the mechanisms of other non-nicotinic medications? Do all existing medications have essentially the same effectiveness? What are the prospects for medications that have a non-CNS base of action, such as a nicotine vaccine or medications that interfere with the metabolism of nicotine? Also, how can we improve the translation of science to practice? Are there realistic ways to proceed today to help move discovery science to development more expeditiously?

Through these five key themes of this symposium, there are a number of overarching issues. The one I would raise at the outset is that we are talking about both nicotine and tobacco. Nicotine addiction may be a large or small part of tobacco addiction. We need to recognize this in medication development. Behavioural influences and sociocultural factors are also important. Is the tobacco-addicted individual in the same situation as a person addicted to cocaine or opioids, for example?

A second issue relevant to the whole is that substantial resources will be needed for us to advance this work. This is an issue both for funding agencies and also for those of us who practise in the field. As a part of the research community, we need to think about ways we can contribute to making progress with existing funding realities. And finally it would be valuable to give some thought to how we as a community can help to effect the substantial agreement that will be required to resolve different points of view? These are some of the questions that I hope we will consider at this meeting.

Reference

Ciba Foundation 1990 The biology of nicotine dependence. Wiley, Chichester (Ciba Found Symp 152)

The hazards of smoking and the benefits of stopping

Richard Peto and Richard Doll[1]

Clinical Trial Service Unit & Epidemiological Studies Unit (CTSU), Richard Doll Building, Old Road Campus, Oxford OX3 7LF, UK

Abstract. In developed countries such as the USA, where cigarette smoking has been widely prevalent for many decades, tobacco is now responsible for about one-third of all cancer deaths, including 90% of the lung cancer deaths and 10–15% of the other cancer deaths. In middle age the proportions are even higher, with tobacco accounting for fully half of all male and a quarter of all female US cancer deaths at ages 0–69. The age-standardized cancer death rates from tobacco have reached their peak in US males, but are still increasing in US females. (There is no good evidence for any other increase in US cancer mortality rates during the past few decades over and above the changes that could plausibly be attributed to tobacco.) In addition, tobacco kills even more people by other diseases than by cancer, and is now responsible for about one-third of all US deaths in middle age. Elsewhere, the epidemic is generally at an earlier stage, but is evolving. For example, current male mortality from tobacco is only three-quarters as great in Spain or Portugal as in the USA, but is still increasing rapidly. Among Spanish and Portuguese women a strange situation exists. Few older women have been persistent cigarette smokers, so at present few are dying from the effects of tobacco. Nowadays, however, about half of the young women become cigarette smokers, and if they persist in the habit then about half will eventually be killed by it. Thus, although the epidemic of death from tobacco may soon be approaching its maximum in men, it is only just beginning in Spanish and Portuguese women. Turning from the world as a whole to the individual, about half of all persistent cigarette smokers are eventually killed by their habit, but stopping works remarkably well. Even in middle age, those who stop before they have incurable lung cancer or some other serious disease avoid most of their subsequent risk of death from tobacco, and for those who stop before middle age the benefits are even greater. A billion people now smoke: hundreds of millions of them will be killed by their habit, but if even a moderate proportion of those who now smoke can manage to escape the habit, many tens of millions of premature deaths will be avoided

2006 Understanding nicotine and tobacco addiction. Wiley, Chichester (Novartis Foundation Symposium 275) p 3–16

---

[1] Sir Richard Doll died in July 2005, after a short illness. He and Sir Richard Peto prepared this article in April 2005, on the occasion of the award to them of the King Faisal International Prize for Medicine in Riyadh, and it appeared posthumously in the proceedings of the King Faisal Award Foundation for 2005.

The smoking of tobacco, particularly in the form of cigarettes, is now generally recognized to be an important cause of disease and to cause a substantially increased risk of death both in middle and old age. What is not generally appreciated is how great the increased risk is and the extent to which it can be avoided by stopping smoking.

Size of risk

The severity of the risk and the large number of diseases that smoking helps to cause are illustrated by the results of two large studies—one in the UK and one in the USA—in which people with known smoking habits have been followed up and the mortality rates of different categories of smokers among them (regular smokers of different numbers of cigarettes, ex-smokers, and life-long non-smokers) are compared. The findings show that the mortality of continuing cigarette smokers is, on average, at least twice that of life-long non-smokers throughout middle and old age. In other words, for those who smoke cigarettes regularly smoking is, in adult life in the UK and the USA, as hazardous as all other causes of death combined, resulting in 1 in 4 of continuing smokers dying because of their habit in middle age (that is, from 35–69 years of age) with those killed by tobacco losing on average 21 years of life, and 1 in 4 dying in old age with those killed by tobacco losing an average of 8 years of life.

This enormous effect is not due to just one chemical or the production of just one disease, but to a wide range of different chemicals—some 4000 having been identified in cigarette smoke—and to a wide range of different diseases. Some 40 diseases are now known to be increased in incidence by smoking, varying from cancer of the lung, the incidence of which is increased so much that at one time over 90% of cases in the UK were due to smoking, through 15 other types of cancer, some of which are only occasionally caused by smoking, myocardial infarction, stroke, and gastric and duodenal ulcers, to the obvious and utterly miserable chronic obstructive lung disease (or chronic bronchitis and emphysema as it is often called).

Two tables illustrate the findings for the diseases most closely related to smoking. Table 1 shows the ratio of the mortality rates in continuous cigarette smokers to those of life-long non-smokers observed in the two studies to which we referred earlier. One study is of 34 000 male British doctors who reported their smoking habits in 1951 and have been followed for 40 years reporting changes in their habits periodically throughout (Doll et al 1994). The other is of a million men and women who reported their smoking habits to the American Cancer Society and have been followed for 10 years. The first two years observations in this study are, however, omitted to reduce the so-called 'healthy respondent effect': that is, the effect of excluding people already known to be ill at the start of a study. Women, it can be

TABLE 1 Ratio of mortality of cigarette smokers and lifelong non-smokers: diseases closely related to smoking

Cause of death	Percentage of all deaths, England and Wales, 2003	British Doctors 1951–1991, men	US Population 1984–1991	
			Men	Women
Cancers of mouth, pharynx and larynx	0.4	24.0	11.4	6.9
Cancer of oesophagus	1	7.5	5.6	9.8
Cancer of lung	5.6	14.9	23.9	14.0
Aortic aneurysm	1.6	4.1	6.3	8.2
Peripheral vascular disease	0.1	—	9.7	5.7
Chronic bronchitis and emphysema	4.5	12.7	17.6	16.2
Pulmonary heart disease	0.3	*	—	—
Peptic ulcer	0.7	3.0	4.6	4.0

*No death reported in non-smokers.

seen, died just like men from diseases caused by smoking when they had smoked as long as men, as they have now done in the USA. Table 2, limited to data from the British study, shows for seven of the same eight diseases (or groups of diseases), the differences in mortality between continuing smokers and ex-smokers and between continuing cigarette smokers with different daily consumptions of cigarettes. The rates are consistently higher in continuing smokers than in ex-smokers and in heavy smokers than in light smokers. For pulmonary heart disease we have had to show mortality rates rather than ratios for smokers compared with lifelong non-smokers as there was no death from this disease in a lifelong non-smoker.

The many other diseases caused in part by smoking are shown in Tables 3 and 4. Some are too rare or too seldom fatal in Western populations nowadays to have been detected in these follow-up studies of mortality, while some are only weakly

TABLE 2   **Diseases closely related to smoking: ex-smokers and current smokers by amount**

		Mortality compared with non-smokers		
			Current smoking per day	
Cause of death	Ex-smoker	Any amount	1–14 cigarettes	25 or more cigarettes
Cancers of mouth, pharynx and larynx	3.0	24.0	12.0	48.0
Cancer of oesophagus	4.8	7.5	4.3	11.3
Cancer of lung	4.1	14.9	7.5	25.4
Aortic aneurysm	2.2	4.1	2.5	5.4
Chronic bronchitis and emphysema	5.7	12.7	8.6	22.5
Peptic ulcer	1.5	3.0	1.4	4.5
Pulmonary heart disease	(7)*	(10)	(5)	(21)

*Mortality rate per 100 00 per year as the rate in non-smokers was zero and the ratios consequently infinite.

related to smoking, so that very large numbers and evidence to exclude confounding have been needed, both of which are most easily obtained in specially designed case-control studies. Ten further types of cancer are listed in Table 3. Their relative importance varies from country to country depending on the background incidence of the disease, as smoking interacts with other causes producing, for example, about a 50% increase in the risk of cancer of the stomach irrespective of whether this disease is uncommon, as in the USA, or very common, as in China.

Fifteen other diseases or groups of disease caused in part by smoking are listed in Table 4, together with four effects on reproductive health. Some are of great importance because the background incidence is so high, and the outcome potentially so serious, as in the case of ischaemic heart disease and stroke. For some the relationship varies greatly with age, the risk of myocardial infarction, being, for example, increased by about 400% under 55 years of age, when the disease is rare among non-smokers, but by only about 20% over 80 years of age, when the disease is common in non-smokers.

TABLE 3   Other cancers related to smoking

Cancers of

Lip	Nose
Nasopharynx	Stomach
Liver	Pancreas
Kidney	Bladder
Cervix	Bone marrow (acute myeloid leukaemia)

TABLE 4   Other diseases and conditions related to smoking

Ischaemic heart disease	Crohn's disease
Hypertension	Osteoporosis
Myocardial degeneration	Periodontitis
Other heart disease	Tobacco amblyopia
Cerebrovascular disease	Macular degeneration
Arteriosclerosis	Impotence
Pulmonary tuberculosis	Reduced fecundity
Asthma	Reduced fetal growth
Pneumonia	Perinatal mortality
Other respiratory diseases	

Much less evidence is available from these studies of the effects of smoking tobacco in other forms, as at the time the studies were conducted cigarettes had largely replaced other tobacco products in most economically developed countries. It is clear, however, that pipe and cigar smoking, as practised in these countries, were, relatively much less harmful. In our study of British doctors they caused only a fifth as much risk as cigarettes (and cigarette smoking did not become common anywhere until the early years of the last century), so that goes a long way to explain why so little attention was paid to the effects of smoking until the middle of the century. The smoke from pipes and cigars is more irritating than the smoke from cigarettes and its different chemical constitution enables the nicotine in it to be absorbed from the mouth. Hence the smoke tends not to be inhaled and the noxious contents other than nicotine, not being carried into the lungs, are not absorbed and distributed throughout the body to anything like the same extent. The effects of pipe and cigar smoking were consequently seen principally in the mouth, pharynx and oesophagus, where they are as capable of causing cancer as cigarette smoking is. Bidis, on the other hand, which are smoked predominantly in India and some other Eastern countries, are like hand-rolled cigarettes and are just as harmful (Gajalakshmi et al 2003).

When all the effects of different methods of smoking are taken into account, Peto et al (2005) have estimated that 30 years ago smoking was responsible for 34% of all deaths in men in the UK. This enormous mortality could not simply be reduced by encouraging a switch from cigarettes back to cigars and pipes, because the ex-cigarette smoker, who has learnt to inhale, might well continue to do so despite the greater irritation that pipe and cigar smoke is likely to cause; the only really effective method of reducing the risk of smoking is by reducing the proportion of smokers who continue. Few people, however, realize how great a benefit cessation can achieve or that some benefit is obtained by stopping at any age, no matter how old. In fact, it is never too late to stop (given that, for example, lung cancer or some other potentially fatal disease has not already been induced); but the sooner it is stopped the greater the benefit.

Benefits of stopping

One set of observations that makes the benefits of stopping smoking very clear, at least for lung cancer, was obtained in a study aimed at assessing the effects of exposure to the radon that is present in the air in all ordinary buildings (Peto et al 2000). The study was carried out in collaboration with Professor Sarah Darby in Devon and Cornwall, where the highest concentrations of radon in house air in the UK tend to occur. Detailed information had to be obtained about people's smoking habits, as these would nearly always cause a much higher risk than the radon and, unless taken into account, would obscure the effect of the radioactive gas that we were seeking to study. Interviews were obtained with nearly 1000 men and women with lung cancer and over 3000 controls, drawn from hospital patients suffering from diseases not caused by smoking and from a random sample of the general population, matched appropriately by sex and age groups.

The study was carried out in the early 1990s by which time a high proportion of men in the UK had stopped smoking for many years and we were able to estimate, from the results of this study and knowledge of the mortality from lung cancer recorded in the national mortality data, just what the risk of dying from lung cancer by 75 years of age would be in the UK if men and women continued to smoke or gave up at different ages. The results for men are shown in Fig. 1. For lifelong non-smokers the risk (in the absence of other causes of death), was about 0.4%; for men who stopped smoking about at 30 years of age, about 1.7%, for men who stopped at about 50 years of age, it was 6%, while for men who continued to smoke it was 16%. These figures, it should be noted, do not imply that only about 20% of the population are liable to develop the disease. On the contrary; twin studies have shown that hereditary factors are of relatively little importance in determining the

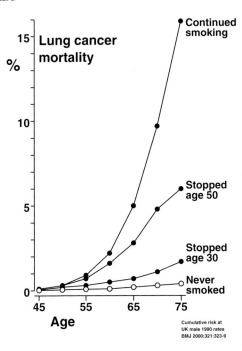

FIG. 1. Cumulative risk of lung cancer by age 75 years at UK male rates 1990 for men who continued to smoke or stopped at different ages.

susceptibility of smokers to lung cancer (Floderus et al 1988, Kaprio & Kosken-vuo 1983, Carmelli & Page 1996). Among smokers with similar patterns of cigarette consumption the difference between those who do and do not develop lung cancer is largely a matter of chance, depending on whether relevant mutations (which are constantly being caused by cigarette smoke in the stem cells of the bronchi) happen to be scattered across different cells or whether one of the stem cells happened, by chance, to accumulate enough mutations to change it into the seed of a growing cancer.

The effect of stopping smoking on the subsequent risk of lung cancer can be seen on a larger scale in the British national data. These show that the prevalence of smoking by men at ages 35–59 years has been progressively reduced since 1950, while it has increased in women of these ages until 1970, before beginning to fall *pari passu* with men (Fig. 2) and that the trends in mortality have followed a few years later until the time came when men and women of these ages had been smoking cigarettes regularly since youth, as is shown for a slightly broader age group (35–69 years) in Fig. 3.

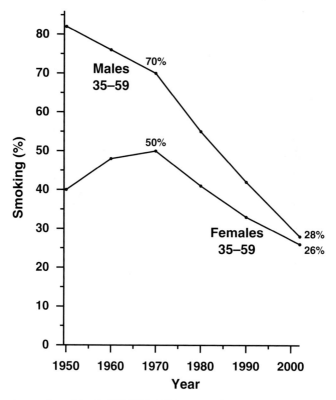

FIG. 2. Prevalence of smoking in UK 1950–2002: men and women aged 35–69 years.

Other diseases

The effect of stopping smoking is not, of course, limited to the risk of lung cancer. We have less precise data for the effect of giving up at different ages on the risk of other diseases. It is seen, however, in Fig. 4 which shows the relative risk of dying from some other diseases or groups of disease in relation to that in non-smokers for men who had given up for different lengths of time. The relative risks are shown for the cancers very strongly related to smoking (lung and larynx) for the other cancers strongly related to smoking (mouth, pharynx, oesophagus, pancreas and bladder) for five cancers weakly related to smoking (nose, stomach, liver, kidney and myeloid leukaemia) and for ischaemic heart disease. All decline progressively, but still remain slightly raised 20 years after stopping. For chronic obstructive lung disease (or chronic bronchitis and emphysema as it used to be called) the trend appears to be different. This, however, is due to the fact that some smokers with

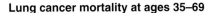

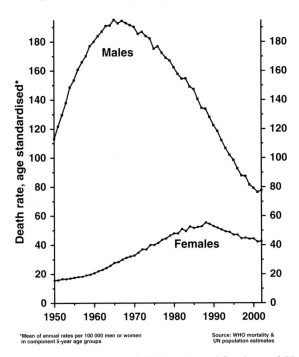

FIG. 3. Mortality from lung cancer UK 1900–2002: males and females aged 35–69 years.

this horrible lung disease stop when disability gets severe, so that the mortality in the first 10 years after stopping is distorted by the inclusion of a number of men who stopped because they were already seriously ill and near to death. We know, however, from a study of transport workers (Fletcher et al 1976, Fletcher & Peto 1977) who were examined every six months over a period of 8 years that the rate of decline of lung function with age among smokers reverts, on average, to the slower rate of decline in non-smokers immediately smoking is stopped.

Total benefit

The total benefit achieved by reducing the risk of all smoking-attributable diseases is seen very clearly in the observations we made of British doctors, whose fate we have followed for 50 years (Doll et al 2004).

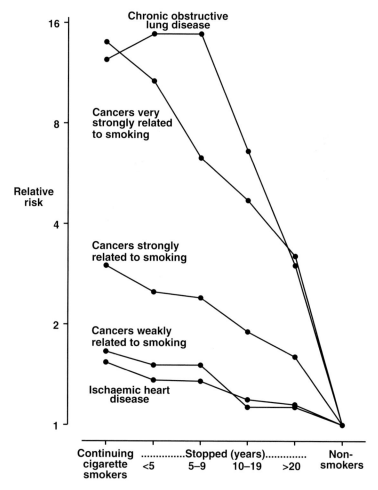

FIG. 4. Relative risk dying of chronic obstructive lung disease, ischaemic heart disease, and three categories of cancer in cigarette smokers who continued to smoke and those who had stopped for different periods of time compared to the risk in life-long non-smokers.

Those who stopped smoking by 35 years of age, in this population at an average age of 29 years, having smoked for not much more than 10 years, had a pattern of survival that did not differ significantly from that of life-long non-smokers. Those who continued smoking lost, on average. 10 years of life expectancy, but those who stopped at ages 60, 50, 40, and 30 years gained by doing so about 3, 6, 9 or the full 10 years respectively.

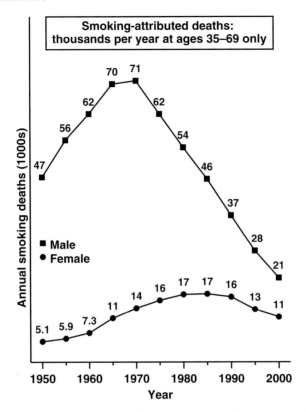

FIG. 5. Annual numbers of deaths attributable to cigarette smoking in males and females aged 35–69 years in the UK between years 1950–2000.

The effect of so many men stopping is seen clearly in the national data. The trend in the prevalence of smoking by men aged 35–69 years of age was shown in Fig. 2 and the trend in the number of deaths at the ages attributed to smoking is shown in Fig. 5. Between 1970 and 2000 the annual number of UK male deaths from smoking fell from about 70 000 to about 20 000 and is still falling, so it is now (2005) only about a quarter of what it was 40 years ago. That among females rose to 17 000 in 1985, since when it too has fallen, and is now (2005) about half of what it was 20 years ago.

Public policy

The findings we have shown have mostly been obtained from observations on men and women in the UK and the USA. There is now, however, ample evidence that much the same overall hazards have been, or will be, observed in all other countries when men and women have been smoking substantial numbers of cigarettes for equally long. This is already clear, for example from studies in China (Lui et al 1999) and India (Gajalakshmi et al 2003). They should, therefore, have a major effect on public policy everywhere.

After the first lecture one of us ever gave on smoking and lung cancer, sometime in the early 1950s, there was a good discussion in the course of which someone said that, if confirmed, our findings with regard to lung cancer were clearly very important. It would, he said, be no good trying to persuade adult smokers to stop as they were already irreversibly addicted to nicotine. The one important thing, he insisted was to discourage young people from starting. On enquiring, this person turned out to be a representative of the tobacco industry. This remains, of course, the industry's policy today. Why? Because as long as adults smoke, children will want to do so too, to show that they are grown-up. It is, however, possible to get many adults to stop smoking. Among adults aged over 50 in Britain, two-thirds of the cigarette smokers have stopped, two-thirds of those who continue say, when interviewed, that they wish they hadn't started and would like to stop, and many of these will eventually succeed in doing so. Most can do it without great difficulty if they really want to. Those most addicted, however, do find it very difficult; but much can now be done to help them. Stopping smoking produces great benefits and, if it can be achieved when smokers are in their 30s, only little harm will have been done. It is, of course, better never to start and if children's role models set the example, there is a good chance that children never will. But adults have to set the example by not smoking themselves.

Acknowledgements

We are very grateful to our colleague Dr Jillian Boreham who has computed for us, over the last 10 years, many of the statistics we have cited and has prepared the figures we have used.

References

Carmelli D, Page WF 1996 Twenty-four year mortality in World War II male veteran twins discordant for cigarette smoking hit. Int J Epidemiol 25:554–559

Doll R, Peto R, Wheatley K, Gray R, Sutherland I 1994 Mortality in relation to smoking: 40 years' observations on male British doctors. Br Med J 309:901–911

Doll R, Peto R, Boreham J, Sutherland I 2004 Mortality in relation to smoking 50 years' observation on male British doctors. Br Med J 328:1519–1528

Fletcher CM, Peto R 1977 The natural history of chronic airflow obstruction. Br Med J 1:1645–1648

Fletcher C, Peto R, Tinker C, Speizer FE 1976 The natural history of chronic bronchitis and emphysema. Oxford University Press, Oxford, UK

Floderus B, Cederlof R, Friberg L 1988 Smoking and mortality: a 21 year follow-up based on the Swedish Twin Registry. Int J Epidemiol 17:332–340

Gajalaksfimi V, Peto R 2003 Smoking and mortality from tuberculosis and other diseases in India. Retrospective study of 43 000 adult male deaths and 35 000 controls. Lancet 362:507–515

Kaprio J, Koskenvuo M 1989 Twins, smoking and mortality: a 12 year prospective study of smoking discordant pairs. Soc Sci Med 29:1083–1089

Liu BQ, Peto R, Chen ZM et al 1998 Emerging tobacco hazards in China: 1. Retrospective proportional mortality study of one million deaths. Br Med J 317:1411–1422

Peto R, Darby S, Deo H, Silcocks P, Whitley E, Doll R 2000 Smoking, smoking cessation and lung cancer in the UK since 1950: combination of national statistics with two case-control studies. BMJ 321:323–329

Peto R, Lopez AD, Boreham J, Thun M 2005 Mortality from smoking 1950–2000. Oxford University Press, Oxford, in press

DISCUSSION

Jarvis: What are your views on the contribution of nicotine to mortality? The focus of this meeting is on nicotine addiction: is there any evidence that it is possible to have populations using nicotine with much lower mortality hazards?

Peto: This is shown clearly by pipe smoking. When it was popular in Britain, it didn't produce anything like the hazard of cigarette smoking, yet it produced comparable nicotine levels. There is a great difference between manufactured cigarettes as nicotine delivery devices and some other devices that have already been tried. The oral tobacco used widely in Sweden seems to give a lot of nicotine with little mortality. The tobacco-containing quids chewed in India cause some risk of oral cancer even among non-smokers, but nothing like the mortality from smoking. Even for cancer of the mouth much the biggest risk is seen with those who both chew and smoke tobacco. As far as I know there is no good evidence that nicotine itself, at the doses used by smokers, is an important toxin. If it could be taken in other ways most of the mortality associated with smoking would be avoided.

Tyndale: One of the controversial areas in the field is smoke exposure reduction, and the benefits of reducing as compared with continuing smoking at the same level or stopping.

Peto: With exposure reduction, the effects depend on whether it is done by using different products. Smokers can try getting their nicotine in ways that are less dangerous, or they can continue to smoke cigarettes and try to reduce the amount they smoke. I think the latter is wholly unrealistic as a strategy. Trying to get people to reduce the number of cigarettes they smoke is hopeless: first they may not keep to it, second they may smoke the remaining cigarettes harder, and third even if you smoke just five cigarettes a day it is probably the most dangerous thing you do. Modification of products available could be important, and the Swedish experience supports this. Ironically, product modification caused the big catastrophe in smoking during the 20th century when people switched from pipes and cigars to manufactured cigarettes.

Tyndale: That's predicated on the idea that we can take someone who is smoking 30 cigarettes per day and have them stop.

Peto: I smoked 30 cigarettes a day and simply stopped, so some people can do it.

Tyndale: But we have a large population who don't seem to be able to do that. So the question is, is there evidence that it is a worthwhile thing to encourage people to cut down, using nicotine or other product alterations to facilitate this?

Peto: For sure, smoking 15 a day is less dangerous than 30 a day.

Tyndale: Do you have data that moving from 30 to 15 cigarettes a day does reduce risk?

Peto: The only data I have seen show that moving from 30 to 15 is a transient state and in that transient state you take more per cigarette and get pretty similar blood levels, and you don't stay at that state very long. It isn't the way to go.

Brody: There is a study on prediction of lung cancer risk (Bach et al 2003) that shows the number of cigarettes smoked during the lifetime is a factor in increased risk.

Shiffman: I don't think there has been a big enough population experiencing this much sustained reduction to even assess the effects.

Jarvis: The best data come from the Multiple Risk Factor Intervention Trial (MRFIT). They used reduced cigarette consumption as one of the design goals of the study. They took the precaution of taking an intake measure, and in men who didn't stop but who cut down over a five year period there was no indication of any reduction in intake markers.

West: In the British doctors' study, in each follow up you have self-reported daily cigarette consumption. You have presumably looked at the pattern of change in this, and whether these changes are related to mortality.

Peto: The problem was that the people who cut down were much more likely next time round to have reported themselves as having stopped. So there is confounding between reduction and cessation. I think reduction is a wrong strategy to pursue, unless it is part of a program that will help people to quit.

Tyndale: Another controversy is the decriminalization of marijuana, and whether that will contribute to the mortality from smoking.

Peto: The problem with marijuana is that it is a gateway drug: it is often smoked with tobacco and people get addicted to nicotine.

Reference

Bach PB, Kattan MW, Thornquist MD et al 2003 Variations in lung cancer risk among smokers. J Natl Cancer Inst 95:470–478

Animal models for nicotine dependence

Ian Stolerman

Section of Behavioural Pharmacology, Institute of Psychiatry P049, King's College London, De Crespigny Park, London SE5 8AF, UK

Abstract. Nicotine dependence is not a consequence of a single psychological or physiological process, but of many different, interacting elements. Many of the concepts that apply to nicotine dependence are applicable to other drugs from diverse pharmacological classes. A case can be made that models for drug dependence are more comprehensive and have greater validity than those for most psychiatric conditions, but they have been targeted largely towards unveiling the mechanisms of dependence. Increasingly, the need is for models to assess the efficacy of aids to smoking cessation and this paper will consider the extent to which the requirements for such models differ from those for models that focus on mechanisms. Different models reflect successive stages of the dependence process (acquisition, maintenance, extinction, relapse) and are assessed in terms of their face, construct and predictive validity. The roles of reinforcement mechanisms, environmental stimuli that accompany drug-taking, cognitive drug effects and drug withdrawal syndromes have to be taken into account. There is no single model that embraces all aspects of dependence and indeed, such a model would not allow the roles of different mechanisms to be isolated and analysed in relation to the genetic and environmental factors relevant for each individual.

2005 Understanding nicotine and tobacco addiction. Wiley, Chichester (Novartis Foundation Symposium 275) p 17–35

Introduction: the current interest in pharmacotherapies for smoking cessation

This paper does not attempt to catalogue the vast range of animal models for nicotine dependence that are available. The features, advantages and limitations of these models have been described previously. Instead the focus is upon a small number of specific aspects of the topic reflecting major changes in the field that have become apparent in recent years. When in about 1988 I first put forward to some pharmaceutical firms the notion that it would be useful to develop an ultra-long-acting nicotine antagonist as an aid for smoking cessation, the idea was politely but rapidly dismissed. The criticisms were unrelated to the scientific basis for the proposal, or the probable efficacy or safety of the product but reflected opinions that there was no way to market a product for smoking cessation, that nobody had ever successfully developed a medication *ab initio* for treating any form of drug dependence,

17

TABLE 1   The diversity of actual and potential pharmacological aids to smoking cessation

Drug class or specific substance	References
Nicotine replacement therapies	Cummings & Hyland (2005), Silagy et al (2004)
Nicotinic partial agonists (Varenicline)	Coe et al (2005)
Antidepressants (bupropion, nortriptyline, moclobemide)	Berlin et al (1995), Hurt et al (1997), Jorenby et al (1999)
Opioid antagonists (naloxone, naltrexone)	Brauer et al (1999)
Glutamate mGluR5 antagonists (MPEP)	Paterson et al (2003)
Cannabinoid CB1 antagonists (Rimonabant)	Cohen et al (2002)
Dopamine D3 receptor ligands (BP 897)	Pilla et al (1999), Le Foll et al (2005)
GABA$_B$ agonists (Baclofen, CGP44532)	Cousins et al (2001), Fattore et al (2002), Paterson et al (2004)
Corticotrophin releasing factor antagonists	Cryan et al (2003)
Glucose	West (2001)
Immunotherapies ('vaccines')	Hieda et al (1997), Cerny et al (2002), de Villiers et al (2002), Keyler et al (1999)

and that it would be damaging for a firm to become associated in any way with drug dependence. At that time the only pharmacotherapy with established efficacy for smoking cessation was nicotine replacement therapy (NRT) and even now bupropion is the only alternative substance that has actually reached the market. Although the concerns that industry had 25 years ago have not been entirely eradicated, the present situation is very different (Cryan et al 2003, George & O'Malley 2004). Table 1 lists agents from the diverse pharmacological classes that are seen as having potential therapeutic value and that are at various stages of development ranging from laboratory animal studies to Phase 3 clinical trials. In view of all this activity directed towards pharmacotherapy of smoking, the availability of appropriate, valid and practical animal models is particularly important.

Defining the targets for animal models

Modelling requires definition of that which is to be modelled. Attention has become increasingly directed towards not simply the demonstration of drug intake by animals, but more specifically upon distinctions between drug-seeking and drug taking. Equally important, drug-directed behaviour needs to be of an impressive strength and power if it is to comply with the 'compulsive behaviour' aspect of influential definitions such as those of the World Health Organization (WHO) and American Psychiatric Association. The WHO, as long ago as 1969, included the words 'compulsion to take a drug' in its definition of dependence (WHO 1969) and paralleling this concept 20 years later, five of seven DSM-IV criteria reflected aspects of compulsive use, such as greater use than intended, much time spent on seeking the substance and continued use despite knowledge of harms caused (American Psychiatric Association 1994).

Drug dependence, nevertheless, has numerous components that work together to engender compulsive intake. The most frequently used models include the assessment of positively reinforcing effects in self-administration procedures and of identifiable cueing (subjective) effects in drug discrimination experiments. It is widely recognized that drug-related environmental stimuli are of profound importance, and that drug intake shows distinguishable phases of acquisition, maintenance and relapse. Different models are required to reflect these diverse aspects of dependence. The range is further extended by procedures for assessing neuroadaptations (tolerance, sensitization and withdrawal) that develop as a result of repetitive and long-term exposure to drugs. It is worth noting that animal models for withdrawal syndromes exist for drugs of virtually all pharmacological classes known to be abused (including nicotine), with the classical hallucinogens being the only exceptions at this time. Underpinning these adaptations seen at the system and whole organism levels are functional changes in cellular and molecular function that may play a crucial role in the future modelling of dependence, once causal relationships with systemic function are more fully identified than is the case now. This article however concentrates on the behavioural features relevant to models of drug intake and does not attempt to deal in an equivalent manner with assessments of neuroadaptations.

It should be apparent from the preceding discussion that the term dependence is used in this article to refer to the full range of processes and mechanisms related to tobacco addiction and not exclusively in relation to the nicotine withdrawal syndrome (so-called 'physical dependence'). It follows that valid models for specific aspects of dependence need not involve subjects that display signs or symptoms of nicotine withdrawal. This is particularly apposite to nicotine self-administration procedures in which animals do not exhibit withdrawal; the model nevertheless retains validity for assessing the reinforcing effects of nicotine independently from the impact of withdrawal.

Implications of the chronic nature of nicotine dependence

Consideration of dependence as a chronic relapsing condition also has implications for models that have not been considered fully. Increasingly it is being recognized that a single treatment or short course of treatment will rarely have permanent or even long-lasting effects, as argued convincingly by McLellan et al (2000). Drug taking and dependence go though clearly distinguishable stages of acquisition, maintenance, detoxification and relapse that comprise the addiction cycle. Models for testing treatments need to take into account the ways in which medications are used clinically and especially the stages of the addiction cycle during which they are applied.

Let us consider the presently approved treatments, NRT and bupropion. These are typically used for a period of several weeks during the detoxification phase yet the criterion for clinical success is based primarily upon abstinence rates six months or even one year later. Long-term abstinence is an entirely appropriate goal, but is there any pharmacological basis for believing that either of these medications has effects that last that long? Most effects of nicotine and bupropion wear off within a few hours. Long-term potentiation induced by nicotine may persist despite receptor desensitization and after the drug has been cleared from the body (Mansvelder & McGehee 2000), but probably not for months! Expecting NRT to have effects after six months may be unrealistic. Do we expect blood pressure to remain low after treatment with antihypertensives is discontinued, or diabetes to be 'cured' by insulin three times a day for a few weeks or schizophrenics by a short course of antipsychotics (McLellan et al 2000)? It is widely agreed that relapse to tobacco use is a major problem that reveals the limitation of current treatments, but does it make sense to test drugs such a bupropion on models for relapse when clinically it is used during detoxification? Yet many of us are in the habit of thinking that as relapse is a major problem, we should test all our treatments on the reinstatement of drug seeking and drug taking. Perhaps this should only be the case for treatments designed to target processes specific to relapse. The current 'launchpad' model of treatment assumes that whatever the distortion to the motivational system caused by chronic drug use, normalization occurs within a few weeks. Perhaps this is true in a small number of cases but the clinical evidence suggests that it is not for most.

Advantages and limitations of some currently used models

Procedures for assessing the effects of drugs desired and sought after by their users are quite diverse. The procedure with most obvious face validity is intravenous self-administration insofar as it reflects most closely the concept of drug-induced reinforcement of behaviour. It also has good construct validity in relation to behavioural approaches to drug-taking and can have high predictive validity with regard to the abuse liability of different classes of drug (Young & Herling 1986). Nevertheless, it is an invasive procedure that requires substantial technical skills and care of animals, and the viability of preparations is inversely related to the size of sub-jects so that lengthy training under ideal and often complex schedules of rein-forcement becomes progressively less feasible as one moves from primate to rat to mouse. Rates of responding are also subject to multiple influences in addition to the reinforcing effects of drugs. These and other limitations have prompted the use of alternative procedures that are claimed also to assess reinforcing effects, but usually less directly and with theoretical limitations that counter, to varying extents, their practical advantages.

Conditioned place preference (CPP) is non-invasive and superficially simpler than self-administration. This method entails the association of the effects of a drug administered by an experimenter with a particular set of environmental stimuli; drug-seeking is then inferred from a tendency of the animal to spend more time in the drug-associated environment than in a control setting. In practice it is also labour-intensive and its relationship to the reinforcing effects of drugs is indirect and subject to at least as many confounding influences as rates of responding. There is also a need to take great care to avoid misleading conclusions due to drug actions on and biases related to the natural preferences or aversions to the different envi-ronments that are integral to the procedure. Carr et al (1989) discussed in detail many of the practical and theoretical limitations of CPP. Intracranial self-stimulation has been increasingly used as a direct marker for drug action on the mesolimbic dopamine system, the most frequently studied of the brain's reward pathways. Drug actions on threshold currents for self-stimulation are relatively independent of confounding effects on rates of responding, construct validity is favourable insofar as the mesolimbic system is the appropriate one for a particular drug, and there appears to be good predictive validity in relation to abuse potential (Esposito et al 1978, Kornetsky & Bain 1992). Changes in thresholds for self-stimulation also serve as a valuable model for quantifying motivationally relevant aspects of the nicotine withdrawal syndrome (Epping-Jordan et al 1998) and studies on the inter-relationships of such effects with patterns of self-administration are beginning to appear (Paterson et al 2004). Nevertheless, it needs to be recognized that the procedure assesses drug actions on a hypothesized mechanism for drug-induced reinforcement rather than directly demonstrating that a drug can serve as a reinforcer; neither drug-taking nor drug-seeking is involved.

Another non-invasive approach, much used by the author of this article, entails the use of drug discrimination methodology for training subjects to obtain non-drug reinforcers by making differential responses according to whether or not they can detect the presence of a drug in the body (Stolerman 1993). In the majority of experiments, it involves training an animal to obtain food reinforcers by pressing one lever when it detects that a drug has been administered and a different lever when only the vehicle for drug delivery has been given. These procedures do not assess reinforcing effects of drugs but their ability to produce recognizable internal states. The ability of a drug to produce an identifiable effect is probably necessary for it to be abused but it certainly is not sufficient because identifiable effects can be motivationally rewarding, neutral or aversive. The major strengths of this non-invasive procedure include its applicability to every class of abused substance including hallucinogens, its pharmacological specificity and an ability to produce highly reproducible, monotonically ascending dose-response curves that facilitate analyses of neuronal mechanisms of drug action. It is limited by uncertainty as to where the ability to recognize drug effects relates to other psychological mechanisms that have a more tightly defined role in dependence and by its complex relationship to reinforcing effects. As in the case of intracranial self-stimulation methodology, neither drug-taking nor drug-seeking is involved. Nevertheless, it is argued here that these procedures should be used more extensively than is presently the case because of their favourable pharmacological characteristics. Self-administration and drug discrimination studies with nicotinic receptor knockout mice agree on the importance of $\beta2$ subunits in the behavioural response to nicotine (Shoaib et al 2002, Maskos et al 2005, 2006).

The relapse stage of the dependence cycle is frequently modelled in laboratory animals by means of reinstatement procedures (Shaham et al 2003). These methods entail first the establishment of drug self-administration and then its suppression by extinction procedures. Reinstatement is then triggered by the presentation of relapse-provoking events of which there are three presently known classes, these being (i) drugs, (ii) drug-associated cues and (iii) environmental stressors. These are elegant experimental techniques but should not be used uncritically. Drug-induced reinstatement may rarely be clinically relevant and human abstinence is not often brought about through extinction procedures that parallel those in current animal reinstatement procedures (Hughes 2002). And as noted earlier, current and most planned pharmacotherapies are not intended for use in the relapse phase but would be applied during detoxification and not used for relapse prevention, although trials have been conducted and this is certainly an option in future years. Reinstatement methodology may become exceptionally important and useful if treatments are developed with a rational basis for a long-term effect. Of the approaches listed in Table 1, only immunotherapy seems targeted to a long-term effect outlasting the period during which the therapeutic agent is administered.

Sophisticated self-administration procedures: measurement issues

As self-administration procedures are the only models that assess directly drug-seeking and drug-taking, it is important to consider whether these methods adequately reflect clinical situations and definitions. How would we know if a self-administration model captures the compulsive nature of dependence? High rates of responding maintained robustly with the drug delivered on simple schedules of reinforcement such as fixed ratio and fixed interval may be a necessary but insufficient criterion because direct drug effects influence response rates. Additionally, more sophisticated techniques than simple rates of responding are needed to explore fully the reinforcing power of non-drug stimuli. A further step therefore is to assess the value of the drug to the animal by increasing the work load for obtaining it (progressive ratio schedules). This approach is being increasingly used for nicotine (Donny et al 1999), as it has proven valuable for drugs from other classes. In addition, models might aim to reflect compulsivity by showing persistent responding despite knowledge of adverse consequences. Thus, aversive events might accompany drug taking and compulsivity would be shown by the extent to which behaviour continued in the face of such punishment. Punishing stimuli can be either unconditioned noxious events or conditioned stimuli that signal the likelihood that unconditioned punishing stimuli will be presented. Models of nicotine dependence have not utilized such approaches.

Sophisticated self-administration procedures: tobacco is more than nicotine

Nicotine is not abused as a pure substance but only in tobacco. Many other substances are present in tobacco and especially tobacco smoke; some of these substances modulate the reinforcing value of nicotine. Monoamine oxidase inhibitors (e.g. Fowler et al 1996a, 1996b) may be such substances and acetaldehyde may also be important as it has been found to enhance nicotine self-administration (Belluzzi et al 2005). Tobacco smoke is also not just a means of dosing with pharmacologically active substances. Smoking is associated with consistent, repetitive exposure to the sight, smell and taste of smoke and such stimuli accompany each dose of nicotine. It is notable that in animal experiments, nicotine alone is rather weakly self-administered; robust self-administration requires non-pharmacological, sensory stimuli to be present along with the nicotine. These stimuli may serve as conditioned reinforcers due to Pavlovian conditioning as a result of their pairing with the effects of nicotine. Nicotine may also potentiate the effectiveness of such non-drug stimuli that themselves are only weakly reinforcing. Recent work by Donny et al (2003) suggests that the latter type of mechanism, whereby there is a synergistic interaction between nicotine and non-drug reinforcers, may be of considerable importance. It is possible that such interactions are much more critical for nicotine than for drugs of other pharmacological classes; studies similar to those of Donny et al (2003), but involving drugs such as cocaine and morphine are needed to examine this issue further. Nevertheless, it now appears essential to examine the effects of putative medications for smoking cessation on this interaction.

Animals motivated to stop nicotine self-administration as models for quit attempts?

The question arises as to whether the traditional approach to the use of self-administration for studying potential therapeutic aids is appropriate. Self-administration was developed to facilitate understanding of various behavioural mechanisms and has also provided a valuable tool in assessments of the abuse liability of drugs and of the neuropharmacological mechanisms underlying drug-induced reinforcement. The aim in such studies is to isolate different aspects of dependence so that mechanisms can be distinguished. However, for studies on treatment efficacy, the situation needs to resemble that for smoking cessation. In animal self-administration, a drug that suppresses self-administration is regarded as a potential treatment, but in the clinic, drugs are not used to induce people to stop smoking! NRT and bupropion are used to assist quit attempts that occur in people who are already highly motivated to stop smoking. Indeed, this motivation is regarded as one of the best predictors of attempts to stop smoking. Therefore, a clinically relevant model for testing pharmacotherapies should utilize subjects who have at least some level of motivation to stop self-administering.

Can there be a rodent analogue of a motivated smoker and, if so, what would it be like? Such a model can be built around behavioural processes in the animal that reflect the events that motivate smokers to attempt to quit. From this perspective, motivation in both humans and animals can be seen as consequence of environmental contingencies. People acquire the motivation to quit through the multiple environmental pressures against smoking. These include the growing range of situations where smoking is socially unacceptable and many smokers also wish to stop due to the aversive medical consequences, the illnesses and disabilities that they are actually experiencing. A further group are aware of the serious nature and frequency of smoking-related diseases, are concerned about potential disability and fatality and realizing that they are at risk, try repeatedly to give up, but with little success.

The motivated rat would be one in which the experimenter arranged the environment in such a way as to apply pressure to the self-administering animal to cut down its drug intake. It has been known for many years that cocaine, amphetamine and morphine self-administration rates can be reduced by using mild electric shocks to punish responding (Grove & Schuster 1974, Smith & Davis 1974). Such a situation may be seen as functionally equivalent to the pressure to stop smoking placed upon a patient who is actually suffering from a smoking-related illness. It is also possible to envisage a situation where responding is punished by presentation of visual or auditory stimuli that have been previously paired with shock or another aversive consequence (such as an encounter with an aggressive animal). Suppression of behaviour by such stimuli might be seen as functionally equivalent to the pressures to stop smoking engendered by fear of future disease. Other approaches can also be considered, including some that do not involve presenting noxious stimuli such as shock. For example, the intake of a drug could be associated with reduced access to a positive reinforcer such as food, so that the opportunity to engage in a concurrent, food-reinforced task is withheld when nicotine is self-administered or the work required to obtain the food is increased. Studies have examined how the availability of an alternative, non-drug reinforcer can reduce the intake of phencyclidine (Campbell & Carroll 2000).

Models of the types discussed above have face validity in the sense that both model and the human situation involve drug-taking. There is a similarity of underlying theoretical construct insofar as both involve the behavioural concept of punishment. But to determine whether there will be predictive validity, it is first necessary to establish such models; then they must be tested by assessing the effects both of drugs that have therapeutic value in the clinic and those that are ineffective clinically (and of non-pharmacological procedure to the extent that it is feasible to do so). It will be essential to tackle this final, critical stage of validation if models using 'motivated rats' are to have practical value.

Studies on the punishment of behaviour that is maintained by the reinforcing properties of nicotine do not seem to have been reported but there is an important recent experiment using a closely related approach with cocaine. Vanderschuren & Everitt (2004) showed if stimuli that had previously been associated with foot-shock were presented during self-administration sessions, then rates of responding for cocaine were reduced selectively. This resembles closely but not precisely the model proposed above because Vanderschuren & Everitt (2004) employed a conditioned suppression paradigm in which the conditioned stimuli were presented independently of responding, rather than as a consequence of it as in punishment procedures. Nevertheless, it is conceivable that application to baselines of nicotine self-administration of procedures similar to those of Vanderschuren & Everitt (2004) may provide the model 'motivated rat' that was suggested above as appropriate for studies relating to smoking cessation. There was a further very interesting finding in Vanderschuren & Everitt (2004) to the effect that after prolonged self-administration of cocaine, there was a reduced magnitude of condition suppression. This finding suggests that there was a progression over time from 'controllable' drug intake to a situation where the behaviour had acquired a compulsive nature such that serious consequences that normally inhibit it were no longer effective. This appears to reflect the 'loss of control' over drug intake that is a critical feature of definitions of dependence. The questions arise (1) as to whether such a transition from controlled to relatively uncontrollable intake would occur with nicotine as it did with cocaine and (2) whether the resulting, unsuccessfully suppressed, responding could be provide the basis for a more appropriate model for the smoking cessation situation than the simple self-administration paradigms that are commonly used at present. Would results with currently used drugs such as NRT and bupropion be different and perhaps more importantly, would any novel substance be found to have the ability to selectively enhance punishment or conditioned suppression of nicotine-reinforced responding?

Summary

Dependence on nicotine resembles dependence on classical drugs of abuse in the sense that it has many aspects. No single model covers all of them and thus there can be no single 'best model'. It is increasingly recognized that methods for nicotine self-administration should have features that reflect the human concepts of compulsive intake, loss of control and progression from drug use to drug dependence. The recent emphasis on reinstatement models may not be appropriate because these models are not relevant to current pharmacotherapy that aims to aid quit attempts and which is usually discontinued before the long-term relapse stage is reached. Non-drug cues and stimuli may be especially important for nicotine as compared with other drugs and future models must take full account of that fact. Then, when we have animals 'motivated to quit' we may be in a better position to assess pharmacotherapies for smoking cessation.

Acknowledgement

I thank Professor Robert West for valuable comments on an earlier version of the paper.

References

American Psychiatric Association 1994 Diagnostic and statistical manual of mental disorders, 4th edn. American Psychiatric Association, Washington, DC

Belluzzi JD, Wang R, Leslie FM 2005 Acetaldehyde enhances acquisition of nicotine self-administration in adolescent rats. Neuropsychopharmacol 30:705–712

Berlin I, Said S, Spreux-Varoquaux O et al 1995 A reversible monoamine oxidase A inhibitor (moclobemide) facilitates smoking cessation and abstinence in heavy, dependent smokers. Clin Pharmacol Ther 58:444–452

Brauer LH, Behm FM, Westman EC, Patel P, Rose JE 1999 Naltrexone blockade of nicotine effects in cigarette smokers. Psychopharmacology 143:339–346

Campbell UC, Carroll ME 2000 Reduction of drug self-administration by an alternative non-drug reinforcer in rhesus monkeys: magnitude and temporal effects. Psychopharmacology 147:418–425

Carr GD, Fibiger HC, Phillips AG 1989 Conditioned place preference as a measure of drug reward. In: Liebman JM, Cooper SJ (eds) The neuropharmacological basis of reward. Clarendon Press, Oxford, p 264–319

Cerny EH, Levy R, Mauel J et al 2002 Preclinical development of a vaccine 'against smoking'. Onkologie 25:406–411

Coe JW, Brooks PR, Vetelino MG et al 2005 Varenicline: an alpha4beta2 nicotinic receptor partial agonist for smoking cessation. J Med Chem 48:3474–3477

Cohen C, Perrault G, Voltz C, Steinberg R, Soubrie P 2002 SR141716, a central cannabinoid CB(1) receptor antagonist, blocks the motivational and dopamine-releasing effects of nicotine in rats. Behav Pharmacol 13:451–463

Cousins MS, Stamat HM, de Wit H 2001 Effects of a single dose of baclofen on self-reported subjective effects and tobacco smoking. Nic Tob Res 3:123–129

Cryan JF, Gasparini F, van Heeke G, Markou A 2003 Non-nicotinic neuropharmacological strategies for nicotine dependence: beyond bupropion. Drug Discov Today 8:1025–1034

Cummings KM, Hyland A 2005 Impact of nicotine replacement therapy on smoking behavior. Annu Rev Public Health 26:583–599

de Villiers SH, Lindblom N, Kalayanov G et al 2002 Active immunization against nicotine suppresses nicotine-induced dopamine release in the rat nucleus accumbens shell. Respiration 69:247–253

Donny EC, Caggiula AR, Mielke et al 1999 Nicotine self–administration in rats on a progressive ratio schedule of reinforcement. Psychopharmacologia 147:135–142

Donny EC, Chaudhri N, Caggiula AR et al 2003 Operant responding for a visual reinforcer in rats is enhanced by noncontingent nicotine: implications for nicotine self-administration and reinforcement. Psychopharmacology 169:68–76

Epping-Jordan MP, Watkins SS, Koob GF, Markou A 1998 Dramatic decreases in brain reward function during nicotine withdrawal. Nature 393:76–79

Esposito RU, Motola AH, Kornetsky C 1978 Cocaine: acute effects on reinforcement thresholds for self-stimulation behavior to the medial forebrain bundle. Pharmacol Biochem Behav 8:437–439

Fattore L, Cossu G, Martellotta MC, Fratta W 2002 Baclofen antagonizes intravenous self-administration of nicotine in mice and rats. Alcohol Alcohol 37:495–498

Fowler JS, Volkow ND, Wang G-J et al 1996a Inhibition of monoamine oxidase B in the brains of smokers. Nature 379:733–736

Fowler JS, Volkow ND, Wang GJ et al 1996b Brain monoamine oxidase A inhibition in cigarette smokers. Proc Nat Academy Sci USA 93:14065–14069

George TP, O'Malley SS 2004 Current pharmacological treatments for nicotine dependence. Trends Pharmacol Sci 25:42–48

Grove RN, Schuster CR 1974 Suppression of cocaine self-administration by extinction and punishment. Pharmacol Biochem Behav 2:199–208

Hieda Y, Keyler DE, Vandevoort JT et al 1997 Active immunization alters the plasma nicotine concentration in rats. J Pharmacol Exp Ther 283:1076–1081

Hughes JR 2002 Is extinction in animals the same as abstinence in humans? Addiction 97:1219

Hurt RD, Sachs DPL, Glover ED et al 1997 A comparison of sustained-release bupropion and placebo for smoking cessation. New Eng J Med 337:1195–1202

Jorenby DE, Leischow SJ, Nides MA et al 1999 A controlled trial of sustained-release bupropion, a nicotine patch, or both for smoking cessation. New Eng J Med 340:685–691

Keyler DE, Hieda Y, St Peter J, Pentel PR 1999 Altered disposition of repeated nicotine doses in rats immunized against nicotine. Nic Tob Res 1:241–249

Kornetsky C, Bain G 1992 Brain-stimulation reward: a model for the study of the rewarding effects of abused drugs. In: Frascella J, Brown RM (eds) Neurobiological approaches to brain-behavior interaction. NIDA Research Monograph 124, US Department of Health and Human Services, Rockville, Maryland, p 73–93

Le Foll B, Sokoloff P, Stark H, Goldberg SR 2005 Dopamine D3 receptor ligands block nicotine-induced conditioned place preferences through a mechanism that does not involve discriminative-stimulus or antidepressant-like effects. Neuropsychopharmacol 30:720–730

Mansvelder HD, McGehee DS 2000 Long-term potentiation of excitatory inputs to brain reward areas by nicotine. Neuron 27:349–357

Maskos U, Molles BE, Pons S et al 2005 Nicotine reinforcement and cognition restored by targeted expression of nicotinic receptors. Nature 436:103–107

Maskos U, Granon S, Faure P, Changeux JP 2006 Nicotinic acetylcholine receptors functions in the central nervous system investigated with a novel method of sterotaxic gene re-expression in knockout mice. In: Understanding nicotine and tobacco addiction. Wiley, Chichester (Novartis Found Symp 275), p 64–82

McLellan AT, Lewis DC, O'Brien CP, Kleber HD 2000 Drug dependence, a chronic medical illness: implications for treatment, insurance, and outcomes evaluation. JAMA 284:1689–1695

Paterson NE, Markou A 2004 Prolonged nicotine dependence associated with extended access to nicotine self-administration in rats. Psychopharmacology 173:64–72

Paterson NE, Semenova S, Gasparini F, Markou A 2003 The mGluR5 antagonist MPEP decreased nicotine self-administration in rats and mice. Psychopharmacology 167:257–264

Paterson NE, Froestl W, Markou A 2004 The GABA(B) receptor agonists baclofen and CGP44532 decreased nicotine self-administration in the rat. Psychopharmacology 172:179–186

Pilla M, Perachon S, Sautel F et al 1999 Selective inhibition of cocaine-seeking behaviour by a partial dopamine D3 receptor agonist. Nature 400:371–375

Shaham Y, Shalev U, Lu L, de Wit H, Stewart J 2003 The reinstatement model of drug relapse: history, methodology and major findings. Psychopharmacology 168:3–20

Shoaib M, Gommans J, Morley A, Stolerman IP, Grailhe R, Changeux J-P 2002 The role of nicotinic receptor beta-2 subunits in nicotine discrimination and conditioned taste aversion. Neuropharmacology 42:530–539

Silagy C, Lancaster T, Stead L, Mant D, Fowler G 2004 Nicotine replacement therapy for smoking cessation. Cochrane Database Syst Rev CD000146

Smith SG, Davis WM 1974 Punishment of amphetamine and morphine self-administration behavior. Psychol Record 24:477–480

Stolerman IP 1993 Drug discrimination. In: Van Haaren F (ed) Methods in behavioral pharmacology. Elsevier, Amsterdam, p 217–243

Vanderschuren LJ, Everitt BJ 2004 Drug seeking becomes compulsive after prolonged cocaine self-administration. Science 305:1017–1019

West R 2001 Glucose for smoking cessation: does it have a role? CNS Drugs 15:261–265

Young AM, Herling S 1986 Drugs as reinforcers: studies in laboratory animals. In: Goldberg SR, Stolerman IP (eds) Behavioral analysis of drug dependence. Academic Press, Orlando, Florida, p 9–67

DISCUSSION

Markou: I would like to discuss nicotine self-administration. I agree with Ian Stolerman that it is a matter of degree as to how reinforcing nicotine administration is. Many of our conceptualizations of the reinforcing effects of drugs come from our experiences with cocaine self-administration. Cocaine is definitely more reinforcing than nicotine and also has a shorter half life than nicotine. As a consequence, cocaine leads to regular and predictable self-administration patterns. Therefore, in comparison to cocaine, nicotine is less reinforcing. However, we can readily obtain self-administration of nicotine in all experimental animals, and the behaviour is well maintained, but with different patterns from those we are used to seeing with cocaine. I think nicotine is a reinforcing drug.

Stolerman: There is no doubt that nicotine can serve as a reinforcer. Whether it is best described as weak or strong depends upon criteria. In many ways, tobacco use appears to be more reinforcing than nicotine alone. The number of people who smoke a few cigarettes a day and become long-term users appears to exceed the percentage of people who try cocaine a few times and develop a cocaine problem. I don't think this is reflected in the animal models that we have. I don't want to imply that nicotine self-administration in the animal models has a trivial effect, but if it is pure nicotine in the absence of any stimuli it is widely accepted to be relatively weak in comparison with cocaine. Would you maintain that nicotine without stimuli is as strong as cocaine?

Markou: I know that Tony Caggiula's data are strong on this. In my lab, when we take the conditioned stimuli away there is a decrease in nicotine self-administration, but not as great as the one that Tony Caggiula sees. This difference in results may be due to the fact that he examined the influence of conditioned stimuli during the acquisition phase of the experiment, while we examined what effect the removal of the conditioned stimuli has after the animals had acquired the response and self-administer nicotine for several weeks. The phase of nicotine self-administration (that is, acquisition versus maintenance) may make a big difference in the role of the conditioned stimuli. The point you make about cocaine is important; studies similar to the ones I described above with nicotine self-administration and conditioned stimuli have not been done with cocaine. Perhaps if we did similar studies with cocaine we would also see the same important role of conditioned stimuli in the acquisition phase of cocaine self-administration.

Picciotto: The studies haven't been done as systematically with cocaine, but it is also the case that if animals self-administer cocaine (or other drugs of abuse that are thought of as very reinforcing), in the absence of cues, the animals self-administer much less. The necessity for cues to drive self-administration behaviour is not unique to nicotine.

Caggiula: I agree with Marina Picciotto; the importance of cues is not restricted to nicotine. Ian asked about whether the nicotine-induced enhancement of the reinforcing properties of other stimuli also occurs for cocaine. There is an old literature showing that stimulants given non-contingently can enhance responding for conditioned reinforcers. We have done some preliminary studies with cocaine using the same self-administration model we used with nicotine, and the same compound visual stimulus. We found that non-contingent cocaine, like non-contingent nicotine, does enhance responding for that stimulus. Our impression is that the difference between nicotine and stimulants such as cocaine is the relative importance of the primary reinforcing effect versus this reinforcement-enhancing effect, with the former being relatively more important for cocaine and the latter being relatively more important for nicotine. It is a difference of degree. You get both effects with both kinds of drugs.

Changeux: How do you react to the distinction between motivational effects and hedonic effects? Does this involve two different systems, two targets and two pharmacological sites of action? Nicotine by itself has very little hedonic effect: people injected with nicotine don't feel high, compared with other drugs where there is a very strong hedonic feeling. People have to learn to smoke, to some extent. Would you make this distinction? Are there different pharmacologies and different targets?

Markou: These are all very good questions. However, experimentally it has not been possible to dissociate, and thus study separately the neurobiology of the motivational and hedonic effects of drugs. Incentive–motivational theories of behaviour conceptualize these two as being the same, with the hedonic properties of drugs providing the motivation for drug administration. Therefore, without us being able to experimentally dissociate the motivational from the hedonic effects of drugs, it is not clear that this question can be addressed systematically. The study of the conditioned stimuli does not get to this issue either because cues associated with smoking acquire motivational/hedonic properties through their predictive associations with smoking.

Stolerman: There are certainly different targets. I understand the main part of your question to be about the relationships between the subjective effects and the behavioural changes. I don't think that self-administration reflects simply subjective effects such as euphoria and I have previously argued this point at some length (Stolerman 1992). The reasons for taking a drug go beyond euphoria. To give one example, which is not reflected in animal self-administration procedures, there is the enhancement of performance of certain tasks that nicotine can bring about, associated with getting more reward. These cognitive enhancing effects may contribute to the reinforcing effects. These effects are frequently quoted by people as a reason for smoking but the normal self-administration procedure doesn't get at this because no attentional demand is placed upon the animal.

Changeux: You say nicotine is weakly self-administered.

Stolerman: Yes, that is true for pure nicotine in the absence of other stimuli. When Spealman and Goldberg (Goldberg et al 1981) demonstrated robust nicotine self-administration behaviour in primates, they used a second-order schedule in which the stimuli presented with nicotine became of profound importance. Their findings seemed to imply that an associative mechanism such as conditioned reinforcement was important. The current data are also saying that it isn't the direct reinforcing effects of nicotine that are the main factor, but rather that its ability to enhance the reinforcing effects of related stimuli that is crucial (Caggiula et al 2002). I think this is a breakthrough because it gives us a new set of ideas as to how to analyse mechanisms in both animal and human studies.

On another point, nicotine is sometimes said not to be euphoric in terms of producing a high. But when nicotine was given to people who were drug abusers, and the subjective responses are assessed, it did produce a euphoric reaction although it was weaker than that of cocaine (Henningfield et al 1985).

Jarvis: As far as I know there is just one study (Jones et al 1999) where cocaine and nicotine were given double blind to people who were users of both drugs. In terms of the subjective experience of drug effects the 'high' from nicotine was rated on a par with cocaine and was frequently confused with cocaine. Without the associated cues, it is not that dissimilar.

Stolerman: For that population, who were not the typical smoking population, it seemed to have quite a marked cocaine-like effect. In other situations, perhaps that effect isn't so strong.

Perkins: One thing of interest there is that the intermediate dose was perceived as cocaine like, while the high dose was perceived as opiate like.

Corrigall: I am not sure why we are focused exclusively on the euphoric effects of nicotine as the reason why humans or animals self administer. There could be many other reasons.

Changeux: The issue is whether self-administration is linked with motivational effects, other than hedonic effects. Perhaps with nicotine self-administration is associated with cues or learning whereas perhaps for other drugs it is associated with the hedonic effects.

Corrigall: Self-administration is, however, a motivational effect.

Changeux: Motivation was not necessarily linked with hedonic effects. This would explain the difference.

Bizarro: If we associate a stimulus with self-administration of nicotine, and then we introduce a fixed ratio schedule for the animal that is rewarded with the presentation of this stimulus, could this be a model for motivation? We might have higher rates of responding to the conditional stimulus than to the nicotine itself.

Stolerman: This is rather like the procedure used by Everitt's group where they make a distinction between drug-seeking and drug-taking. The seeking is essentially rewarded by a conditioned, nicotine-associated stimulus. This has been shown most clearly with cocaine; precisely this model hasn't been used with nicotine.

Picciotto: Peter Olausson and Jane Taylor have done experiments in rat that are close to this. They have shown that there is not a lot of difference between nicotine and cocaine pre-treatment on responding for a conditioned reinforcer (Taylor & Jentsch 2001, Olausson et al 2004).

Bizarro: Are the rates higher for the conditioned stimulus?

Picciotto: I'm not sure they can be compared directly.

Bizarro: I think this is an interesting approach. If we think about the unique aspects of nicotine use, one of them is that people can use nicotine everywhere and at almost all times. It is a unique drug because of this. How many stimuli will be associated with the drug over 30 years of use? This approach to the motivation of the user is more on the conditional stimulus than the drug itself. Perhaps this is a line of research that should be pursued. We need to look more closely at different conditional stimuli. Economy and reward could be concepts that fit better with the use of nicotine.

Shiffman: We should think hard about the human context in which people use nicotine. The comparison of the addictive properties of nicotine, opiates and cocaine is complicated by the issue of availability. We have such free access to nicotine, and this makes the role of conditioned stimuli much more powerful. The pairing with all kinds of stimuli may have a powerful effect. That said, it is compelling in a clinical context that people don't report much subjective effect from nicotine. This is quite a contrast to people who take opiates and cocaine. One may be able to set up artificial situations in which people obtain something called euphoria from nicotine, but this is not typical of normal smoking. Nor do people report anything that looks like a subjectively experienced effect of the conditioned stimuli. What is remarkable is that people persist in smoking behaviour in the absence of any subjectively recordable reinforcement.

Stolerman: I do not entirely agree. Ken Perkins' drug-discrimination experiments (Perkins et al 1994) show that smokers and non-smokers can identify the effects of nicotine. But I agree with your comment in the sense that the striking profile of subjective effects seen with other drugs isn't there with nicotine. It is not the subjective effects and mood changes (if any) that matter; it is the strong tobacco-seeking and taking behaviour that is the problem and must be the target for investigators.

Walton: You pointed out that people who take tobacco only a few times then become hooked, and that this doesn't happen as often with cocaine. There must be a relative paucity of non-drug reinforcers for cocaine in the environment. We are also fortunate to live in a society where we don't have advertising for cocaine! There is a huge amount of advertising still going on for tobacco which I would have thought is adding to these non-drug reinforcers in the environment.

Shiffman: Another way of thinking of this is that because cocaine is illegal and expensive, cocaine ends up being used in a limited range of circumstances and with certain people. There are paraphernalia associated with it, and certain behaviours and stimuli are involved in acquiring it. To the extent that cocaine use is driven by associated stimuli, this will constrain the use and stimulation of use. Nicotine generally has the opposite profile. It is available everywhere and it is used in all kinds of company and all kinds of contexts. This is changing. As we impose tobacco control restrictions we are starting to see a change in the pattern of self administration. In the USA, it is startling to learn that 1 out of 4 current smokers report that they don't smoke every day. This is inconsistent with our withdrawal-based models of tobacco smoking and dependence. When we have correlated the prevalence of intermittent smoking with state tobacco control policies, the correlation has been high. In the context of unrestricted smoking, it is the use across almost all contexts that drives the behaviour.

Perkins: I want to second Ian's point about the inadequacy of the self-administration models in the motivated animal. I would extend this to the human: I'm not sure we have good human models (in the laboratory at least) that simulate the clinical situation. If you administer the original FDA-approved doses of nicotine replacement to humans and then measure *ad lib* smoking behaviour, you don't see a change (see Perkins et al 2005). There are animal data in which the same thing is done (nicotine pre-treatment) and no change is seen in nicotine self-administration. I think that the human laboratory model predicts very well the pre-clinical model with other species, but does not predict the human clinical model. We have a problem with laboratory-based human research if we are trying to predict what is going to happen in the clinical situation.

Shiffman: This is not the only disanalogy between these laboratory procedures and the human situation. When people fail in smoking cessation it is often in the presence of very powerful associated stimuli.

Chiamulera: Nicotine is not only a reinforcing drug, it also has other pharmacological effects. It is a cognitive enhancer, an anxiolytic and has analgesic effects. In animal models such as self-administration, or human experiments, we don't know exactly what mixed pharmacological effects lie behind the behaviour. My concern is that a negative result with the self-administration paradigm could be a false negative result. We should all make more effort to develop other models which includes those different pharmacological effects of nicotine that may be relevant for tobacco addiction, so as to have a more global approach.

Picciotto: One of the striking things about nicotine is that although it is a weak reinforcer, it has remarkable extinction properties. In experiments where animals have to press a lever to receive cocaine, if you switch for cocaine for saline there is the extinction burst where the animals seem to be looking for the drug, and then there is extinction of behaviour. In mice, if you leave nicotine-associated cues available there is no extinction at all when nicotine is switched with saline.

Markou: I don't agree with the statement that extinction does not occur readily to nicotine self-administration in either rats or mice. It may take a few days, but extinction does occur eventually.

Picciotto: This is the striking difference. The self-administration, the operant behaviour itself is perhaps weaker for nicotine, but the extinction phase is very different. This is probably why we have so few papers on relapse models, because it is such a pain to get the animals to extinguish that it is hard to get relapse.

Markou: We can definitely get extinction in our animals on a regular basis. I don't have experience with cocaine extinction, so I can't readily compare them, but we can do extinction and reinstatement with no difficulty in rats.

Picciotto: How long does it take?

Markou: No more than two weeks.

West: One of the reasons for putting this meeting together was that as a consumer of this basic research, I felt there were a lot of contradictions and conflicts in some very basic statements about nicotine. One of the things that has already come up is how powerful nicotine is as a primary reinforcer. I had come to the view that it isn't as powerful as we had originally thought, but this is an issue that I would like to see some resolution of. If people are getting different results, what is the reason for this? Now we hear another issue, which is the extent to which responding for nicotine extinguishes relatively quickly or slowly in animals. Also, the model that Ian Stolerman has concentrated on is a positive reinforcement model. To what extent is negative reinforcement involved in nicotine addiction? This is something that merits discussion. In the case of human clinical situations we get more of a sense that negative reinforcement is important, to the extent that although they are weak there are relationships between withdrawal symptoms such as depression and subsequent relapse. How is it that something that provides no positive reinforcement at all, such as a nicotine patch, can suppress craving for a cigarette? This is an interesting phenomenon that we tend to take for granted. Ian, do you see any role in the animal literature for more advanced negative reinforcement-type models of nicotine dependence?

Stolerman: There are many examples in the animal literature of nicotine withdrawal signs. Some of these studies, notably the ones carried out by Markou and colleagues relate to motivational effects of this withdrawal (Epping-Jordan et al 1998). Such findings imply that relief from withdrawal contributes to the self-administration of nicotine but what we lack is a way of quantifying such effects and distinguishing then from direct reinforcing actions. Some research has moved towards the establishment of a modified self-administration procedure that is associated with the development of nicotine withdrawal signs, but this has not yet been achieved (e.g. Paterson et al 2004). Success in this area would resolve the issue raised by Robert West. This is difficult with many types of drug in animal models and needs to be the focus of more attention in the future.

Clarke: Small procedural differences can make a huge difference to results. No one has mentioned the fact that animal nicotine self-administration studies all use very short pulses of nicotine. Nicotine is typically injected in 1–2 s. This in no way models the pharmacokinetics of smoking where arterial levels peak at around 20–25 s after the end of the pulse. What does intravenous self-administration in animals really model? I have a horrible feeling that a nicotine-free animal given a quick pulse of nicotine may be getting a large burst of dopamine release that is simply not seen in a smoker.

References

Caggiula AR, Donny EC, White AR et al 2002 Environmental stimuli promote the acquisition of nicotine self-administration in rats. Psychopharmacology (Berl) 163:230–237

Epping-Jordan MP, Watkins SS, Koob GF, Markou A 1998 Dramatic decreases in brain reward function during nicotine withdrawal. Nature 393:76–79

Goldberg SR, Spealman RD, Goldberg DM 1981 Persistent behavior at high rates maintained by intravenous self-administration of nicotine. Science 214:573–575

Henningfield JE, Miyasato K, Jasinski DR 1985 Abuse liability and pharmacodynamic characteristics of intravenous and inhaled nicotine. J Pharmacol Exp Ther 234:1–12

Jones HE, Garrett BE, Griffiths RR 1999 Subjective and physiological effects of intravenous nicotine and cocaine in cigarette smoking cocaine abusers. J Pharmacol Exp Ther 288:188–197

Olausson P, Jentsch JD, Taylor JR 2004 Repeated nicotine exposure enhances responding with conditioned reinforcement. Psychopharmacology (Berl) 173:98–104

Paterson NE, Markou A 2004 Prolonged nicotine dependence associated with extended access to nicotine self-administration in rats. Psychopharmacology 173:64–72

Perkins KA, DiMarco A, Grobe JE, Scierka A, Stiller RL 1994 Nicotine discrimination in male and female smokers. Psychopharmacology (Berl) 116:407–413

Perkins KA, Stitzer M, Lerman C 2005 Medication screening for smoking cessation: a proposal for new methodologies. Psychopharmacology (Berl) 15:1–9

Stolerman IP 1992 Drugs of abuse: behavioural principles, methods and terms. Trends Pharmacol Sci 13:170–176

Taylor JR, Jentsch JD 2001 Repeated intermittent administration of psychomotor stimulant drugs alters the acquisition of Pavlovian approach behavior in rats: differential effects of cocaine, d-amphetamine and 3,4-methylenedioxymethamphetamine ('Ecstasy'). Biol Psychiatry 50:137–143

Defining and assessing nicotine dependence in humans

Robert West

Cancer Research UK Health Behaviour Unit, Department of Epidemiology and Public Health, University College London, Brook House, 2-16 Torrington Place, London WC1E 6BT, UK

Abstract. 'Addiction' and 'dependence' are used synonymously by most researchers and defined as a reward-seeking (usually drug taking) behaviour that has become out of control. The diagnosis has been based on the alcohol dependence syndrome identified 30 years ago by Edwards and Gross and includes tolerance, craving, withdrawal symptoms, difficulty controlling use, important activities given up, and continuation despite harmful consequences. A substantial proportion of smokers are addicted by reference to these criteria. However, it is possible to improve on both the definition and its assessment. This paper proposes that addiction is more usefully regarded as a symptom of potentially a range of underlying pathologies involving the 'motivational system'. Even among smokers there is heterogeneity in the pathology that makes it difficult for them to abstain voluntarily and this has important implications for treatment. For example, there will be smokers for whom the pathology involves a largely reversible effect of nicotine in creating an 'acquired drive', others for whom nicotine has induced long-term changes that make life less comfortable in its absence, and others whose smoking is more situationally driven. Assessment of addiction should first quantify the degree to which the behaviour dominates the individual's repertoire and then assess the underlying pathology in the motivational system. A framework for doing this is discussed.

2005 Understanding nicotine and tobacco addiction. Wiley, Chichester (Novartis Foundation Symposium 275) p 36–58

'Nicotine as delivered by cigarettes is addictive.' There are two common interpretations of this statement. One is that a substantial proportion of people who experiment with cigarettes go on to exhibit a syndrome that meets the DSM-IV (Diagnostic and Statistical Manual IV of the American Psychiatric Association) or ICD-10 (Intenational Classification of Diseases 10) criteria for dependence (RCP 2000, USDHHS 1988). The second is that many smokers have lost control over their smoking behaviour. These two interpretations are related but they are not the same because some items in the diagnostic criteria are not necessarily indicative of loss of control. To complicate things further, some researchers use the term 'dependence' to refer to a physiological condition in which abstinence from nicotine results in adverse withdrawal symptoms. Most researchers use the term 'nico-tine addiction' and 'nicotine dependence' synonymously.

Addiction is a socially defined construct so there are no objective criteria by which to judge the correctness of any definition (for a fuller discussion see West 2006). It is also open to multiple interpretations each being slightly different from the other. However, the label is important because it has significant implications for policy, research, clinical practice and litigation. It is therefore worth trying to clarify the concepts to derive a consistent terminology.

This article examines the phenomena that come under the rubric of nicotine dependence and addiction and argues for an approach to assessment in which first the severity of addiction in terms of the single concept of loss of control is iden-tified followed by an examination of the various possible pathologies that are con-tributing to this phenomenon.

Revisiting the DSM and ICD dependence criteria

DSM and ICD criteria were derived from the alcohol dependence syndrome char-acterized by Edwards & Gross (1976). The syndrome was not intended to act as a template for dependence syndromes for other substances (G. Edwards, personal communication) and indeed it was thought that others would apply the methods to other substances and arrive at syndromes specific to them. The alcohol dependence syndrome was a carefully observed characterization of the clinical presentation of alcohol dependence and many of its features were related to the pharmacology of that particular drug.

Neither was it intended that the dependence syndrome would necessarily define addiction. Addiction is currently regarded as a concept involving impaired control over a reward-seeking (usually drug-taking) behaviour. The field has come to con-sider that it can be assessed by reference to the dependence syndrome criteria but the two need not be related in this particular way. Thus there is a distinction between construing the DSM or ICD criteria as 'indices of a behaviour that has become out of control' and as 'a collection of symptoms that can be empirically shown to fit together as a syndrome'.

In the event, the application of the DSM and ICD criteria to smoking leads to classification of some 60–80% of current smokers in countries such as Germany and the USA as addicted (Hoch et al 2004, Grant et al 2004). Similar findings are observed with other drugs (e.g. Shaffer & Eber 2002). One might imagine, there-fore, that the dependence syndrome originally based on alcohol is performing satisfactorily in what it sets out to do, which is to determine how far smoking fits a common model of dependence.

There are problems, however. On the face of it, not all the criteria are equally rel-evant to smoking (Table 1). Of the DSM criteria the only ones that clearly have high

TABLE 1   DSM-IV criteria and their apparent relevance to nicotine addiction

Diagnostic and Statistical Manual—IV (APA 1995)
A maladaptive pattern of substance use leading to clinically significant impairment or distress as manifested by
three (or more) of the following, occurring at any time in the same 12-month period:

Criterion	*Relevance to nicotine from cigarettes*
Substance is often taken in larger amounts or over longer period than intended	Variable: It is not clear what proportion of smokers formulate clear intentions to smoke for just a limited time when they start and then find they cannot stop. Neither is it clear how far smoking a cigarette on a particular occasion stimulates a binge of smoking that is hard to control.
Persistent desire or unsuccessful efforts to cut down or control substance use	High: This is a strong feature of smoking with a large majority having tried unsuccessfully to stop before middle age (RCP 2000).
A great deal of time is spent in activities necessary to obtain the substance (e.g. visiting multiple doctors or driving long distances), use the substance (e.g. chain smoking), or recover from its effects	Variable: Smoking is an activity that does not require a great investment in time because relative to other addictions it is relatively inexpensive and can be performed while doing other things. However, with smokers for whom cigarettes are expensive relative to income this may be relevant (e.g. Marsh & MacKay 1994).
Important social, occupational, or recreational activities given up or reduced because of substance abuse	Variable: Smoking does not cause intoxication or need for recovery and can be carried out alongside other activities. Therefore there is little reason to give up activities in order to smoke unless one lives in a society where there are substantial smoking restrictions.
Continued substance use despite knowledge of having a persistent or recurrent psychological, or physical problem that is caused or exacerbated by use of the substance	Variable: Whereas the adverse effects of high levels of alcohol use are typically concurrent, the adverse effects of smoking usually start to become serious only in later life. A belief that one might experience a smoking-related disorder is not the same as experiencing marital break-up, loss of job etc. in the present. Once the health effects start to manifest themselves, this criterion starts to become more relevant.
Tolerance, as defined by either: need for increased amounts of the substance in order to achieve intoxication or desired effect; or markedly diminished effect with continued use of the same amount	Unknown: There is evidence that some subjective effects of nicotine reduce over months or years of smoking (Perkins et al 1994) but little evidence yet of chronic tolerance to the hedonic effects. It is, however, subject to acute tolerance within the span of a day (West & Russell 1988). Chronic tolerance seems to be primarily manifest to the aversive properties of nicotine. While of interest and possibly playing a role in enabling people to smoke comfortably, that is not in the spirit of this item.

TABLE 1   *(Continued)*

Diagnostic and Statistical Manual — IV (APA 1995)
A maladaptive pattern of substance use leading to clinically significant impairment or distress as manifested by three (or more) of the following, occurring at any time in the same 12-month period:

Criterion	Relevance to nicotine from cigarettes
Withdrawal, as manifested by either: characteristic withdrawal syndrome for the substance; or the same (or closely related) substance is taken to relieve or avoid withdrawal symptoms	High: There is a characteristics nicotine withdrawal syndrome that becomes manifest on cessation of smoking and is relieved at least partially by nicotine patches and other nicotine preparations (USDHHS 1988, RCP 2000). Where there are nicotine products that are widely available at low cost to the user, as in the UK, they are heavily used. For example, more than 60% of quit attempts in the UK involve use of nicotine products (West et al 2005b).

---

relevance are persistent desire or unsuccessful attempts to control use and withdrawal symptoms. Of the ICD criteria only the difficulties controlling use and desire/urge criteria could, on current evidence, be considered to be of high relevance.

At the same time, in neither the DSM nor the ICD criteria is there mention of smoking immediately after waking which would appear to be an important element demonstrating a compulsive pattern of behaviour, nor is there mention of awakening in the night to smoke, titration of nicotine intake, brand preference (indicating an increasing stereotypy) and other factors that arguably form part of the syndrome observed with smokers.

It is worth noting that it is not just that smoking does not fit all the ICD and DSM criteria well; neither do many other drugs of dependence. Thus while traditional factor analytic techniques have led to claims that most of the illicit drugs fit well with a single dimension model based on DSM criteria (Morgenstern et al 1994), factor analysis is not well suited to assessing the applicability of particular criteria and a more appropriate item-response theory approach has raised doubts about the broad applicability of some items to all the drug classes (Langenbucher et al 2004).

Additionally, where research has been conducted to develop new dependence questionnaires based on the alcohol dependence syndrome concept, it has encountered problems with some items (e.g. Topp & Mattick 1997), although conclusions about the applicability of the dependence syndrome concept have sometimes glossed over this (see Topp & Darke 1997). It seems that there is a general problem when attempting to define a single set of criteria for drugs that have very different pharmacological properties and societal norms governing use (Table 2).

TABLE 2   ICD-10 criteria and their apparent relevance to nicotine addiction

International Classification of Diseases 10 (WHO 1992)
Three or more of the following must have been experienced or exhibited at some time during the previous year:

Criterion	*Relevance*
Difficulties in controlling substance-taking behaviour in terms of its onset, termination, or levels of use	High: there is clear evidence that a majority of smokers have difficulty in cutting down or stopping.
A strong desire or sense of compulsion to take the substance	High: strong desire to smoke and powerful urges are a dominant part of the smoker's experience (RCP 2000).
Progressive neglect of alternative pleasures or interests because of psychoactive substance use, increased amount of time necessary to obtain or take the substance or to recover from its effects	Low: smoking in most societies is compatible with daily activities, even if time needs to be taken out of these activities where there are smoking restrictions.
Persisting with substance use despite clear evidence of overtly harmful consequences, depressive mood states consequent to heavy use, or drug related impairment of cognitive functioning	Moderate: smokers are aware of the health risks of smoking and this is the most commonly cited reason for wanting to stop (Lader & Goddard 2004). However, serious health effects do not become manifest until later life and a possibility of future health effects is not as powerful a balancing force as current effects that would rapidly be mitigated if the addictive activity were to cease (for a discussion see West 2006).
Evidence of tolerance, such that increased doses of the psychoactive substance are required in order to achieve effects originally produced by lower doses	Unknown: although there is chronic tolerance to some of the effects of nicotine (Perkins et al 1994), most of this appears to be to be the aversive effects. There is acute tolerance to the hedonic effect but this does not lead smokers to ingest more nicotine after the first one of the day to compensate; in fact they ingest less (Benowitz & Jacob 1984). It has also been found that young smokers who have been smoking for just a year or so take in as much nicotine per cigarette as do adult smokers (McNeill et al 1989).
A physiological withdrawal state when substance use has ceased or been reduced, as evidence by: the characteristic withdrawal syndrome for the substance; or use of the same (or a closely related) substance with the intention of relieving or avoiding withdrawal symptoms	Moderate: the emphasis on the physiological reduces the relevance of this criterion. Cigarette withdrawal symptoms have been shown to be affected by expectancies and inhalation of an irritant vapour (Hughes et al 1989, Rose & Behm 1994).

It is also important to recognize that depending on how the criteria are interpreted, they can sometimes set a low threshold for addiction. This is particularly apparent when trying to apply them to adolescent smoking where adolescents who smoke infrequently and at a low rate can be defined as addicted depending on their responses on DSM-based questionnaires (for a fuller discussion see Tiffany et al 2004). There is no question of the fact that many smokers are highly addicted but an inappropriate application of the DSM-IV criteria can undermine the credibility of the assessment.

Focusing on assessment of loss of control

If we are to construe addiction as distinct from a dependence syndrome (i.e. as a behaviour that has become out of control), then assessing severity of dependence should focus more than the DSM and ICD criteria do on ways in which this manifests itself. Thus tolerance and withdrawal symptoms would not be included as markers because they are not necessarily linked to loss of control, merely symptoms that could, depending on the pharmacology of the drug, contribute to it.

A scale that was derived from all the DSM and ICD criteria may not relate well to addiction in terms of loss of control because of inclusion of items of less relevance to that construct. In fact a recent test of this found that a dependence questionnaire based on a combination of DSM and ICD criteria did very poorly in predicting abstinence; a higher scores was associated with greater likelihood of abstinence (Etter 2005) even though it did predict withdrawal symptoms.

Of the DSM and ICD criteria, failure of attempts to stop would seem to be the most important. However, someone could in theory be so addicted that s/he would never even contemplating trying to stop. Therefore, a practical marker would need to be something that did not require an attempt at abstinence.

One possible marker would be the person's subjective level of dependence; that is, how addicted s/he feels. This does form part of some dependence scales (e.g. the Severity of Dependence Scale; Gossop et al 1995). The problem with this is that it requires a degree of insight that the person might not have. On the other hand, at least with other drugs this approach has been shown to yield assessment scores that relate to behaviours that are considered indicative of addiction (Gossop et al 1995, 2002).

The other obvious approach is to use a set of behavioural markers. In the case of smoking, this has been a very popular approach. The Fagerstrom Test for Nicotine Dependence (FTND) contains six items as shown in Table 3 (Heatherton et al 1991). Four of the items are reports of behaviour and would be expected to be reasonably easy to answer: cigarettes per day, time to first cigarette of the morning, smoking more in the morning and smoking even when ill. One is subjective but still focused on the issue of loss of control (difficulty not smoking in non-smoking

TABLE 3   The Fagerstrom Test for Nicotine Dependence (Heatherton et al 1991)

	Response options	*Score*	*Relevance to addiction*
How soon after you wake up do you smoke your first cigarette? *(Circle one response)*	Within 5 minutes 6–30 minutes More than 30 min	3 2 0	High: this is a simple semi-quantitative behavioural marker of compulsion to smoke
Do you find it difficult to stop smoking in no-smoking areas? *(Circle one response)*	No Yes	0 1	High: this is a subjective marker of compulsion to smoke
Which cigarette would you hate most to give up? *(Circle one response)*	The first of the morning Other	1 0	Unknown: this is based on the assumption that the first cigarette of the morning has special significance in more addicted smokers
How many cigarettes per day do you usually smoke? *(Write the number on the line **and** circle one response)*	__ per day 10 or less 11 to 20 21 to 30 31 or more	 0 1 2 3	High: frequency of an activity is a simple behavioural marker, though smokers can smoke cigarettes more heavily to get a desired dose of nicotine so this will be affected by price and smoking restrictions
Do you smoke more frequently in the first hours after waking than during the rest of the day? *(Circle one response)*	No Yes	0 1	Unknown: this is related to item 3. but using a behavioural marker
Do you smoke if you are so ill that you are in bed most of the day? *(Circle one response)*	No Yes	0 1	High: this is a behavioural marker of compulsion

areas) and the other relates to a presumption about the need to smoke for withdrawal relief (which cigarette would hate to give up).

Because it is more clearly targeted at the manifestations of loss of control, and uses simple behavioural markers, the FTND might be expected to provide a better marker of addiction than questionnaires based on self-rated addiction or the DSM or ICD criteria.

The FTND has been widely studied and regularly predicts success of cessation attempts (see West et al 2001). However, it has been noted that the items cannot readily be mapped on to a single dimension (see Richardson & Ratner 2005). This is not necessarily a problem if the purpose of the scale is to provide a quantitative assessment of loss of control. It is conceivable that loss of control could be manifest in different people in different ways. The net result would be that they are less likely to be able to stop smoking were they to try.

Focusing on smoking motivation

Another approach is to consider smoking as a 'rational addiction' (for a discussion see West, 2006). Under this view of addiction, what seems to be loss of control, is in fact a series of choices that addicts make in which on some occasions they choose to try and abstain and then, once the consequences of their abstention becomes evident, they choose to resume the behaviour.

Under this view, it would be appropriate to consider the explicit motives that smokers report for their smoking. Smoking motivation questionnaires date back to the 1960s and there are many variants. All the published scales use factor analysis to determine a number of dimensions representing smoking motives (e.g. Berlin et al 2003, West & Russell 1985). In principle this approach provides for a more robust measurement of underlying dimensions of motivation that is independent of the wording of particular questions. However, it suffers from the problem that items can be correlated with each other for a number of reasons—it may be because they measure the same underlying dimension or that they measure two distinct dimensions that happen to be relate to each other. One example is anxiety and depression which are distinct yet correlated dimensions of mood.

Another approach is simply to use single ratings for each of a set of putative motives. Findings using this approach have been briefly reported but the approach has not been fully explored (West 1995). It was noted that reported enjoyment of smoking was not related to likelihood of success at stopping whereas saliva cotinine as a marker of frequency and intensity of smoking behaviour was. It could be argued that motives for smoking are not very good markers of loss of control because the rational addiction model does not apply to smoking.

The nicotine dependence syndrome and assessment of addiction

The DSM and ICD criteria were derived from the alcohol dependence syndrome concept but in revisions moved to some degree away from it to focus more on evidence of compulsion. A recent study has derived a nicotine dependence syndrome scale based on the original criteria (Shiffman et al 2004). These criteria are: (a) narrowing of the repertoire of drug use behaviour, (b) increased salience of the drug-seeking behaviour, (c) increased tolerance to the drug, (d) repeated withdrawal symptoms, (e) repeated relief or avoidance of withdrawal symptoms by drug use,

(f) awareness of compulsion to the use the drug, and (g) rapid 'reinstatement' of the syndrome after a lapse.

Shiffman developed a questionnaire-based self-report scale that sought to assess these elements of the syndrome and found through factor analysis that they did not cohere into one dimension. In fact five dimensions were postulated. None of the five dimensions was individually related to time to relapse. However, in smokers attempting to stop a single total score weighted in favour of items that related to manifestations of loss of control were predictive of cravings during abstinence and of time to relapse (Shiffman et al 2004). On the other hand, while the scale showed evidence of adding to the ability to predict the adverse experiences associated with abstinence, it did not provide clear evidence of incremental predictive validity over cigarettes per day in its relationship with time to relapse.

Elements of the dependence syndrome, smoking motivation and loss of control: a more detailed examination

This section presents some new data on individual features of smoking and smoking motivation and their ability to predict ability to maintain abstinence in a sample of smokers undergoing treatment. The aims are: (1) to examine the extent to which smokers seeking help with stopping smoking endorse a range of dependence-related items, including those based on DSM-IV and a smoking motives scale, and (2) to assess the relationship between these and ability to maintain complete abstinence up to 6 months.

The sample consisted of 452 smokers smoking 10 or more cigarettes per day, attending a group treatment programme. The mean (SD) age was 43.1 (12.5). Sixty-one percent (276) were female. None received any medication to help them stop. They were taking part in a trial examining the effect of glucose tablets as an aid to smoking cessation. They completed a questionnaire approximately one week prior to their designated quit date and were followed up weekly for 4 weeks after the quit date and then at 6 months. They were asked about any smoking and claims of abstinence were checked by means of expired air carbon monoxide concentrations at each assessment. In accordance with usual practice, participants who did not attend assessments were regarded as having smoked (West et al 2005a).

In a sample such as this, it would be expected that items that reflect addiction are endorsed by the large majority of participants. In cases where a significant proportion do not endorse that item, it is of interest to know whether those that do are less likely to be successful at maintaining abstinence.

Table 4 shows the frequencies of endorsement of items related to the dependence syndrome as well as mean ratings of motives for smoking and self-perceived dependence and responses on the FTND. It also shows the partial point-biserial or tetrachoric correlation coefficients (depending on whether the dependence item was

TABLE 4 Endorsement/ratings of items relating to addiction and associations of these with continuous abstinence for 6 months

Item DSM-IV related items	Percent 'Yes'/mean (SD)	Partial correlations with 1 month and 6 months of abstinence	
		1 month	6 months
1. Compared with when you first started smoking, do you smoke more now in order to be satisfied?	82.5%	−0.011	0.03
2. Do you get less of an effect from your smoking than when you first started?	70.8%	−0.06	0.06
3. Do you smoke more than you had intended to when you first started?	91.6%	—	—
4. When you started smoking did you intend to stop before now?	80.0%	−0.07	−0.05
5. Have you at any time tried to quit or cut down on smoking cigarettes and found you could not?	90.4%	—	—
6. Have you spent a great deal of time doing nothing other than smoking?	53.8%	−0.14*	−0.04
7. Have you wished many times that you could quit or cut down on smoking cigarettes?	99.6%	—	—
8. Have you at any time spent money on cigarettes instead of food or other necessities?	53.4%	−0.10	−0.18**
9. Do you believe that your continued smoking is damaging your health?	98.4%	—	—
10. Have you at any time started smoking again to keep from having problems caused by quitting or cutting down?	67.3%	0.00	−0.03
DSM total (range 0–10)	7.8 (1.7)	−0.17*	−0.06
FTND items			
1. How soon after you wake up do you smoke your first cigarette?	<5 min 37.7% 6–30 min 44.2% >30 min 17.9%	−0.11*	−0.01
2. Do you find it difficult to stop smoking in no-smoking areas?	37.7%	−0.11*	−0.06
3. Which cigarette would you hate most to give up? (First of the morning)	55.9%	−0.16***	−0.12**
4. How many cigarettes per day do you usually smoke?	22.9 (8.3)	−0.12**	−0.05
5. Do you smoke more frequently in the first hours after waking than during the rest of the day?	51.5%	−0.12**	−0.17***
6. Do you smoke if you are so ill that you are in bed most of the day?	51.8%	−0.05	−0.03
FTND total	5.5 (2.3)	−0.24***	−0.12*

TABLE 4 (*Continued*)

Item *DSM-IV related items*	Percent 'Yes'/mean (SD)	Partial correlations with 1 month and 6 months of abstinence	
		1 month	*6 months*
Severity of Dependence Scale Items **(0 = never or almost never, 3 = always or** **nearly always)**			
1. Have you at any time thought that your smoking was out of control?	1.7 (0.9)	−0.12	−0.03
2. Has the prospect of not smoking made you anxious or worried?	1.4 (0.9)	−0.19**	−0.15*
3. Have you worried about your smoking?	2.1 (0.7)	−0.11	−0.04
4. Have you wished that you could stop smoking?	2.4 (0.6)	−0.03	0.06
5. How difficult would you have found it stop or go without cigarettes? (0, easy; 3, impossible)	1.9 (0.6)	−0.11	−0.09
SDS total (range 0 to 15)	9.5 (2.5)	−0.18**	−0.08
Smoking Motives Scale (1 = not at all, **5 = very much)**			
1. Do you use smoking to help you cope with stress?	3.9 (1.0)	0.00	0.00
2. Do you use smoking to help you socialize?	2.8 (1.3)	0.02	0.03
3. Do you use smoking to give you something to do when you are bored?	3.7 (1.1)	0.02	0.06
4. Do you use smoking to help you to concentrate and stay alert?	3.0 (1.2)	0.04	0.07
5. Do you smoke because you feel uncomfortable if you don't?	2.9 (1.3)	0.03	0.05
6. Do you use smoking to help you to keep your weight down?	2.1 (1.3)	0.05	0.08
7. Do you enjoy smoking?	3.7 (1.7)	−0.02	0.02
SMS total (range 7 to 45)	22.1 (4.2)	−0.03	0.04

Note: In the case of DSM-related items the *n* is reduced to 251 because this questionnaire was introduced after the study had begun. *n*s vary slightly by analysis because of missing data.

Where percent endorsement is greater than 90% no correlation is given because of lack of variance.

quantitative or binary respectively) with abstinence from the quit date to one month and to six months controlling for whether they received glucose or not.

Correlations are used here to provide a simple quantitative index of association. Even where the odds ratios are moderate the correlations will be low because of the nature of the distributions so one should not read a great deal into to their absolute size. Although glucose did not affect abstinence in this group it was controlled for in the partial correlations. It would also be expected that where there is substantial variation in the quantitative items, this would predict abstinence.

There are many different ways of characterizing abstinence and each one may yield different results. For present purposes continuous abstinence up to 4 weeks and up to 6 months were used as markers of loss of control. It was of interest to determine whether there was a major discrepancy between the pattern of correlations using these two markers.

The findings of any questionnaire-based assessment of addiction must be interpreted in the light of the context. In this the smokers were seeking treatment to help them stop smoking so one might imagine that endorsement of items related to addiction would be biased towards the positive. Even so, it is of note that most of the DSM-related items were endorsed by a large majority of the participants. The two items that were endorsed by fewer smokers showed some association with abstinence either at one month or 6 months. A total score that simply counted the number of endorsements was significantly associated with one month but not 6 month abstinence.

The FTND items showed a more consistent relationship with abstinence and the endorsement rate was sufficiently low to allow variation within this sample. It has generally been thought that cigarettes per day and time to first cigarette of the day are the two key items when it comes to assessing addiction but in this data set the two most consistent items related to morning smoking. The total scale score which was derived using the recommended formula was associated with both short and long-term abstinence even within this dependent sample. The total FTND score significantly improved the prediction of both 4 week and 6 month abstinence over and above what could be achieved by daily cigarette consumption and time to first cigarette of the day (partial correlations were 0.15 and 0.18, respectively, $P < 0.005$ in both cases).

The Severity of Dependence Scale items showed sufficient variation in this sample for there to be an opportunity for an association with abstinence but only one item was related to abstinence and that was anxiety about stopping smoking. Perceived difficulty in abstaining showed no evidence of a relationship.

It was particularly noteworthy that although the items relating to smoking motivation showed sufficient variation to allow the possibility of an association with abstinence there was no suggestion that such as association was present. As had been previously found, enjoyment of smoking bore no detectable relationship to ability to maintain abstinence.

It is important not to read too much into findings from one sample in one context, but these data point to a number of useful conclusions.

- First, although DSM-IV criteria differ in relevance to smoking, it is possible to operationalize them all in terms that have relevance for smokers who are seeking treatment. Even those that have more modest relevance may turn out to be indicative of loss of control. In particular, prioritising smoking over other needs may be an important marker.
- Secondly, FTND items relating to morning smoking, beyond the time to first cigarette of the day, can be useful in the assessment of dependence and the scale as a whole is more predictive of abstinence than just cigarettes per day and time to first cigarette of the day.
- Thirdly, subjective ratings of addiction in a sample that could be presumed to be in the more addicted range are not predictive of ability to maintain abstinence, with the exception of an item that relates to feelings of anxiety about giving up smoking.
- Fourthly, a rational addiction model of addiction in which expressed motives for smoking such as enjoyment did not prove helpful in stratifying smokers in this kind of sample who were or were not able to sustain abstinence.

The data presented and the preceding analysis suggest that there is some way to go before we could confidently claim to have an optimal set of markers for the severity of addiction. Arguably, a factor analytic approach will not be very helpful in this enterprise because there may be many different manifestations of addiction that do not correlate well with each other. In the meantime, the FTND continues to perform well and it is not just cigarettes per day and time to first cigarette of the day that are important.

Pathologies underlying nicotine addiction

The foregoing discussion has not touched on the question of the potential variety of pathologies that may give rise to nicotine addiction. It seems likely that there are many of these.

West (2006) has argued that pathologies underlying addiction may fall into three classes: those that exist independent of the addictive behaviour itself but which make the behaviour more compulsive (e.g. anxiety, depression, impulsivity); those that arise from an interaction between the activity and a susceptibility in the individual (e.g. sensitivity to the rewarding nature of the activity or to its capacity to create an acquired drive); and those that exist in the person's environment so that what might be considered a 'normal' motivational system would have difficulty in controlling the behaviour (e.g. strong norms promoting the behaviour in the person's micro-culture or the wider social environment).

This suggests that there will be smokers whose smoking seems to them to satisfy needs that will remain once they stop, those who might have acquired a drive to smoke because of the way their motivational system has responded to nicotine but whose drive will reduce if they abstain for long enough, those who have acquired a drive to smoke and for whom the drive will remain strong even after an extensive period of abstinence, those for whom a strong cue-related habit has developed, those who have formed powerful expectancies relating to their smoking and what it does for them, those whose identity is strongly tied into being a smoker, those whose environment will continue to promote nicotine use even when they are strong enough to resist internally generated forces arising from the above—and any combination of these.

The assessment of nicotine addiction *per se* is unlikely to be enough to determine how far each of these pathologies is operating in a particular case. Neither is the characterization of a dependence syndrome. Neither is it likely that the classic typological approach will bear fruit because the number of permutations arising from the importance of different elements is too great and the motivational system is interconnected and likely to revert to its former state following specific interventions directed at just one element.

Clinical implications

From the clinical perspective, the above analysis suggests assessing in detail the pathologies within the different parts of the motivational system, then attempting to determine which, if any, are amenable to change with interventions that are at our disposal. Following this a treatment plan would be formulated that recognizes the realities of what can be changed with a short intervention, what requires a continuing intervention and what requires repeated interventions.

Current psychological treatments are primarily geared towards using motivational techniques (such as group support, bolstering reasons for not smoking) to suppress smoking, practical advice (such as avoiding cues) to minimize impulses to smoke in the face of underlying habit mechanisms, and reshaping the smokers' evaluative beliefs (e.g. persuading them that it does not help with stress) to try to stop them wanting to smoke. Pharmacological treatment is primarily geared towards reducing the acquired drive to smoke.

This treatment model assumes that the pathologies will diminish if the smoker manages to maintain abstinence so that in time his or her normal restraint mechanisms will be enough to cope with any residual motivation to smoke. Experience shows that this is unrealistic except in a few cases. In most cases, the underlying pathologies remain strong enough after the end of treatment to cause relapse. If we can develop better assessment methods we should be able to work out more individualized treatment plans—both in terms of content and duration.

Research implications

From the research perspective, we need continually to remind ourselves that we are dealing with social constructs. Hence, when we talk about nicotine addiction having a particular heritability or a particular relationship with other measures of interest we are talking about a particular index of a particular definition of addiction (Lessov et al 2004). For the purposes of research it is probably better to use more specific measures where issues of semantics are less important, such as saliva cotinine concentration, time to relapse from a quit attempt or likelihood of success of quit attempts.

Conclusions

This paper has argued that some clarification is required concerning the concept of nicotine addiction and how far the nicotine dependence syndrome and DSM and ICD criteria for dependence provide a means of measuring its severity or are clinical phenomena of interest in their own right.

It has been argued that if we take addiction as a reward seeking behaviour that has become out of control, then its assessment should be undertaken using manifestations of that lack of control rather than features of a clinical syndrome, some of which may not be relevant to it. The internal coherence of a scale that does this is not relevant—only its ability to predict which smokers are unable to exercise control. In this regard the FTND has performed well and provides value beyond cigarettes per day and time to first cigarette of the day.

The paper has also argued that, while a clinical syndrome of nicotine dependence is of interest, it is less useful when attempting to determine how best to treat smokers wanting to stop than an assessment of the specific pathologies underlying their loss of control.

Finally, the paper has argued that for research purposes, it may be better to focus on more objectively defined markers of the behaviour or at least a measure such as the FTND that has gained common currency, than to get embroiled in measures that rely on potentially differing interpretations and operationalizations of the concept of dependence.

References

APA 1995 Diagnostic and statistical manual of mental disorders, 4th edn. Washington, DC, American Psychiatric Association

Benowitz NL, Jacob P 3rd 1984 Daily intake of nicotine during cigarette smoking. Clin Pharmacol Ther 35:499–504

Berlin I, Singleton EG, Pedarriosse AM et al 2003 The Modified Reasons for Smoking Scale: factorial structure, gender effects and relationship with nicotine dependence and smoking cessation in French smokers. Addiction 98:1575–1583

Edwards G, Gross MM 1976 Alcohol dependence: provisional description of a clinical syndrome. Br Med J 1:1058–1061

Etter JF 2005 A comparison of the content-, construct- and predictive validity of the cigarette dependence scale and the Fagerstrom test for nicotine dependence. Drug Alcohol Depend 77:259–268

Gossop M, Darke S, Griffiths P et al 1995 The Severity of Dependence Scale (SDS): psychometric properties of the SDS in English and Australian samples of heroin, cocaine and amphetamine users. Addiction 90:607–614

Gossop M, Marsden J, Stewart D 2002 Dual dependence: assessment of dependence upon alcohol and illicit drugs, and the relationship of alcohol dependence among drug misusers to patterns of drinking, illicit drug use and health problems. Addiction 97:169–178

Grant BF, Hasin DS, Chou SP, Stinson FS, Dawson DA 2004 Nicotine dependence and psychiatric disorders in the United States: results from the national epidemiologic survey on alcohol and related conditions. Arch Gen Psychiatry 61:1107–1115

Heatherton TF, Kozlowski LT, Frecker RC, Fagerstrom KO 1991 The Fagerstrom Test for Nicotine Dependence: a revision of the Fagerstrom Tolerance Questionnaire. Br J Addict 86:1119–1127

Hoch E, Muehlig S, Hofler M, Lieb R, Wittchen HU 2004 How prevalent is smoking and nicotine dependence in primary care in Germany? Addiction 99:1586–1598

Hughes JR, Gulliver SB, Amori G, Mireault GC, Fenwick JF 1989 Effect of instructions and nicotine on smoking cessation, withdrawal symptoms and self-administration of nicotine gum. Psychopharmacology (Berl) 99:486–491

Lader D, Goddard E 2004 Smoking related attitudes and behaviour, 2003. London, Office of National Statistics

Langenbucher JW, Labouvie E, Martin CS et al 2004 An application of item response theory analysis to alcohol, cannabis, and cocaine criteria in DSM-IV. J Abnorm Psychol 113:72–80

Lessov CN, Martin NG, Statham DJ et al 2004 Defining nicotine dependence for genetic research: evidence from Australian twins. Psychol Med 34:865–879

Marsh A, MacKay S 1994 Poor smokers. London, Policy Studies Institute

McNeill AD, Jarvis MJ, Stapleton JA, West RJ, Bryant 1989 Nicotine intake in young smokers: longitudinal study of saliva cotinine concentrations. Am J Public Health 79:172–175

Morgenstern J, Langenbucher J, Labouvie EW 1994 The generalizability of the dependence syndrome across substances: an examination of some properties of the proposed DSM-IV dependence criteria. Addiction 89:1105–1113

Perkins KA, Grobe JE, Fonte C et al 1994 Chronic and acute tolerance to subjective, behavioral and cardiovascular effects of nicotine in humans. J Pharmacol Exp Ther 270:628–638

RCP 2000 Nicotine addiction in Britain. Royal College of Physicians, London

Richardson CG, Ratner PA 2005 A confirmatory factor analysis of the Fagerstrom Test for Nicotine Dependence. Addict Behav 30:697–709

Rose JE, Behm FM 1994 Inhalation of vapor from black pepper extract reduces smoking withdrawal symptoms. Drug Alcohol Depend 34:225–229

Shaffer HJ, Eber GB 2002 Temporal progression of cocaine dependence symptoms in the US National Comorbidity Survey. Addiction 97:543–554

Shiffman S, Waters A, Hickcox M 2004 The nicotine dependence syndrome scale: a multidimensional measure of nicotine dependence. Nicotine Tob Res 6:327–348

Tiffany ST, Conklin CA, Shiffman S, Clayton RR 2004 What can dependence theories tell us about assessing the emergence of tobacco dependence? Addiction 99 Suppl 1:78–86

Topp L, Darke S 1997 The applicability of the dependence syndrome to amphetamine. Drug Alcohol Depend 48:113–118

Topp L, Mattick RP 1997 Validation of the amphetamine dependence syndrome and the SAmDQ. Addiction 92:151–162

USDHHS 1988 The health consequences of smoking: nicotine addiction. A report of the Surgeon General. United States Department of Health and Human Services, Rockville, MD

West R 1995 Nicotine is addictive: the issue of free choice. In: Clarke P, Quik M, Adlkofer P, Thuraux P (eds) The effects of nicotine on biological systems II. Berlin, Birkhauser p 265–272

West R 2006 Theory of addiction. Blackwell, Oxford, in press

West RJ, Russell MA 1985 Pre-abstinence smoke intake and smoking motivation as predictors of severity of cigarette withdrawal symptoms. Psychopharmacology 87:334–336

West R, Russell MA 1988 Loss of acute nicotine tolerance and severity of cigarette withdrawal. Psychopharmacology 94:563–565

West R, McEwen A, Bolling K, Owen L 2001 Smoking cessation and smoking patterns in the general population: a 1-year follow-up. Addiction 96:891–902

West R, Hajek P, Stead L, Stapleton J 2005a Outcome criteria in smoking cessation trials: proposal for the common standard. Addiction 100:299–303

West R, DiMarino M, Gitchell J, McNeill A 2005b The impact of UK policy initiatives on use of medicines to aid smoking cessation. Tob Control 14:166–171

WHO 1992 International classification of diseases and related health problems, tenth revision (ICD-10). Geneva, World Health Organization

DISCUSSION

Shiffman: The issue of restriction of range is important. If you are looking at people who are dependent enough to seek treatment, which is a high bar, this is going to severely constrain the correlations. I fear to get at the kind of analysis you are proposing, we need to look at a broader range of people. From an Item Response Theory perspective, it is a bit like testing maths ability in maths graduate students by giving them long division. It will be uninformative. If you do it in sixth graders, however, you will get a nice curve. Also, I have a more generous interpretation of DSM-IV than you do. Constructs in DSM-IV are meant to be measures of compulsion. The question becomes one of how do we measure compulsion? Do we just ask someone whether they feel compelled? These are all ways of getting at loss of control by looking at variables and stimuli that *ought to* control behaviour, such as whether you lose your life and health if you do this. If we see that behaviour is not affected by those forces, we then say it is out of control. This is what it means to be out of control.

West: On the methodological side I agree. What I would like to see is population level studies. This can't be done cross-sectionally, obviously, but we can do longitudinal studies in which we have good comprehensive assessments of the kinds of things that interest us. We then identify people who make quit attempts, and look at the success of those quit attempts. We don't have those kinds of studies at the moment. We do have some range restriction, I agree. Bear in mind, though, that people come into clinics with all sorts of motivation, and while the bar is set high in that they feel they need help in quitting smoking, it is not necessarily that high in terms of dependence. It's 10+ cigarettes per day, average FTND of about 5.6. Although those parameters are from a subset of the population, relative to each other I would expect this subpopulation to show the same kind of pattern unless there is some discontinuity; that is, unless the things that affect probability of stopping in the whole population are not the same as those affecting this in the upper half of the distribution. It is striking that the FTND consistently does well in population studies as well as in clinical samples of this kind.

Shiffman: The issue is that it is a 'difficult' set of items (in the Item Response Theory sense), and therefore is discriminating only at the high end. Taking the analogy of long division for maths graduate students, conversely if there was a test of advanced calculus you could get a nice distribution in advanced graduate students. It is striking in the data that all the items that are discriminating are ones with low relevance. These are completely related: whenever you have 85% of people endorsing and 85% relapsing, how could that item be discriminating? It is masked out.

West: My other area of research is traffic accidents, and we see similar skewed distributions. There, as here, even where you have anything about 85% there is enough variation to show relationships. My argument is that if what we are interested in is loss of control, then all of our markers should be focused on that. This leads to your second point: this is where I think that DSM-IV hasn't gone far enough away from the alcohol-dependence syndrome, because it still has tolerance in there. I don't think tolerance is relevant to loss of control. I would be arguing for DSM-IV and ICD-10 to go the rest of the way in focusing on loss of control.

Tyndale: We have also been struggling with how to define and use dependence in these contexts. We work on relative rates of nicotine metabolism. In our populations we see very similar plasma nicotine levels targeted by very different amounts of smoking behaviour; identified by groups of slow and fast nicotine metabolizers (Rao et al 2000, Schoedel et al 2004). The existence of these two groups can confound the use of FTND based on the two main questions, amount smoked each day and time to first cigarette, although we see similar scores on not wanting to give up the first cigarette. The slow metabolizers are under-represented in smoking populations if you have a 10 cigarettes per day cut-off. In Caucasians this is probably just noise in the kind of data you are talking about, where just 5–10% the population will be slow or fast metabolizers. But well above 50% of Japanese, for example, carry these variants resulting in slow metabolism, and this changes the relationship to the outcomes you used. If you are using these FTND questions in mixed populations you need to pay attention to the fact that they may have different validity and meaning across those different ethnic groups for a variety of reasons. In our studies we struggle with how to define dependence. If someone is smoking to generally get to similar plasma nicotine levels (Rao et al 2000) but is using a different amount of behaviour to achieve this, are they more or less dependent? Thus we capture most of these people with DSM-IV, where we find that FTND is confounded by metabolism. This may be a fairly minor component of clinical studies if you have 10 cigarettes per day cut-offs and are talking about Caucasians, but it will be different in other populations.

Shiffman: The biggest screening in Robert West's study is not the formal criterion of 10+ cigarettes per day, but the fact that it is a treatment sample. By definition, these are people who have asked for help. Almost always, these are people with histories of repeated failure.

Tyndale: We also see relatively high rates of spontaneous quitting among slow metabolizers, so they may be at lower frequency in this group.

Shiffman: Our clinics are so aversive, it is very few who can drag themselves in!

Walton: I want to address this point about the rate of nicotine metabolism confounding some of these issues. If we sample for slow metabolizers it would help us to take the metabolic variables out of the equation. This might help to identify the questionnaire elements that are important but not dependant on rate of nicotine metabolism. I predict that the first cigarette of the day might not be so important. This might allow other elements to come out. The other way to do this is by stratifying according to genotype, but then you'd need a large study to do this.

Tyndale: A more practical way of doing this may be to look at the 3-hydroxycotinine/cotinine levels in smokers. This would give a pretty good estimate of the range of rates of metabolism across the population. If you over-sampled into the slower rates of metabolism you would knock out at least the component based on this. We see longer times to first cigarette in the morning for slow metabolizers on the FTND, but other elements may be different. This sampling is one way of reducing the impact of the metabolism rates without genotyping. On the other hand, whether you want to reduce this impact or not depends on who you are trying to treat.

Balfour: There is another issue we need to bear in mind when comparing nicotine with other drugs of abuse. For most drugs defined as addictive in DSM-IV there is a dose–response curve: the more you take, the bigger the effect. With nicotine, there is an optimum dose and some issues with desensitization of receptors. As a result, there isn't a simple dose–response relationship.

Jarvis: I have been thinking about the questionnaire items you mentioned, and the use of nicotine intake as an indicator. We know that all of these, and in particular time to first cigarette of the day, correlate quite well with nicotine intake. In a way, it is worth thinking about whether one can explore simply nicotine intake as one's addiction indicator. It doesn't in itself incorporate all those subjective elements which are in the questionnaire items, but it may do just as well in predicting outcomes. It may be a good way of defining the extent of the problem that individuals have.

Changeux: You have used loss of control, which you defined as longer than intended use despite knowledge of harmful effects. I am not a blunt behaviourist, but you have to rely on introspection for these definitions. This is a highly subjective kind of assessment. Do you think you can approach this in a more quantitative way? Can you be more specific about how we can make these assessments more scientific?

West: As a recovering radical behaviourist, I agree with the sentiment of what you say, but what people find in a clinical situation is that you cannot move away from the experience of the addict as an addict. The emotional side of what addicts experience is a major part of the problem itself. From a scientific point of view we can assess this using operational definitions and markers as best we can. We just have to recognize that this is not very good; we are doing our best with a limited set of instruments. If what we are talking about is something that has got out of control, we can define this and not just in a metaphysical sense. We can say that here are individuals who are seriously attempting to control their behaviour and are failing. I think we ultimately use failure of abstinence as our criterion, but our measure of dependence is something we take while the person is still smoking. I think Martin is right: we have data to indicate that cotinine, as one objective measure, is highly predictive of failure of abstinence. But what is of interest to know is whether it adds to or is added to by these kind of questionnaire type measures, some of which are subjective but some of which are also self-reports of behaviours which people can report accurately, such as when you have your first cigarette of the day.

Changeux: Can you assess these subjective criteria compared with other more objectively controlled behaviours? Can you distinguish between effects unique to nicotine and effects due to the temperament of the person?

West: I think we can. Part of the problem with defining addiction is that we want to include some non-drug-taking behaviours. Gambling is a good example. It is easy to define addiction if we limit ourselves to compulsive drug-seeking behaviour. But as soon as you start to incorporate other behaviours it starts to get difficult. It is possible, though. We also have to recognize that addiction is a socially defined construct which has no fixed boundaries. There are addiction-like behaviours that aren't addiction; there are behaviours which are hard to say are or aren't; and there are behaviours which definitely are addiction.

Corrigall: What would you see as valuable work from the basic end of the field to address this?

West: I was impressed with Ian Stolerman's suggestions for ways in which animal models might develop. I thought he might raise an issue that the behavioural economists are looking at, which is the response options and to what extent animals will prioritize nicotine as opposed to other reinforcers.

Hajek: Coming back to defining and assessing dependence, one productive approach could be seeing the core of dependence in the inability to quit, and then looking for predictors of that outcome. Our knowledge on this is meagre. The current questionnaire measures seem to predict successful smoking cessation with a correlation of around 0.2, which even for behavioural science is rather pathetic. What other predictors could we use? Living with a smoker could predict outcome more accurately than this, which could give a hint about the nature of dependence. Other predictors include mental illness, age and low socioeconomic status. Another popular idea concerns polarization of smokers into those who smoke for pleasure versus those who smoke to cope. Robert's motivational scale doesn't suggest that there is much mileage in this, but there is another related way of cutting the cake: some people smoke primarily in response to their falling blood nicotine levels, whereas others smoke more in response to external cues. Looking at examples of people from both extremes makes me think this may deserve attention.

Corrigall: How much of this breaks down according to nicotine biology versus other biology and behaviour? We don't have an answer.

Chiamulera: I noticed that one of your points was for us to identify objective measures. This is fine for research but to try to put this into practice in the setting of a GP's survey is not practical. GPs have very little time: the only question they are taught to ask is 'do you smoke?' This is the way they assess. We need to find a compromise between what we would like to ask people for research purposes and what is actually used in practice. Knowing the way GPs work, I would strongly recommend the use of an easy-to-use diagnostic test for objective evaluation of smoking status, such as a dipstick or breath analyser. Perhaps even a questionnaire could be used, but it would have to be faster than the Fagerstrom, whilst remaining as valid.

Shiffman: It is not clear that GPs should be assessing dependence. The algorithm is: if you smoke, you should quit. The incremental value of assessing dependence is very small. Treatment matching is only worth doing when there is a high cost to the treatment. In this case we optimize the outcome by saying that if you smoke you should be treated.

Chiamulera: Within the dimension of the smoker group there is a wide range of different patient types.

Shiffman: What is the treatment implication of that range? What should a GP do differently? I don't think there are any data suggesting that differential treatment based on assessment optimizes the outcomes.

Perkins: One more question is useful: 'Are you interested in quitting now?'

West: That is true for brief interventions, but if we buy into the idea that nicotine addiction is a serious, life threatening, chronic relapsing condition, we need to put more effort into the assessment of patients and clients who we are treating. One of the things that we are seeing more of in the clinical world is recognition of the fact that there will be some patients who can be launched into 'orbit' with a short programme of treatment. There are others who will need longer treatments and those who need episodic treatments. We need to identify these subgroups as early as possible, and we need to know what it is about their pharmacology or social environment that will enable us to target the optimum interventions. This is not assessing the severity of nicotine addiction; it is assessing the mechanism that leads to loss of control for that individual.

Corrigall: Alternatively, one could question which parts of this dependence one could treat. Not everyone is chronically relapsing. There are phases of the disease which we could treat.

Picciotto: You have been focusing on compulsion, but the measures you have that correlate best are still measures of nicotine dependence on the Fagerstrom scale. How does this capture the compulsion of use in the chippers that are becoming an increasing percentage of current smokers and who may not be represented in your population of treatment seekers? How do you reconcile this with the clear compulsion of the person whose last cigarette is the hardest to give up? That is, they no longer need these degrees of nicotine dependence as captured by first cigarette in the morning, but clearly have compulsive behaviour that they can't stop.

Jarvis: We need to be careful about equating this non-daily use with chippers. In the US data the non-daily users, on average, say they are smoking 25 days a month and consuming about 5–10 cigarettes per day. We are not talking about chippers.

Shiffman: It has become an increasing proportion. In the USA, the non-daily users are now 25% of all smokers. The distribution runs down to people who are just smoking just one or two days per week. In a lot of the developing world the dominant pattern of smoking is intermittent.

Jarvis: There's an important question about whether the way nicotine dependence manifests itself will change as these social rules get more tight. At the moment we don't have the intake data which enables us to know whether it is changing.

Shiffman: Robert West mentioned how important Griffifth Edwards' alcohol dependence syndrome model has been, but the early development of dependence constructs around opiates has also been influential. So our dominant implicit model is that the dependent person tries to maintain a constant blood level of the abused substance all day. It turns out that daily smoking is the only drug abuse behaviour that fits that model! What's happening now is that nicotine users aren't all doing this. There is something fundamentally wrong with the model which worked pretty well when people were smoking 20 cigarettes a day every day. This can't explain this new pattern of smoking, and it also doesn't explain most cocaine and opiate use.

West: We need some objective marker of addiction. I have said that we should achieve this by taking a group of people who try to stop, and then look at the proportion that fails. The reasons people will fail in an attempt to stop won't just be about addiction. There will be a whole range of other factors that are not addiction-related which will contribute to that. It isn't that failure to stop smoking *is* dependence: it is a criterion for assessing the *relative* validity of different measures that we might have of dependence. It will be interesting to see that, if it is the case that a higher proportion of the population are becoming intermittent smokers, to what extent is their failure to stop related to dependence as we are construing it, or the fact that their motivation to stop is less because they recognize that the health effects they will be suffering are less great as well.

Powell: I want to revert to the issue of other indicators of the severity of dependence. We have recruited 150 smokers who were willing to try to quit. We assessed them prior to their quit attempt under two conditions: one after administering them with nicotine via lozenge, and once after administering a placebo. In addition to assessing them on the Fagerstrom we have also assessed them on a range of cognitive and behavioural indicators, which we have derived from the incentive sensitization model of addiction. We wanted to see whether any deficits that are apparent during acute abstinence would resolve, and functioning recover to the levels of non-smokers. We would also like to know whether a smoker's level of impairment on these tasks in the placebo condition has any bearing on whether or not they succeed in abstaining over the first week, as verified by cotinine levels. It turns out that there is a predictive relationship.

Three of the indices of cognitive impairment at baseline jointly accounted for about 20% of the variance in outcome at seven days, which is more than accounted for by severity of dependence as assessed by the Fagerstrom. The particular cognitive indices that we found during the placebo condition to predict seven day outcome are interesting. One of them was attentional bias to smoking-related cues, confirming a finding in one or two other studies. Another was deficits of response inhibition, which we looked at using an oculomotor task; those participants less able to inhibit a reflexive response were less likely to be abstinent at seven days. The third measure was a simple psychomotor speed variable. These findings were in a sample of 100–150 smokers whose use ranged from light up to heavy.

References

Rao Y, Hoffmann E, Zia M et al 2000 Duplications and defects in the CYP2A6 gene: identification, genotyping, and in vivo effects on smoking. Mol Pharmacol 58:747–755

Schoedel K, Hoffmann E, Rao Y, Sellers E, Tyndale RF 2004 Ethnic Variation in CYP2A6 and association of genetically slow nicotine metabolism and smoking in adult Caucasians. Pharmacogenetics 14:615–626

General discussion I

Jarvis: I want to say something about nicotine use in populations and how it manifests itself: the phenomenology of nicotine addiction. We are using nicotine intake as our marker of nicotine dependence and exploring this, rather than questionnaire measures. What determines nicotine intake preferences in individuals? We think individuals show characteristic nicotine preferences, but we don't know what sets the level or how stable those preferences are over a person's smoking career. We know something about how nicotine intakes escalate in novice users: it seems to be quite quick, but we don't have a huge amount of data. Do people's preferred nicotine intakes change with age? I have some data to show on this. The phenomenon of compensation—people changing the way they inhale in response to changes in nicotine availability from products—is well established. Whether people completely compensate or not is unknown. We don't know whether smokers can successfully adapt to lower nicotine intakes. There is an issue about how social and other factors impact on the level of dependence. A key question to me is how nicotine dependence presents itself in different populations in different countries. Finally, do product characteristics determine nicotine intake? The answer to this is a clear no: it is smokers who determine the intakes they get from different products.

If we use cotinine as our measure of nicotine intake and dependence, we see a good relationship between cigarette consumption and cotinine up to about 15 cigarettes per day, and then it asymptotes. This hides enormous between-individual variability in nicotine intake. Different people take in vastly different amounts of nicotine at any given level of smoking. In relation to intake and average consumption, we can estimate how much smokers are taking in from the cigarettes they smoke. Overall, smokers take in just over a milligram of nicotine on average from each cigarette. The higher the reported cigarette consumption the lower the nicotine intake is per cigarette. We have been discussing the emergence of occasional smoking: what is going on with low-level smokers? The estimated nicotine per cigarette goes up. For people who say they are smoking less than one cigarette per day, if we simplify this by saying they smoke one per day, their estimated nicotine intake from that cigarette is 5 mg. We should therefore be careful about drawing too many conclusions from the number of cigarettes and from daily or non-daily smoking. People tend to take in more nicotine per cigarette if they smoke less. A second example of the significance of nicotine compensation is the different nicotine yields of different brands. There is essentially no relationship between nominal brand yield and measured nicotine intake. This is powerful evidence for compensation. People who self-select to smoke low yielding brands take up to 10 times more nicotine per cigarette than the nominal machine-smoked yield, whereas those smoking higher yielding brands take only 1–1.5 times the nominal yield.

What about stability of nicotine intake over time in a population of smokers? Data from the UK, going from 1980–2000, show that there has been a 40% decline in nicotine yield from cigarettes over that period as measured by machine. What is seen in measured cotinine levels in comparable samples of the population over that period is that there has been no change at all. I don't know whether this would extend back to smokers in the 1950s when yields were much higher. This raises the question as to whether it is realistic to think that it might be possible to get a population of smokers to adapt to lowered nicotine intakes over time by changing the characteristics of the product smoked. The issue of nicotine intake across the lifetime of a smoker is another important issue. From cross-sectional data we see that on average measured nicotine intakes go up with age, peaking in middle age, and then they decline again in older people. This might be because smokers gradually become more dependent as they age and then lose a bit of interest. But it is equally possible that all this is showing is selection factors operating on who is in the smoking population. If it is true that through the early adult years it is the lighter smokers who are quitting, then you are left with a population of heavier smokers. Of these, the heavier smokers will be selectively leaving the population later through premature death. It could be that smokers have intake preferences which are set for that individual and which stay the same across time.

Are there other factors influencing nicotine dependence? I find this a fascinating question. We think of nicotine intake as being biologically determined, yet there is clear evidence that social factors are important in determining the level of nicotine dependence that individuals attain to. If we go across levels of socio-economic status from affluent to the most deprived, we know smoking prevalence increases greatly in poorer groups, but comparing poor smokers with more affluent smokers, the more deprived you are the higher the nicotine intake. Social circumstances are in some way determining the level of nicotine dependence. I mentioned cross-national difference. One example is that across levels of socioeconomic status (SES), there is clear evidence that Scottish smokers take in more nicotine than English smokers. More dramatically, smokers in Britain (predominantly white) show slightly higher levels of nicotine intake than US white smokers, but within the USA there are striking differences by ethnic group. African American smokers take in substantially more nicotine than the white smokers, and the US Hispanics seem to be happy with much lower nicotine intakes. We don't have data on French, German or Japanese smokers. What we can see is that smokers regulate their nicotine intake, and that smokers not products determine intake, and nicotine intake is an excellent marker of nicotine dependence. But there are some gaps: we lack the information we need to understand what the phenomena we are trying to explain are.

Perkins: I would caution against the conclusion that the comparison across yields reflects compensation. I think the smokers are taking cigarettes that have had the paper manufactured to deliver low yields, and then converting it into a regular nicotine cigarette. The content is the same across all those different yields. We can't really address this until we have cigarettes with lowered amounts of nicotine in the tobacco itself. In this case perhaps the product can alter the amount of nicotine intake by the smoker.

Jarvis: Then the question becomes whether the smokers will live with it.

Perkins: I don't think the comparison across yield is a good test of the compensation theory. It is easy to defeat that manufacturing process.

Jarvis: Yes, but compensation occurs. Almost all these smokers will have started on a high-yield brand.

Perkins: Compensation assumes that it is more difficult to obtain the nicotine so they are over-smoking somehow. I am not so sure that is occurring, because the content is not different.

Jarvis: The evidence is clear that people do over-smoke in a variety of ways, and the end product is that the observed nicotine intake is the same across all brands. If it were not for nicotine need driving smoking, then one wouldn't predict that this would occur.

Picciotto: The nicotine metabolite is standing in as a marker for all the other constituents of cigarette smoke. They might be smoking for something else, and by getting more of the nicotine they are getting more of that as well. What I think Ken Perkins is saying is that if it is purely the nicotine, then you have to vary the ratio of nicotine to the other constituents to demonstrate this properly.

Perkins: Yes, that would be a much better test.

Clarke: If we assume that nicotine is the key determinant in regulating smoking behaviour, do we feel that people are smoking for nicotine, or is there some aversive threshold that people are smoking up to?

Corrigall: The study done by Neal Benowitz in which people were treated with nicotine in the lab (Benowitz et al 1998) addresses this in part. The subjects did continue to smoke, although they smoked less when their nicotine load was substantially higher. Mike Russell proposed that the amount of nicotine in cigarettes be increased to foster reduced smoking. But before we advocate this, we need to have better data about exactly what is going on.

Jarvis: The Neal Benowitz study gave people a plateau level of nicotine through a very slow route. The smoking is then superimposed on that level. It may not be the systemic level that is important but the acute spikes. It is clear that too high levels of nicotine are aversive for smokers. I don't think we know quite how close to the aversive level the levels that smokers achieve are.

Clarke: In your Hispanic populations, has anyone tried to see whether they find lower levels aversive than other populations?

Jarvis: If you express those population nicotine intakes on a per cigarette basis, Hispanics seem to take the same nicotine dose from each cigarette as UK smokers; they just have a much lower cigarette consumption. African American smokers in the USA seem to take almost twice as much from each cigarette.

Shiffman: Hispanic smokers also have a much higher prevalence of non-daily smoking.

Balfour: If smokers learn to smoke with conditioned stimuli present in the smoke, then in one sense the blood nicotine level is not that important. They are smoking primarily for the conditioned sensory stimuli present in the smoke rather than the pharmacological properties of nicotine *per se.*

Caggiula: In self-administration studies where the animal has to perform the same response in order to get nicotine and the stimuli that are standing in for the stimuli that we are talking about in smoking. They take a lot of nicotine, and they get a lot of exposure to the stimuli. But when you give the animal an opportunity to control the nicotine and the stimuli separately, they take much less nicotine to produce exactly the same enhancement of the stimulus effect. In the normal self-administration procedure where the stimuli and the nicotine intake are confounded, they take much more nicotine than when they are able to unconfound the two effects.

Jarvis: How does this link in with the observation that the lower the cigarette consumption the larger the nicotine intake per cigarette?

Caggiula: What you need to do is unconfound the nicotine intake from the other smoking-associated stimuli.

Corrigall: In a scientific sense I agree that the proper experiment needs to be done. But logically, there seems to be a conundrum with those animal data. They show that a bit of nicotine will increase the reinforcing value of weak stimuli, versus the fact that people will up-regulate their smoking when faced with low-yield cigarettes.

Shiffman: People can't disentangle the two. If they are seeking the stimuli, they will take in more nicotine.

Corrigall: That holds true only if the stimuli are cigarette-based.

Tyndale: In some ways we have the ability to look at this with altering nicotine metabolism. We have been able to rapidly increase and also slow the rate of nicotine metabolism. Within a subject you can then look at how they compensate during smoking. We get nice compensation with some components, but not complete compensation in either direction. When we block nicotine metabolism, reducing the rates of nicotine inactivation, their nicotine plasma levels do go higher while their smoking decreases. They decrease their smoking substantially but it is not a complete compensation. If we increase their rates of nicotine metabolism people increase their smoking to keep nicotine levels up.

Shiffman: That contradicts Tony Caggiula's conclusion.

Tyndale: It is consistent in the sense that if you block nicotine metabolism, you should see much more down-regulation of the behaviour than we do, suggesting that some smoking is driven by components other than nicotine.

Bertrand: Along the same lines, there are fast and slow nicotine metabolizers, and the latter find it easier to quit. You would assume, therefore, that just using nicotine replacement therapy would allow everyone to quit. Are we missing something and what is the best way of helping people to quit?

Jarvis: The missing element here is the route and speed of administration of nicotine. The available replacement therapies give lower doses of nicotine and more slowly, in a less rewarding way.

Reference

Benowitz NL, Zevin S, Jacob P 3rd 1998 Suppression of nicotine intake during ad libitum cigarette smoking by high-dose transdermal nicotine. J Pharmacol Exp Therap 287:958–962

Nicotinic acetylcholine receptor functions in the CNS investigated with a novel method of stereotaxic gene re-expression in knockout mice

Uwe Maskos, Sylvie Granon, Philippe Faure and Jean-Pierre Changeux[1]

URA CNRS 2182 Récepteurs & Cognition & Institut Pasteur, 25 rue du Dr Roux, 75724 Paris Cedex 15, France

Abstract. Nicotinic receptors (nAChR) are important targets of the neurotranmitter and modulator acetylcholine. Ten neuronal nAChR subunits have been identified that assemble to form a variety of pentameric oligomers possessing diverse physiological and pharmacological properties and different distributions in the CNS. We investigated the role of the different subunits in knockout mice constructed by homologous recombination. Among other features, in $\beta2^{-/-}$ mice nicotine no longer stimulates dopamine release in vivo and elicits electrical responses of mesencephalic dopaminergic neurons. Moreover, the $\beta2^{-/-}$ mice show deficits in nicotine self-administration and in executive functions. Thus the $\beta2$ subunit is necessary, but has not yet been shown to be sufficient for these functions. We have therefore developed a novel strategy to selectively re-express the β_2 subunit on a knockout background using a lentiviral vector. Fully functional high-affinity nAChRs are recovered in the ventral tegmental area (VTA) and are shown to be *sufficient* to restore nicotine-elicited dopamine release and nicotine self-administration *in vivo*. Moreover, slow exploratory behaviour of these mice was restored in a sequential locomotor task testing executive function. These data highlight the critical role of endogenous cholinergic regulation mediated by nicotinic receptors on higher cognitive functions. In a more general manner, the method makes possible the differential analysis of the neuronal circuits involved in nicotine addiction.

2005 Understanding nicotine and tobacco addiction. Wiley, Chichester (Novartis Foundation Symposium 275) p 64–82

The nicotinic acetylcholine receptors (nAChRs) are well characterized transmembrane allosteric proteins involved in the physiological responses to acetylcholine (Changeux & Edelstein 1998, 2005). They are pentameric oilgomers composed of five identical (homopentamers) or different (heteropentamers) polypeptide chains

---

[1]This paper was presented at the Symposium by Jean-Pierre Changeux, to whom correspondence should be addressed

arranged symmetrically around an axis perpendicular to the membrane. The agonist binding sites are located in the synaptic domain at the interface between adjacent subunits and the ion channel lies along the axis of symmetry in the transmembrane region (Corringer et al 2000, Unwin 2005). Their distance is larger than 3 nm at the molecular scale: the interaction between the neurotransmitter site and ion channel is thus a typical 'allosteric' interaction and mediated by a conformational transition of the protein molecule (Changeux 1980). nAChRs may spontaneously exist under several discrete interconvertible conformational states: basal or resting (closed), active (open) or desensitized (closed) (Heidmann & Changeux 1979a, b, 1980, Edelstein et al 1996). Nicotinic ligands, agonists or competitive antagonists, but also allosteric effectors binding to sites distinct from the ACh binding site, may differentially affect the equilibrium established between the various conformations (Changeux 1980).

CNS nuclei with ACh-containing neurons (such as the pedunculopontine nucleus, medial septal nucleus and nucleus basalis) send widespread projections to most areas in the brain (Mesulam et al 1983). In addition to their primordial role in neuromuscular and motor autonomous transmission, nAChRs are involved in several central functions including control of voluntary motion, memory and attention, sleep and wakefulness, reward and pain, anxiety, and sensory gating (Cordero-Erausquin et al 2000, Robbins 2000). Nicotinic agonists thus exhibit multiple pharmacological actions when they bind to neuronal nAChRs.

Several human neuropathologies have recently been shown to be caused by genetic alterations on nAChR genes, including congenital myasthenia, autosomal frontal lobe nocturnal epilepsy, and possibly schizophrenic or autistic syndrome (Lena & Changeux 1997, Lindstrom 1997, Bertrand 2002, Perry et al 1999, Levin & Rezvani 2002). These receptors may also be involved in several neuropathologies such as Parkinson and Alzheimer's diseases and Gilles de la Tourette syndrome (Zoli et al 1999, Picciotto & Corrigall 2002). However, the most widespread human pathology associated with nAChRs is the addiction to nicotine (Peto et al 1996, Di Chiara 2000, Dani & De Biasi 2001, McGehee 2002).

Yet, because of the limited specificity of the available agonists and antagonists, it has been difficult to assess, on pharmacological grounds, the contribution of defined nAChR subunits and oligomers to specific behaviours. Here, we review how the generation of mice that lack one or more nAChR subunits has provided a powerful experimental approach to elucidate the relationships between the subunits composition, the physiological and pharmacological properties of nAChRs and the associated behaviours. The first part thus focuses on recent observations related to nAChR subunit composition and pharmacology that have been derived from the analysis of knockout mice and provide the basis for the analysis of the contribution of defined nAChRs to behaviour. Thus the deleted subunit is *necessary*, but has not been demonstrated to be *sufficient* for these functions. We have therefore developed a novel strategy to selectively re-express the deleted subunit on the knockout background using a lentiviral vector. New perspectives on the endogenous role of nicotinic receptor function and nicotine-elicited electrophysiological and behavioural effects will also be highlighted.

Pharmacology and subunit composition

Among the broad diversity of nAChR oligomers present in the brain (LeNovère et al 2002), equilibrium binding, physiological and pharmacological studies have distinguished two principal categories of nAChR pentamers. High affinity nAChRs are formed by the assembly of $\alpha 4$ and $\beta 2$ subunits ($\alpha 4^*\beta 2^*$-nAChRs): they bind nicotine with affinity but do not interact with α-bungarotoxin (α-BgT). On the other hand, $\alpha 7$ homo-oligomers ($\alpha 7^*$-nAChRs) bind nicotine with low affinity but α-bungarotoxin with high affinity. Alkondon & Albuquerque (1993) and Zoli et al (1998) have compared agonists (such as nicotine, cytisine and choline) and antagonists (such as α-BgT) potencies, and nAChR response kinetics in electrophysiological and binding experiments to distinguish these nAChR subtypes. The authors propose that $\alpha 7^*$-nAChRs exhibit low affinity for ACh and nicotine, rapidly desensitize and are involved in *phasic* synaptic responses, whereas $\alpha 4\beta 2^*$-nAChRs possess a high affinity for ACh and nicotine, desensitize slowly and are engaged in *tonic* paracrine-like transmission (Descarries 1997).

In other territories of the brain, the situation can be rather more complex, as for instance, for the dopaminergic (DA) reward neurons of the ventral tegmental area (VTA) (Klink et al 2001, Champtiaux et al 2002, 2003). DA neurons indeed express mRNAs coding for most, if not all, neuronal nAChR subunits. Immunoprecipitation experiments performed on mouse striatal extracts lead to the identification of three main types of heteromeric nAChRs ($\alpha 4\beta 2^*$, $\alpha 6\beta 2^*$ and $\alpha 4\alpha 6\beta 2^*$) in DA terminal fields and nicotine-elicited DA release in striatal synaptosomes and recordings of ACh-elicited currents in DA neurons from $\alpha 4$, $\alpha 6$, $\alpha 4\alpha 6$ and $\beta 2$ knockout mice establish that $\alpha 6\beta 2^*$ nAChRs are functional and sensitive to α-conotoxin MII inhibition but do not contribute to DA terminal release caused by systemic nicotine administration. In contrast, (non-$\alpha 6$)$\alpha 4\beta 2^*$ nAChRs represent the majority of functional heteromeric nAChRs on DA neuronal soma and most likely contribute to nicotine reinforcement (Champtiaux et al 2002, 2003).

Physiological and behavioural analysis of mice with the nAChR $\beta 2$ subunit deleted

Human disorders with symptomatic cognitive impairments linked to abnormalities of the neurotransmitter system for ACh, as well as a wealth of animal experiments, support a role of the cholinergic system mediated through nAChRs in learning and memory (Levin 1992, Perry et al 1999).

Mice lacking the β2-subunit have been constructed (Picciotto et al 1995) and show an almost complete disappearance of high affinity nicotine binding. Furthermore they display abnormal passive avoidance, impaired nicotine self-administration and drug discrimination, exhibit a reduced nociceptive response to nicotine and decreased visual acuity. On the other hand, general spatial memory tested in the water-maze task is not affected (Picciotto et al 1998, Marubio et al 1999, Rossi et al 2001).

The β2 subunit is involved in passive avoidance learning

Learning and memory in β2 subunit knockout mice were examined using the passive avoidance test (Picciotto et al 1998). This test measures the animal latency to perform a highly probable behaviour (entry into a dark chamber) for which it had previously been punished during the training session. β2 knockout mice showed enhanced latency of entry (i.e. more stable memory of the punishment) compared with wild-type littermates. This implies that some β2*nAChRs are endogenously active, and directly or indirectly exert a negative effect in the circuits involved in passive avoidance response. Surprisingly, low doses of nicotine normally increase the retention of the avoidance response (see next paragraph).

The β2 subunit is involved in executive functions and social behaviour

We have explored the contribution of nAChRs to complex cognitive functions referred to as executive processes. The management of these processes provides the maintenance of goal representation, the appropriate adaptation of behaviour in a changing environment, the organization of sequences of actions over time, and the inhibition of prepotent or previous responses. Previous modelling studies (Dehaene et al 1998, Schultz et al 1997) and former work in humans and animals has shown that these processes require prefrontal and/or cingulate activation. Behavioural protocols known to rely on the integrity of these structures (see Granon et al 1994, 1995) were adapted to mice (Granon et al 2003, Maskos et al 2005).

We have developed an automated analytical procedure for locomotor behaviour in the mouse (Faure & Korne 2001, Faure et al 2003, Granon et al 2003). This method makes possible the distinction and quantitative evaluation of high-level executive components from low-level motor behaviour. Furthermore, to study an index of adapted responses to a context that potentially leads to conflict resolution, we designed procedures aimed at the distinction between several types of sequential behaviours in a social learning context. Interestingly, the 'supervisory planning' *exploratory* organization of mouse locomotor behaviour and conflict resolution were found selectively impaired in the $\beta2^{-/-}$ mice challenged in different spatial learning and social paradigms (Granon et al 2003, Maskos et al 2005). On the other hand more automatic *navigatory* behaviours were not modified accounting for paradoxical 'gains of function' in some behavioural tests (see above).

$\beta2$ subunit mediates the reinforcing properties of nicotine

Addictive drugs, such as cocaine, ethanol, amphetamine and nicotine, interact with the mesotelencephalic dopaminergic system, which is classically assumed to mediate their reinforcing properties. Nicotine administered systemically causes an increase in extracellular dopamine levels in the dorsal and, preferentially, ventral striatum. The nAChRs involved are plausibly located on dopamine containing neurons of the ventral tegmental area (VTA) and substantia nigra (SN), and in terminal fields of those neurons in the striatum and nucleus accumbens (see above). Microdialysis experiments showed that nicotine elicited a dose-dependent increase in striatal dopamine release in wild-type but not in knockout mice, which implicates $\beta2^*$-nAChRs in these effects. *In vitro*, low concentrations of nicotine (similar to those found in the arterial blood of smokers when they are smoking) elicited an increase in the discharge frequency of dopamine-containing neurones of the SN and VTA in wild-type animals, but not in knockout mice. Finally, nicotine self-administration has been tested in wild-type and knockout mice. Both demonstrated cocaine self-administration during the training session and were clearly capable of learning this behaviour. However, knockout mice progressively ceased self-administration when switched to nicotine, whereas wild-type mice continued, which demonstrate that $\beta2^*$-nAChRs contribute to the reinforcing properties of nicotine (Picciotto et al 1998).

A novel method for the targeted re-expression of nAChR subunits

The midbrain VTA is considered the principal brain region mediating the reinforcement properties of multiple drugs of abuse, including nicotine, but its precise contribution is still challenged (Laviolette & van der Kooy 2004). To further understand the specific role of $\beta2^*$-nAChRs in mediating the effects of nicotine and endogenous acetylcholine on reinforcement and cognition, we selectively re-expressed the $\beta2$ subunit in the VTA of $\beta2^{-/-}$ mice. Our approach was to generate a lentiviral expression vector containing a bi-cistronic cassette simultaneously expressing the $\beta2$ subunit and the enhanced green fluorescent protein (eGFP) facilitating efficient detection of transduced cells (Maskos et al 2002). Despite their growing use in gene therapy and animal models, no functional neurotransmitter receptor had been expressed *in vivo* using this system.

Lentiviral vectors

Lentivirus-based expression systems (Naldini et al 1996), initially developed for gene therapy purposes, provide several advantages over other virus-based *in vivo* transgene expression strategies. First, as with all retroviruses, they are capable of stable integration into the genome of the host cell, facilitating the potential for long-term, stable transgene expression. Second, once the viral transgene has been stably integrated, continued expression of viral proteins (and the accompanying potential for destructive immune responses) is avoided. Third, lenti-retroviruses are capable of genomic integration into non-dividing cells, such as neurons and other terminally differentiated cells.

The lentiviral expression vectors used are derived from the pHR' expression vectors first described by Naldini et al (1996), with several subsequent modifications (Fig. 1A). To increase the safety of the expression vector, the U3 region of 3' long terminal repeat (LTR) was deleted (ΔU3), rendering the integrated viral DNA replication-incompetent. Furthermore, abolishing the promoter activity of the 3' LTR prevents potential promoter interference with the transgene promoter and increases transgene expression. The central polypurine tract (cPPT) and the central termination sequence (CTS) of the wild-type HIV-1 have been added, thus creating the 99 base pair central DNA 'flap'. This feature, unique to lentiviruses, likely enhances infection of non-dividing cells by facilitating transport of the pre-integration complex through the nuclear membrane pores, rather than requiring nuclear membrane destruction during mitosis and significantly enhances HIV vector-mediated cell transduction of different types of brain cells. Finally, the woodchuck hepatitis B virus post-transcriptional regulatory element (WPRE) has been added to increase RNA stability and transgene expression.

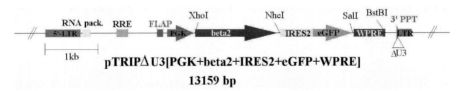

pTRIPΔU3[PGK+beta2+IRES2+eGFP+WPRE]

13159 bp

FIG. 1A. (A) Map of lentiviral expression vector. Diagram of transgene lentiviral vector between and including the LTR regions. LTR, long terminal repeat; RNA pack, genomic RNA packaging signal; RRE, rev response element; FLAP, sequence comprising central polypurine tract, and central termination sequence; PGK, promoter of the mouse phosphoglycerate kinase gene; beta2, mouse wild-type β2 nicotinic acetylcholine receptor subunit cDNA; IRES2, internal ribosome entry sequence; eGFP, enhanced green fluorescent protein; WPRE, woodchuck hepatitis B virus post-transcriptional regulatory element; 3'PPT, 3'polypurine tract; ΔU3, deletion of U3 portion of 3'LTR.

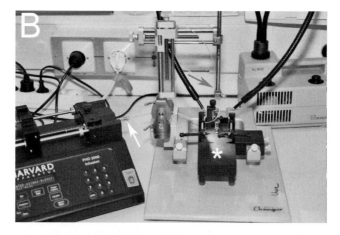

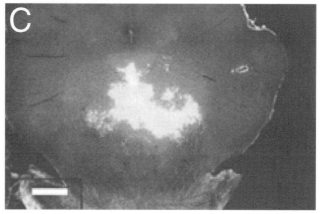

FIG. 1B,C.   (B) Set-up used for the efficient, reproducible injection of lentivirus. The mouse rests on a specialized adaptor (Cunningham & McKay 1992, asterisk). The injection needle (Cooper Needle Works, UK, arrow) is attached to a microelectrode holder, and connected via Teflon tubing to a $5\,\mu l$ Hamilton syringe (white arrow) driven by an infusion pump at $0.2\,\mu l/min$. (C) Lentiviral transduction of the posterior ventral tegmental area (VTA). This is an image taken on an upright Zeiss microscope using standard FITC filters. Scalebar, $300\,\mu m$.

Analysis of 'local stereotaxic transgenics'

We specifically re-expressed the nAChR $\beta2$ subunit by stereotaxically injecting such lentiviral vector into the VTA of mice carrying $\beta2$ subunit deletions (Fig. 1BCD). We first demonstrated the efficient re-expression of ligand-binding nicotinic acetyl-choline receptors in dopamine-containing neurons of the VTA. nAChR functionality was then assessed by recording the effect of nicotine on the *in situ* electrophysiological activity of DA neurons in the VTA. In wild-type (WT), intravenous injection of $30\,\mu g/kg$ of nicotine caused the well-established rapid 1.5-fold increase in firing frequency lasting nearly 10 min (Fig. 2A). Knockout (KO) produced either no or, in a few cases, short duration responses, in agreement with previous *in vitro* observations on midbrain slices. $\beta 2^{-/-}$ mice with the $\beta 2$ + eGFP bi-cistronic vector (VEC) showed responses to nicotine characterized by the same rapid increase in firing frequency observed in WT, demonstrating re-expression of functional nAChRs. However, unlike neurons from WT, this effect did not persist for more than 2 min on average. These data show that the re-expression of the $\beta 2$ subunit exclusively in the VTA is sufficient to recover an effect of nicotine on DA neurons. Remarkably, the sustained (up to 10 min) increase in firing rate recorded in WT mice was not observed in the VEC mice. This suggests that the sustained firing of DA neurons in the VTA could be dependent on $\beta 2$ subunit expression in other—exci-

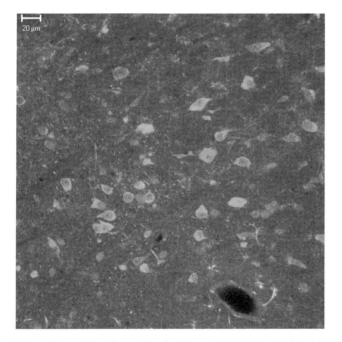

FIG. 1D.   (D) Detailed analysis of transduced cell types in the VTA. Double-label immunohistochemistry with an anti-TH antibody reveals dopaminergic neurons. GABAergic neurons lack TH immunoreactivity, and glial processes can be discerned around the ventricle (lower right).

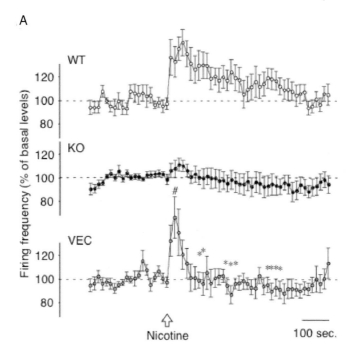

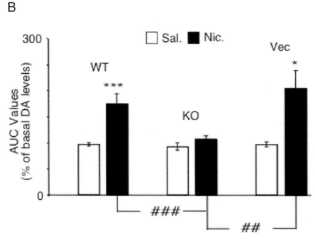

FIG. 2. Restoration of electrophysiologically responsive nAChRs and of nicotine elicited dopamine release. *In vivo* recordings in the VTA demonstrate a partial restoration of the nicotine elicited firing rate in dopaminergic neurons (A). *In vivo* microdialysis in freely moving mice shows complete restoration of nicotine elicited dopamine release in the nucleus accumbens. WT, wild-type C57BL/6J mice injected with the eGFP-only lentivector; KO, $\beta2^{-/-}$ mice injected with the eGFP-only lentivector; VEC, $\beta2^{-/-}$ mice injected with the $\beta2$ + eGFP bi-cistronic vector.

tatory—structures, such as glutamatergic prefrontal cortex or ponto-tegmental afferents (Mansvelder et al 2003). In addition, the precise subunit stoichiometry of the VEC mice may also be slightly different from WT, as most nAChR subunits are expressed in VTA neurons (Klink et al 2001) and no molecular tool exists so far to definitively identify nAChRs of known composition.

To determine whether the re-expressed $\beta 2^*$-nAChR with a different DA firing rate could still mediate normal levels of nicotine-elicited dopamine release, we used *in vivo* intracerebral microdialysis in awake, freely moving mice. In both VEC and WT, we observed a statistically significant increase in dopamine release in the nucleus accumbens (NuAcc) following 1 mg/kg intraperitoneal nicotine injection (Fig. 2B). No nicotine-elicited dopamine release was observed in KO, as described for uninjected $\beta 2^{-/-}$ mice (Picciotto et al 1998). These data confirm a complete restoration of nicotine-elicited dopamine release from the NuAcc by the re-expressed $\beta 2$ subunit in the intact behaving animal. Moreover, comparison between the effects of nicotine on electrophysiological activity and dopamine release, although obtained under different conditions, confirms that the long-term release of dopamine (more than 2 h) in VEC is independent of the time course of the nicotine-elicited increase in firing rate of VTA DA neurons.

To assess whether the nicotine-elicited responses observed in the VTA and NuAcc in VEC were sufficient to support nicotine reinforcement, we developed an intra-VTA nicotine self-administration paradigm in the mouse, as described for morphine self-administration. Mice (7 WT, 10 KO, 9 VEC) were implanted and tested in a Y maze. WT exhibited a clear nicotine-seeking behaviour from the second learning session, as measured both by the increasing choice of the nicotine-reinforced arm (Fig. 3A) and decreasing latency to trigger the injections over time (Fig. 3B). In contrast, KO did not acquire nicotine self-administration behaviour. Their arm choice remained at chance level during the experiment, whereas latency to trigger injections gradually increased under nicotine sessions. This particular combination of parameters (no arm choice, long latency) is typically observed in non-reinforced animals. As observed for WT mice, VEC mice also acquired intra-VTA nicotine self-administration behaviour and improved their performance over learning sessions. However, they displayed a delay in the acquisition of self-administration, differing from KO mice from the fourth learning session, and their discrimination performance was slightly lower than that observed for WT mice at the end of the experiment. As observed for WT, self-injection latency decreased over nicotine sessions in VEC, confirming nicotine-seeking behaviour. Therefore, we conclude that re-expression of $\beta 2^*$-nAChR in the VTA is not only *necessary* but also *sufficient* to re-establish sensitivity to nicotine reward in drug-naïve mice. The neuronal structures and molecules involved in nicotine addiction have remained a debated issue; our data provide decisive evidence that the $\beta 2^*$-nAChR in neurons originating in the VTA play a crucial role.

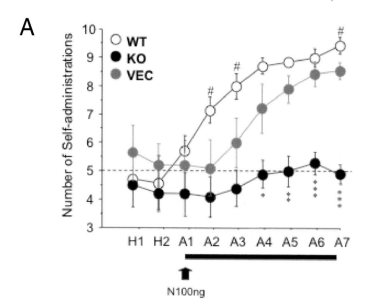

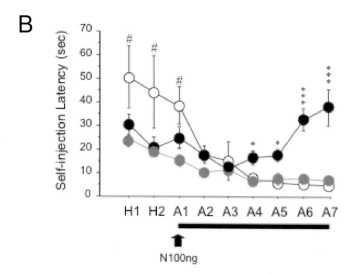

FIG. 3.   Intra-VTA self-administration of nicotine. Re-injected $\beta2^{-/-}$ KO mice (VEC) efficiently self-administer nicotine with the same self-injection latency as WT.

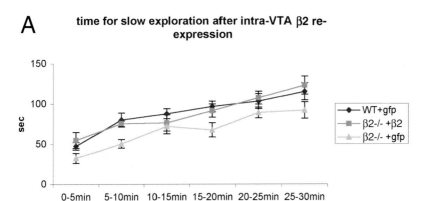

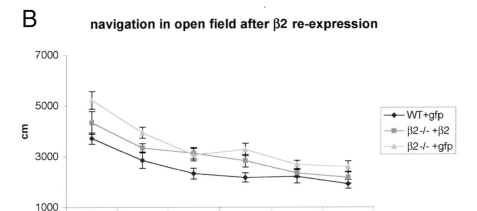

FIG. 4. Exploration and navigation of animals in an open field. Exploration (A) and navigation (B) was quantified for the three experimental groups, and plotted for each 5 min interval. A statistically significant restoration of exploration was observed for VEC when compared with WT.

Having established that re-expressed $\beta2^*$-nAChR respond to nicotine *in vivo*, we investigated the potential role of endogenous ACh in cognitive behaviours: the circuit containing the VTA, NuAcc and ventral pallidum is involved in translation of environmental stimuli into adaptive responses, and therefore is involved in exploratory and novelty-seeking behaviours (Fig. 4). Exploratory behaviours, in rodents and other mammals, contribute to the acquisition of environmental knowledge and give rise to a variety of cognitive processes including spatial and non-spatial memory, spontaneous adaptation and strategy set-up (Bardo et al 1996). Alterations in exploratory activity can be quantitatively analysed in rodents via detailed decompositions of the speed and location of trajectories of the animal in an open field. Motor function, spatial and non-spatial memory systems, and anxiety processes are normal in $\beta 2^{-/-}$ mice. However, $\beta 2^{-/-}$ mice exhibit modified spatiotemporal organization of displacements, with increased *navigatory* and decreased *exploratory* behaviour (Granon et al 2003).

We thus tested whether the features of behaviour distinguishing wild-type from $\beta 2^{-/-}$ mice were rescued in VEC. Three experimental groups were placed in a circular open field and their trajectories measured by a video tracking system. WT and KO differed significantly for the two components, confirming our published results on uninjected mice and demonstrating the absence of any LV injection-related effect on these behaviours. However, VEC showed a selective restoration of exploration, bringing this measure up to the level of WT without a significant modification of navigation. In addition, the quantitative decomposition of trajectories showed that the sequencing of movements in VEC is differentially restored, depending on the type of movements evaluated. VEC exhibited transitions between fast and slow movements in the central portion of the arena that were similar to WT. This form of slow exploratory behaviour allows animals to gather spatial information external to the open field by making rearings and head movement. Conversely, VEC mice exhibited KO-like sequencing of fast navigatory movements. The targeted expression of $\beta 2^*$-nAChR in the VTA thus generated a *dissociation* between exploratory and navigatory behaviour.

Our results demonstrate that nAChRs in neurons originating in the VTA and/or their axonal projections suffice for the differential restoration of the cognitive function as studied in our paradigm. This behaviour therefore appears to be mediated by endogenous acetylcholine released either by projections from the pedunculopontine and latero-dorsal tegmental nucleus (Laviolette & van der Kooy 2004), or by endogenous local acetylcholine acting on $\beta 2^*$-nAChR expressed on axonal projections from the VTA to the NuAcc. It suggests the implication of dopamine or GABA as the neuro-modulatory substance for this executive function, as there is also an important projection of GABA-ergic neurons to the prefrontal cortex (Carr & Sesack 2000).

Conclusion

Nicotine reinforcement has been postulated to mobilize multiple intricate networks including ascending DA, cholinergic and serotonergic pathways together with glutamatergic and GABA-ergic neurons from multiple brain regions. The present study reveals, for the first time, that restoration of $\beta 2^*$-nAChRs specifically in the VTA and its axonal projections restores the self-administration of nicotine, i.e. that the nAChR system in the VTA and its axonal projections is a major factor of nicotine reinforcement. Even more unexpected is the selective recovery of cholinergic action on a complex cognitive behaviour, for which we provide a molecular ($\beta2^*$-nAChRs) and anatomical basis (neurons originating in the VTA).

This work further illustrates the efficiency of the lentiviral vector technique *in vivo* in the analyses of the neural bases of spontaneous cognitive behaviours, their regulation by endogenous neurotransmitters and a specific receptor species in the absence of external intervention. In a general manner, a molecular dissection of higher brain functions henceforth becomes accessible to *in vivo* investigation at the cellular and neuronal network level.

Acknowledgments

This work was supported by Collège de France, AFM, ARC, MILDT and CEE contracts.

References

Alkondon M, Albuquerque EX 1993 Diversity of nicotinic acetylcholine receptors in rat hippocampal neurons. I. Pharmacological and functional evidence for distinct structural subtypes. J Pharmacol Exp Ther 265:1455–1473

Bardo MT, Donohew RL, Harrington NG 1996 Psychobiology of novelty seeking and drug seeking behavior. Behav Brain Res 77:23–43

Bertrand D 2002 Neuronal nicotinic acetylcholine receptors and epilepsy. Epilepsy Curr 2:191–193

Carr DB, Sesack SR 2000 GABA-containing neurons in the rat ventral tegmental area project to the prefrontal cortex. Synapse 38:114–123

Changeux JP 1980 The acetylcholine receptor: an 'allosteric' membrane protein. Harvey Lect 75:85–254

Changeux JP, Edelstein SJ 1998 Allosteric receptors after 30 years. Neuron 21:959–980

Changeux JP, Edelstein SJ 2005 Allosteric mechanisms of signal transduction. Science 308:1424–1428

Champtiaux N, Han ZY, Bessis A et al 2002 Distribution and pharmacology of alpha 6-containing nicotinic acetylcholine receptors analyzed with mutant mice. J Neurosci 22:1208–1217

Champtiaux N, Gotti C, Cordero-Erausquin M et al 2003 Subunit composition of functional nicotinic receptors in dopaminergic neurons investigated with knock-out mice. J Neurosci 23:7820–7829

Cordero-Erausquin M, Marubio LM, Klink R, Changeux JP 2000 Nicotinic receptor function: new perspectives from knockout mice. Trends Pharmacol Sci 21:211–217

Corringer PJ, Le Novere N, Changeux JP 2000 Nicotinic receptors at the amino acid level. Annu Rev Pharmacol Toxicol 40:431–458

Dani JA, De Biasi M 2001 Cellular mechanisms of nicotine addiction. Pharmacol Biochem Behav 70:439–446

Descarries L, Gisiger V, Steriade M 1997 Diffuse transmission by acetylcholine in the CNS. Prog Neurobiol (Oxf) 53:603–625

Dehaene S, Kerszberg M, Changeux JP 1998 A neuronal model of a global workspace in effortful cognitive tasks. Proc Natl Acad Sci USA 95:14529–14534

Di Chiara D 2000 Role of dopamine in the behavioural actions of nicotine related to addiction. Eur J Pharmacol 393:295–314

Edelstein SJ, Schaad O, Henry E, Bertrand D, Changeux JP 1996 A kinetic mechanism for nicotinic acetylcholine receptors based on multiple allosteric transitions. Biol Cybern 75:361–379

Faure P, Korn H 2001 Is there chaos in the brain? I. concepts of nonlinear dynamics and methods of investigation. C R Acad Sci Serie III Sci Vie 324:773–793

Faure P, Neumeister H, Faber D, Korn H 2003 Symbolic analysis of swimming trajectories reveals scale invariance and provides a model for fish locomotion. Fractals 11:233–243

Granon S, Vidal C, Thinus-Blanc C, Changeux JP, Poucet B 1994 Working memory, response selection, and effortful processing in rats with medial prefrontal lesions. Behav Neurosci 108:883–891

Granon S, Poucet B, Thinus-Blanc C, Changeux JP, Vidal C 1995 Nicotinic and muscarinic receptors in the rat prefrontal cortex: differential roles in working memory, response selection and effortfull processing. Psychopharmacology (Berl) 119:139–144

Granon S, Faure P, Changeux JP 2003 Executive and social behaviors under nicotinic receptor regulation. Proc Natl Acad Sci USA 100:9596–9601

Heidmann T, Changeux JP 1979a Fast kinetic studies on the allosteric interactions between acetylcholine receptor and local anesthetic binding sites. Eur J Biochem 94:281–296

Heidmann T, Changeux JP 1979b Fast kinetic studies on the interaction of a fluorescent agonist with the membrane-bound acetylcholine receptor from Torpedo marmorata. Eur J Biochem 94:255–279

Heidmann T, Changeux JP 1980 Interaction of a fluorescent agonist with the membrane-bound acetylcholine receptor from Torpedo marmorata in the millisecond time range: resolution of an 'intermediate' conformational transition and evidence for positive cooperative effects. Biochem Biophys Res Commun 97:889–896

Klink R, de Kerchove d'Exaerde A, Zoli M, Changeux JP 2001 Molecular and physiological diversity of nicotinic acetylcholine receptors in the midbrain dopaminergic nuclei. J Neurosci 21:1452–1463

Lena C, Changeux JP 1997 Pathological mutations of nicotinic receptors and nicotine-based therapies for brain disorders. Curr Opin Neurobiol 7:674–682

Levin ED 1992 Nicotinic systems and cognitive function. Psychopharmacology 108:417–431

Levin ED, Rezvani AH 2002 Nicotinic treatment for cognitive dysfunction. Curr Drug Targets CNS Neurol Disord 1:423–431

Laviolette SR, van der Kooy D 2004 The neurobiology of nicotine addiction: bridging the gap from molecules to behaviour. Nat Rev Neurosci 5:55–65

Le Novere N, Corringer PJ, Changeux JP 2002 The diversity of subunit composition in nAChRs: evolutionary origins, physiologic and pharmacologic consequences. J Neurobiol 53:447–456

Lindstrom J 1997 Nicotinic acetylcholine receptors in health and disease. Mol Neurobiol 15:193–222

McGehee DS 2002 Nicotinic receptors and hippocampal synaptic plasticity . . . it's all in the timing. Trends Neurosci 25:171–172

Mansvelder HD, De Rover M, McGehee DS, Brussaard AB 2003 Cholinergic modulation of dopaminergic reward areas: upstream and downstream targets of nicotine addiction. Eur J Pharmacol 480:117–123

Marubio LM, del Mar Arroyo-Jimenez M, Cordero-Erausquin M et al 1999 Reduced antinociception in mice lacking neuronal nicotinic receptor subunits. Nature 398:805–810

Maskos U, Kissa K, St Cloment C, Brulet P 2002 Retrograde trans-synaptic transfer of green fluorescent protein allows the genetic mapping of neuronal circuits in transgenic mice. Proc Natl Acad Sci USA 99:10120–10125

Maskos U, Molles BE, Pons S et al 2005 Recovery of nicotine reinforcement and cognitive functions by targeted expression of nicotinic receptors. Nature 436:103–107

Mesulam MM, Mufson EJ, Wainer BH, Levey AI 1983 Central cholinergic pathways in the rat: an overview based on an alternative nomenclature (Ch1–Ch6). Neuroscience 10:1185–1201

Naldini L, Blomer U, Gallay P et al 1996 In vivo gene delivery and stable transduction of non-dividing cells by a lentiviral vector. Science 272:263–267

Perry E, Walker M, Grace J, Perry R 1999 Acetylcholine in mind: a neurotransmitter correlate of consciousness? Trends Neurosci 22:273–280

Peto R, Lopez AD, Boreham J et al 1996 Mortality from smoking worldwide. Br Med Bull 52:12–21

Picciotto MR, Corrigall WA 2002 Neuronal systems underlying behaviors related to nicotine addiction: neural circuits and molecular genetics. J Neurosci 22:3338–3341

Picciotto MR, Zoli M, Lena C et al 1995 Abnormal avoidance learning in mice lacking functional high-affinity nicotine receptor in the brain. Nature 374:65–67

Picciotto MR, Zoli M, Rimondini R et al 1998 Acetylcholine receptors containing the beta2 subunit are involved in the reinforcing properties of nicotine. Nature 391:173–177

Robbins TW 2000 Chemical neuromodulation of frontal-executive functions in humans and other animals. Exp Brain Res 133:130–138

Rossi FM, Pizzorusso T, Porciatti V, Marubio LM, Maffei L, Changeux JP 2001 Requirement of the nicotinic acetylcholine receptor beta 2 subunit for the anatomical and functional development of the visual system. Proc Natl Acad Sci USA 98:6453–6458

Schultz W, Dayan P, Montague PR 1997 A neural substrate of prediction and reward. Science 275:1593–1599

Unwin N 2005 Refined structure of the nicotinic acetylcholine receptor at 4A resolution. J Mol Biol 346:967–989

Zoli M, Lena C, Picciotto MR, Changeux J-P 1998 Identification of four classes of brain nicotinic receptors using beta2 mutant mice. J Neurosci 18:4461–4472

Zoli M, Picciotto MR, Ferrari R, Cocchi D, Changeux J-P 1999 Increased neurodegeneration during ageing in mice lacking high-affinity nicotine receptors. EMBO J 18:1235–1244

DISCUSSION

Markou: Can you tell us about the nAChR up-regulation in nicotine addiction?

Changeux: The up-regulation of acetylcholine binding sites was initially discovered in smokers' brains as an increase of high affinity nicotine binding sites. In mice and in rats, after chronic exposure to nicotine a 10–20-fold increase in acetylcholine binding sites takes place in the brain. Lindstrom has shown that this increase is not due to transcriptional regulation. It is some kind of post-transcriptional regulation. This was investigated in my laboratory by Jerome Sallette and Pierre-Jean Corringer using the gene chimeras method (Sallette et al 2004). Systematic analysis of $\beta2/\beta4$ chimeras demonstrates that (i) the extracellular domain of the nicotinic receptor molecule critically contributes to up-regulation, (ii) only residues belonging to two $\beta2$ segments, 74–89 and 106–115, confer up-regulation to $\beta4$, and (iii) on an atomic three-dimensional model these residues form a compact microdomain that mainly contributes to the subunit interface but also faces the acetylcholine binding site. We have also demonstrated that nicotine acts intracellularly (Sallette et al 2005). To address the molecular mechanism of up-regulation, we transfected HEK293 cells with human $\alpha4\beta2$ receptors and traced the subunits throughout their intracellular biosynthesis, using metabolic labelling and immunoprecipitation techniques. We show that high-mannose glycosylated subunits mature and assemble into pentamers in the endoplasmic reticulum and that only pentameric receptors reach the cell surface following carbohydrate processing. Nicotine is shown to act inside the cell and to increase the amount of β subunits immunoprecipitated by the conformation-dependent mAb290, indicating that nicotine enhances a critical step in the intracellular maturation of these receptors. This wasn't anticipated. Many of us thinking in terms of drug receptors considered that all the effects of drugs were due to the interaction with receptors exposed to the cell surface! This work was done *in vitro* in HEK293 cells, and confirmed with neuronal cell cultures.

Balfour: In vivo there is marked regional variation in the degree of up-regulation, and in whether or not up-regulation is seen. In some parts of the brain the up-regulation of receptors doesn't seem to be accompanied by an up-regulation of function. Are you arguing for a functionally significant up-regulation?

Changeux: In the system we have been using, yes. We have followed the up-regulation *in situ* by autoradiography. In agreement with what you say, we find that some regions of the brains up-regulate more than others (I. Cloëz, unpublished results). This may be due to the subunit composition of the receptor in these different locations.

Bertrand: What is still unclear is how much functional up-regulation contributes to the addiction mechanisms. Similarly, we are still debating the importance of receptor desensitization caused by chronic nicotine exposure. These questions are difficult to answer because they can only be addressed if we understand the receptor function and contribution to the neuronal network. Even if we dispose of a selective PET ligand we would still need to determine the receptor function.

Clarke: Is it clear whether up-regulation of nicotinic receptors by nicotine plays any role in nicotine dependence?

Changeux: There is a correlation. In our experience there is clearly an increase of the response of the cells to nicotine. Whether this has to do with nicotine addiction or not is a question we hope that we will be able to answer soon.

Stolerman: I'd like to address the lentiviral re-expression studies that you have done. As well as the technical feat in terms of manipulations at the molecular level, there is a remarkable achievement of obtaining intra-VTA self-administration of the drug in mice. This line of work strengthens the case for $\beta2$-containing receptors being involved in dependence. Where does this leave $\alpha7$? Is it the case that $\alpha7$ has no role in dependence?

Changeux: These studies (Maskos et al 2005) were done using a broad variety of techniques including single-cell extracellular recordings in the VTA *in vivo*, with anaesthetized animals. If addiction has to do with subjective states of motivation, we have to make the studies with animals in a conscious state. This is currently being done. The present data clearly indicate that the $\beta2$ subunit has the dominant role. Yet, something is happening with the $\alpha7$ knockout which is under study. At that stage one cannot say that $\alpha7$ has no role in dependence.

Corrigall: It looks like the VTA is the sole site involved: if you remove the $\beta2$ receptors you decrease nicotine self-administration to virtually zero. If you replace the $\beta2$ subunit, it presumably combines with $\alpha4$ and it looks like nicotine self-administration has been restored completely.

Changeux: I don't like to use the word 'completely', but the restoration of function is very significant. This is quite an interesting finding in the case of self-administration. I am personally more interested by the fact that a restoration of cognitive functions goes together with that of self-administration. This would mean that the systems involved in learning and cognitive behaviour are biased by nicotine at the level of the reward systems. This is consistent with the models of cognitive learning that Dehaene and myself proposed for delayed response tasks linked with the prefrontal cortex (Dehaene & Changeux JP 1991). In this model we proposed a critical role of the dopamine reward systems in cognitive learning by the prefrontal cortex. In mice, the prefrontal cortex is tiny. In the rat, the contribution of the prefrontal cortex is easier to look at. But the link between prefrontal cortex and reward system had to be established. I hope the present data contribute to that. During the discussion this morning, the issue was raised of the validity of animal models. Between rats and humans there are clearly differences, but these also exist between mice and rats! We have to be aware of this.

Picciotto: Can you speculate on the role of the $\beta2$ receptors in the dopaminergic versus the GABAergic neurons? You showed it was expressed in both, and showed rescue data for dopamine. Do you think there is an important role for GABA neurons, and more specifically is there a difference in the ratio in the rescue versus the wild-type that might explain the delay in the self-administration?

Changeux: That is an interesting question, and I hope we will be able to answer it next year! There is a very interesting pattern of nicotinic receptor subunits in the GABAergic interneurons of the VTA. It seems that there is more diversity in the GABAergic neurons than there is in the dopaminergic neurons (Klink et al 2001). There is an interesting possible role for computation of the inhibitory neurons in the VTA. If we look at the cerebral cortex, the network of inhibitory neurons plays a crucial role in oscillation and the state of wakefulness/consciousness why not in the VTA for nicotine addiction.

Chiamulera: I have a comment on the loss of executive top-down control in the $\beta2$ knockout mice, with decrease of prefrontal cortex control. This is important. It is another good example showing that we can improve the 'basic' self-administration/mesolimbic paradigm. We can still have an operant behavioural measure that is relevant not only for the effect of nicotine on reward/drug taking function, but also for associated cognitive phenomena. For example, the loss of top-down control could change the attentional process towards smoking related cues and trigger drug-seeking behaviour.

Picciotto: It is interesting that it is still dependent on the VTA. You can rescue it despite the fact that it is clearly a cortical function in the circuit that's initiated in the VTA.

Changeux: This is an interesting and original aspect. As I mentioned already, Dehaene and myself did extensive modelling of delayed-response tasks: these are computer models of behaviour. In these models the reward system is playing a crucial role for the selection of a given plan of action. This idea has also been used by Sejnowski, Schultz and others, but in the more complex paradigm of reward learning or anticipation of reward. But I don't know how far we can generalize to a higher organism from these mouse experiments.

Walton: The folding of the protein is facilitated by the ligand. What do you envisage is happening in nicotine naïve people? Could acetylcholine have a similar function?

Changeux: This is an interesting question. We have speculated that up-regulation through nicotine binding to the immature receptor can unravel a possible mechanism of neuronal plasticity. Acetylcholine or its precursor choline may penetrate through the membrane and have a similar effect as nicotine. Acetylcholine and/or choline could be the natural physiological effectors for this kind of plasticity.

References

Dehaene S, Changeux JP 1991 The Wisconsin Card Sorting Test: theoretical analysis and modeling in a neuronal network. Cereb Cortex. 1991 1:62–79

Klink R, de Kerchove d'Exaerde A, Zoli M, Changeux JP 2001 Molecular and physiological diversity of nicotinic acetylcholine receptors in the midbrain dopaminergic nuclei. J Neurosci 21:1452–1463

Maskos U, Molles BE, Pons S et al 2005 Nicotine reinforcement and cognition restored by targeted expression of nicotinic receptors. Nature 436:103–107

Sallette J, Bohler S, Benoit P et al 2004 An extracellular protein microdomain controls upregulation of neuronal nicotinic acetylcholine receptors by nicotine. J Biol Chem 279:18767–18775

Sallette J, Pons S, Devillers-Thiery A et al 2005 Nicotine upregulates its own receptors through enhanced intracellular maturation. Neuron 46:595–607

Nicotine-mediated activation of signal transduction pathways

Marina R. Picciotto

Department of Psychiatry, Yale University School of Medicine, 34 Park Street—3rd Floor Research, New Haven, CT 06508, USA

Abstract. Activation of nicotinic acetylcholine receptors (nAChRs) results in depolarization and entry of calcium into neurons. These processes initiate signal transduction cascades likely to be important for changes in synaptic strength that may underlie the development of nicotine addiction. Nicotine can activate a number of protein kinases and phosphatases *in vitro* and *in vivo*, including protein kinases A and C and the MAP kinase pathway. Of particular interest are signalling molecules, such as the protein phosphatase calcineurin, that can be activated by calcium entry. In addition, chronic nicotine exposure can result in circuit level changes in quantity and activation of proteins involved in signal transduction. Transcription factors such as the cyclic-AMP response element binding protein (CREB) are attractive candidates for initiating long-term changes downstream of nAChRs. A better understanding of the signalling pathways activated by nicotine administration will be critical in understanding the transition between nicotine exposure and addiction.

2005 Understanding nicotine and tobacco addiction. Wiley, Chichester (Novartis Foundation Symposium 275) p 83–95

Although several neural circuits involved in acute nicotine action have been defined, less is known about changes in cellular and molecular signalling following chronic exposure to nicotine. Chronic administration of drugs of abuse is known to alter the activity and expression of many gene products (reviewed in Nestler 2004). It is now widely accepted that these neuroadaptations underlie the long-term behavioural consequences of chronic drug exposure, including dependence, withdrawal and relapse to drug taking. A better understanding of the particular molecular adaptations that are important for these behavioural changes, and the time-course of their appearance and resolution will be critical for understanding how acute drug taking can result in the transition to drug dependence and addiction.

Nicotine, acting through nicotinic acetylcholine receptors (nAChRs) can depolarize and increase the firing rate of dopamine neurons in the mesolimbic dopamine (DA) system (Grenhoff et al 1986) and can stimulate release of DA from nerve terminals (Rowell et al 1987). Many of the neuroadaptive changes resulting from nico-

tine exposure are common to other drugs of abuse and are likely to be downstream
of dopamine signalling. For example, chronic nicotine self-administration results in
elevation of fos-related antigen-like immunoreactivity in DA terminal regions in
rats (Merlo Pich et al 1997), as has also been shown for cocaine and opiates (Nye
& Nestler 1996, Kelz et al 1999). Like cocaine and opiate administration (Beitner-
Johnson & Nestler 1991), nicotine treatment increases levels of tyrosine hydroxylase (TH), the rate limiting enzyme for catecholamine synthesis, in the ventral
tegmental area (VTA) following repeated nicotine injection (Smith et al 1991).
Increases in TH have also been observed in the LC, the hippocampus, the hypo-
thalamus, and adrenal medulla (Naquira et al 1978, Mitchell et al 1993), suggesting
that nicotine exposure can result in widespread changes in catecholamine levels and
function.

While adaptations in the mesolimbic dopamine system are likely to be critical for
many addictive processes, nicotine-induced changes in gene expression have also
been identified in several other brain areas. Neuroadaptations unique to nicotine
may explain why it appears to be less reinforcing than other drugs of abuse in some
animal models while still potently driving smoking behaviour and very high rates of
relapse to smoking. For example, nicotine exposure results in many molecular
changes in the hypothalamic–pituitary–adrenocortical (HPA) axis, which is a critical mediator of stress responses (Matta et al 1998). Similarly, while all drugs of abuse
were able to stimulate the mitogen-activated protein kinase (MAP kinase) pathway
in the nucleus accumbens (NAc), nicotine was particularly potent at inducing
extracellular-regulated kinase (ERK) activity in the frontal cortex (FC) (Valjent et al
2004). Adaptations in the HPA axis and FC are intriguing given the literature suggesting an interaction between stress and smoking behaviour (Swan et al 1988) and
the responsiveness of FC to smoking-related cues (Due et al 2002).

A number of studies also demonstrate that chronic nicotine treatment results
in activation of signalling pathways in cell culture. For example, chronic nicotine
exposure increases protein kinase A (PKA) activity in PC12 cells leading to an
increase in expression of the $\alpha3$ nAChR subunit (Madhok et al 1995). Similarly,
nicotine increases PKA-mediated phosphorylation of the $\alpha4$ but not the $\alpha3$ subunit
in *Xenopus* oocytes (Hsu et al 1997). Nicotine can stimulate the MAP kinase pathway
in PC12 cells (Tang et al 1998) and protein kinase C (PKC) activity in both
PC12 (Messing et al 1989) and bovine adrenal chromaffin cells (Tuominen et al
1992).

Clearly, nicotine can influence signalling both directly in particular cell types, as
well as indirectly through stimulation of the release of other neurotransmitters. This
review will summarize some recent findings related to the ability of nicotine to influence calcium-dependent signal transduction pathways in primary neuronal cultures,
as well as recent studies of the effects of chronic nicotine exposure *in vivo* on signalling pathways in the brain.

Regulation of calcium signalling

Calcium is a critical messenger for regulation of synaptic plasticity. Nicotine can increase intracellular calcium by activating nAChRs permeable to calcium (McGehee & Role 1996), as well as by depolarizing the cell, leading to activation of voltage-gated calcium channels or release of calcium from intracellular stores (Tsuneki et al 2000). Nicotine treatment can reduce glutamate-mediated calcium influx into primary cortical neurons (Stevens et al 2003), suggesting that signalling downstream of nAChRs can affect responses to other neurotransmitters. Alteration of glutamate-mediated calcium influx in cortical neurons by nicotine involves activation of $\beta2$ subunit-containing nAChRs and transient activation of voltage-gated calcium channels (Stevens et al 2003). Calcium influx then activates calcineurin leading to L-type calcium channel inactivation. This results in decreased calcium entry into the neuron upon glutamate stimulation (Stevens et al 2003).

The ability of nicotine to modulate glutamate-mediated calcium entry is likely to vary depending on neuronal cell type and nAChR subtype. While knockout of the $\beta2$ subunit abolished the effect of nicotine on glutamate-mediated calcium entry, blockade of $\alpha7$ nAChRs with α-bungarotoxin did not alter calcium entry (Stevens et al 2003). In addition, activation of $\alpha7$ nAChRs did not result in alteration of glutamate-mediated calcium entry in the hippocampus (Dajas-Bailador et al 2000).

These studies strongly implicate calcineurin as a signalling molecule downstream of nAChR activation in some neuronal cell types. Calcineurin is a high-affinity calcium sensor (Yakel 1997) that has been hypothesized to be important for setting the threshold between calcium signals that decrease synaptic strength and those that increase synaptic strength (Lisman 1989). It is known that both long-term depression (LTD) and long-term potentiation (LTP) rely on calcium entry, and one hypothesis is that low levels of calcium might be sufficient to activate calcineurin leading to LTD, while higher levels of calcium that result in LTP recruit lower affinity calcium kinases leading to increased synaptic efficacy (Lisman 1989). Activation of nAChRs results in calcium entry into neurons, but the rapid desensitization of these receptors makes it likely that only low levels of calcium will enter the cell following nicotine administration (Fenster et al 1999). This low level calcium entry makes a high affinity calcium-dependent enzyme, such as calcineurin, a very attractive candidate for transducing the calcium signal generated by nicotine. Since both glutamate signalling and calcineurin activation are important for LTP and LTD (Malenka & Nicoll 1999), activation of calcineurin could also be important for effects of nicotine on processes such as learning or addiction.

MAP kinase signalling following nicotine administration

The ability to activate ERK in the mesolimbic DA system is a common property of drugs of abuse (Valjent et al 2004). ERK is also activated by nicotine (Nakayama et al 2001) and is important in mediating neuronal plasticity in several neuronal cell types (Sweatt 2001). MAP kinase signalling is therefore another attractive candidate for contributing to synaptic changes that may be important for development of nicotine addiction. ERK activity is necessary for the ability of nicotine to activate TH in bovine adrenal chromaffin cells (Haycock 1993) and for nicotine-mediated activation of CREB in PC12 and ciliary ganglion cells (Nakayama et al 2001). Thus, it seems to be an important signalling molecule in mediating long-term effects of nicotine *in vitro*.

Studies *in vivo* demonstrate that acute nicotine treatment activates ERK in the NAc indirectly through increased dopamine release and subsequent signalling through DARPP-32 (Valjent et al 2005). In mice, chronic nicotine exposure altered the levels and phosphorylation state of ERK in the frontal cortex (Brunzell et al 2003). This is consistent with changes seen following acute nicotine treatment in rats that were particularly marked in frontal cortex and were not dependent on DARPP-32 (Valjent et al 2004, 2005). In contrast, total ERK levels were significantly decreased in the amygdala following chronic nicotine exposure (Brunzell et al 2003), a brain area that could contribute to effects of nicotine on emotionality (reviewed in (Picciotto et al 2002), or on drug seeking (Taylor et al 1998) and withdrawal behaviours (Schulteis et al 2000).

Several pathways could be involved in the ability of nicotine to activate ERK. Nicotine could stimulate ERK through increased release of neurotrophic factors and subsequent activation of their receptors (Belluardo et al 1999). Alternatively, calcium entry through nAChRs (Nakayama et al 2001), or release from internal stores (Chang & Berg 2001) may be necessary for ERK activation. Increased calcium levels can activate PYK2, which in turn activates RAS, an activator of ERK (Tahara et al 2001). PYK2 is up-regulated following chronic administration of cocaine (Freeman et al 2002), although regulation of PYK2 has not yet been observed following nicotine administration (Brunzell et al 2003). Finally, ERK can be activated in response to increased neuronal activity (Murgia et al 2000); thus chronic nicotine treatment may stimulate ERK indirectly by modulating neuronal firing in circuits stimulated by nicotine. Similarly, ERK phosphorylation could be a marker of circuits activated by nicotine *in vivo*.

Nicotinic modulation of CREB signalling

The transcription factor CREB can be activated as a result of calcium signalling (Kornhauser et al 2002) as well as through activation of the MAP kinase pathway (Adams et al 2000). CREB is also critical for long-term changes in synaptic efficacy (Bourtchuladze et al 1994). Thus, CREB activation has been investigated as a potential mediator of long-term changes resulting from chronic drug administration (Carlezon & Konradi 2004). CREB and the active, phosphorylated form of CREB

(P-CREB) are regulated in the NAc and frontal cortex following chronic nicotine exposure. In mouse cortex the ratio of P-CREB to total CREB was increased following nicotine exposure, although overall levels of CREB were decreased (Brunzell et al 2003). These data are consistent with the idea that nicotine activates CREB in cortex acutely, but that down-regulation of CREB protein may be an adaptive response to chronic activation following chronic exposure. In rat cortex, P-CREB- and CREB were decreased during nicotine withdrawal (Pandey et al 2001), whereas levels of CREB returned to normal following withdrawal in mice (Brunzell et al 2003). Despite potential species and dosing differences, both studies demonstrate adaptations in CREB signalling in cortex following nicotine treatment.

In NAc chronic nicotine exposure resulted in a dramatic decrease in P-CREB despite an overall increase in total CREB levels, indicating that CREB activity was greatly decreased. This is likely to be the result of chronic activation of DA signalling, since this adaptation is common to several drugs of abuse, including morphine, ethanol and cocaine (Widnell et al 1996, Carlezon et al 1998, Misra et al 2001). In addition, decreased CREB activity is likely to have functional consequences on nicotine reinforcement. Viral-mediated expression of mCREB, a dominant-negative construct that decreases CREB activity, increased cocaine and morphine place preference whereas over-expression of CREB attenuated place preference (Carlezon et al 1998, Barrot et al 2002). Taken together, these data suggest that decreased CREB activity might regulate the reinforcing efficacy of nicotine following chronic administration. In addition, since CREB in the NAc increases stress-like responses (Barrot et al 2002), and an increased level of CREB is present following chronic nicotine treatment, this could contribute to dysphoria associated with nicotine withdrawal.

Nicotine can increase the activity of several protein kinases that activate CREB (Shaywitz & Greenberg 1999) including PKA, PKC, ERK and calcium-dependent protein kinases (CAM kinases) (Messing et al 1989, Madhok et al 1995, Damaj 2000, Nakayama et al 2001). It is possible that nicotine-dependent changes in CREB phosphorylation in the NAc are mediated through PKA activation, as has been reported for cocaine (Self et al 1998). In contrast, changes in FC CREB phosphorylation may be dependent on ERK activation, since levels of ERK phosphorylation are increased in parallel with CREB phosphorylation in this brain region following chronic nicotine exposure (Brunzell et al 2003).

Conclusions

A large number of molecular alterations have been identified in the mesolimbic dopamine system and in other brain areas following chronic administration of drugs of abuse. Some of these alterations have been validated functionally in behavioural paradigms after treatment with other drugs of abuse (Carlezon & Konradi 2004);

however, a great deal of work remains to be done to determine which of these molecular changes have consequences on nicotine-related behaviours, particularly those related to reward or reinforcement. A more complete characterization of the signalling pathways altered by chronic nicotine administration and a better understanding of their behavioural consequences is critical for developing novel treatment strategies targeting long-term adaptations in response to chronic nicotine intake from smoking.

Acknowledgements

M.R.P. is supported by grants from NARSAD and the National Institutes of Health (DA00436, DA14241, DA10455 and AA15632).

References

Adams JP, Roberson ED, English JD, Selcher JC, Sweatt JD 2000 MAPK regulation of gene expression in the central nervous system. Acta Neurobio Exp 60:377–394

Barrot M, Olivier JD, Perrotti LI et al 2002 CREB activity in the nucleus accumbens shell controls gating of behavioral responses to emotional stimuli. Proc Natl Acad Sci USA 99:11435–11440

Beitner-Johnson D, Nestler EJ 1991 Morphine and cocaine exert common chronic actions on tyrosine hydroxylase in dopaminergic brain reward regions. J Neurochem 57:344–347

Belluardo N, Mudo G, Caniglia G, Cheng Q, Blum M, Fuxe K 1999 The nicotinic acetylcholine receptor agonist ABT-594 increases FGF-2 expression in various rat brain regions. Neuroreport 10:3909–3913

Bourtchuladze R, Frenguelli B, Blendy J, Cioffi D, Schutz G, Silva AJ 1994 Deficient long-term memory in mice with a targeted mutation of the cAMP-responsive element-binding protein. Cell 79:59–68

Brunzell DH, Russell DS, Picciotto MR 2003 In vivo nicotine treatment regulates mesocorticolimbic CREB and ERK signaling in C57Bl/6J mice. J Neurochem 84:1431–1441

Carlezon WA, Konradi C 2004 Understanding the neurobiological consequences of early exposure to psychotropic drugs: linking behavior with molecules. Neuropharmacology 47:47–60

Carlezon WA, Thome J, Olson VG et al 1998 Regulation of cocaine reward by CREB. Science 282:2272–2275

Chang KT, Berg DK 2001 Voltage-gated channels block nicotinic regulation of CREB phosphorylation and gene expression in neurons. Neuron 32:855–865

Dajas-Bailador FA, Lima PA, Wonnacott S 2000 The alpha7 nicotinic acetylcholine receptor subtype mediates nicotine protection against NMDA excitotoxicity in primary hippocampal cultures through a Ca(2+) dependent mechanism. Neuropharmacology 39:2799–2807

Damaj MI 2000 The involvement of spinal Ca(2+)/calmodulin-protein kinase II in nicotine-induced antinociception in mice. Eur J Pharmacol 404:103–110

Due DL, Huettel SA, Hall WG, Rubin DC 2002 Activation in mesolimbic and visuospatial neural circuits elicited by smoking cues: evidence from functional magnetic resonance imaging. Am J Psychiatry 159:954–960

Fenster CP, Beckman ML, Parker JC et al 1999 Regulation of alpha4beta2 nicotinic receptor desensitization by calcium and protein kinase C. Mol Pharmacol 55:432–443

Freeman WM, Brebner K, Lynch WJ et al 2002 Changes in rat frontal cortex gene expression following chronic cocaine. Mol Brain Res 104:11–20

Grenhoff J, Aston-Jones G, Svensson TH 1986 Nicotinic effects on the firing pattern of midbrain dopamine neurons. Acta Physiol Scand 128:351–358

Haycock JW 1993 Multiple signaling pathways in bovine chromaffin cells regulate tyrosine hydroxylase phosphorylation at Ser19, Ser31 and Ser40. Neurochem Res 18:15–26

Hsu YN, Edwards SC, Wecker L 1997 Nicotine enhances the cyclic AMP-dependent protein kinase-mediated phosphorylation of alpha4 subunits of neuronal nicotinic receptors. J Neurochem 69:2427–2431

Kelz MB, Chen J, Carlezon WA et al 1999 Expression of the transcription factor Delta FosB in the brain controls sensitivity to cocaine. Nature 401:272–276

Kornhauser JM, Cowan CW, Shaywitz AJ et al 2002 CREB transcriptional activity in neurons is regulated by multiple, calcium-specific phosphorylation events. Neuron 34:221–233

Lisman J 1989 A mechanism for the Hebb and the anti-Hebb processes underlying learning and memory. Proc Natl Acad Sci USA 86:9574–9578

Madhok TC, Matta SG, Sharp BM 1995 Nicotine regulates nicotinic cholinergic receptors and subunit mRNAs in PC 12 cells through protein kinase A. Mol Brain Res 32:143–150

Malenka RC, Nicoll RA 1999 Long-term potentiation–a decade of progress? Science 285:1870–1874

Matta SG, Fu Y, Valentine JD, Sharp BM 1998 Response of the hypothalamo-pituitary-adrenal axis to nicotine. Psychoneuroendocrinology 23:103–113

McGehee DS, Role LW 1996 Presynaptic ionotropic receptors. Curr Opin Neurobiol 6:342–349

Merlo Pich E, Pagliusi SR, Tessari M, Talabot-Ayer D, Hooft van Huijsduijnen R, Chiamulera C 1997 Common neural substrates for the addictive properties of nicotine and cocaine. Science 275:83–86

Messing RO, Stevens AM, Kiyasu E, Sneade AB 1989 Nicotinic and muscarinic agonists stimulate rapid protein kinase C translocation in PC12 cells. J Neurosci 9:507–512

Misra K, Roy A, Pandey SC 2001 Effects of voluntary ethanol intake on the expression of Ca(2+)/calmodulin-dependent protein kinase IV and on CREB expression and phosphorylation in the rat nucleus accumbens. Neuroreport 12:4133–4137

Mitchell SN, Smith KM, Joseph MH, Gray JA 1993 Increases in tyrosine hydroxylase messenger RNA in the locus coeruleus after a single dose of nicotine are followed by time-dependent increases in enzyme activity and noradrenaline release. Neurosci 56:989–997

Murgia M, Serrano AL, Calabria E, Pallafacchina G, Lomo T, Schiaffino S 2000 Ras is involved in nerve-activity-dependent regulation of muscle genes. Nature Cell Biol 2:142–147

Nakayama H, Numakawa T, Ikeuchi T, Hatanaka H 2001 Nicotine-induced phosphorylation of extracellular signal-regulated protein kinase and CREB in PC12 cells. J Neurochem 79:489–498

Naquira D, Zunino E, Arqueros L, Viveros H 1978 Chronic effects of nicotine on catecholamine synthesizing enzymes in rats. Eur J Pharmacol 47:227–229

Nestler EJ 2004 Molecular mechanisms of drug addiction. Neuropharmacology 47:24–32

Nye HE, Nestler EJ 1996 Induction of chronic Fos-related antigens in rat brain by chronic morphine administration. Mol Pharmacol 49:636–645

Pandey SC, Roy A, Xu T, Mittal N 2001 Effects of protracted nicotine exposure and withdrawal on the expression and phosphorylation of the CREB gene transcription factor in rat brain. J Neurochem 77:943–952

Picciotto MR, Brunzell DH, Caldarone BJ 2002 Effect of nicotine and nicotinic receptors on anxiety and depression. Neuroreport 13:1097–1106

Rowell PP, Carr LA, Garner AC 1987 Stimulation of [3H]dopamine release by nicotine in rat nucleus accumbens. J Neurochem 49:1449–1454

Schulteis G, Ahmed SH, Morse AC, Koob GF, Everitt BJ 2000 Conditioning and opiate withdrawal. Nature 405:1013–1014

Self DW, Genova LM, Hope BT, Barnhart WJ, Spencer JJ, Nestler EJ 1998 Involvement of cAMP-dependent protein kinase in the nucleus accumbens in cocaine self-administration and relapse of cocaine-seeking behavior. J Neurosci 18:1848–1859

Shaywitz AJ, Greenberg ME 1999 CREB: a stimulus-induced transcription factor activated by a diverse array of extracellular signals. Ann Rev Biochem 68:821–861

Smith KM, Mitchell SN, Joseph MH 1991 Effects of chronic and subchronic nicotine on tyrosine hydroxylase activity in noradrenergic and dopaminergic neurones in the rat brain. J Neurochem 57:1750–1756

Stevens TR, Krueger SR, Fitzsimonds RM, Picciotto MR 2003 Neuroprotection by nicotine in mouse primary cortical cultures involves activation of calcineurin and L-type calcium channel inactivation. J Neurosci 23:10093–10099

Swan GE, Denk CE, Parker SD, Carmelli D, Furze CT, Rosenman RH 1988 Risk factors for late relapse in male and female ex-smokers. Addictive Behav 13:253–266

Sweatt JD 2001 The neuronal MAP kinase cascade: a biochemical signal integration system subserving synaptic plasticity and memory. J Neurochem 76:1–10

Tahara S, Fukuda K, Kodama H, Kato T, Miyoshi S, Ogawa S 2001 Potassium channel blocker activates extracellular signal-regulated kinases through Pyk2 and epidermal growth factor receptor in rat cardiomyocytes. J Amer Coll Cardiol 38:1554–1563

Tang K, Wu H, Mahata SK, O'Connor DT 1998 A crucial role for the mitogen-activated protein kinase pathway in nicotinic cholinergic signaling to secretory protein transcription in pheochromocytoma cells. Mol Pharmacol 54:59–69

Taylor JR, Punch LJ, Elsworth JD 1998 A comparison of the effects of clonidine and CNQX infusion into the locus coeruleus and the amygdala on naloxone-precipitated opiate withdrawal in the rat. Psychopharmacology 138:133–142

Tsuneki H, Klink R, Léna C, Korn H, Changeux JP 2000 Calcium mobilization elicited by two types of nicotinic acetylcholine receptors in mouse substantia nigra pars compacta. Eur J Neurosci 12:2475–2485

Tuominen RK, McMillian MK, Ye H, Stachowiak MK, Hudson PM, Hong JS 1992 Long-term activation of protein kinase C by nicotine in bovine adrenal chromaffin cells. J Neurochem 58:1652–1658

Valjent E, Pages C, Herve D, Girault J, Caboche J 2004 Addictive and non-addictive drugs induce distinct and specific patterns of ERK activation in mouse brain. Eur J Neurosci 19:1826–1836

Valjent E, Pascoli V, Svenningsson P et al 2005 Regulation of a protein phosphatase cascade allows convergent dopamine and glutamate signals to activate ERK in the striatum. Proc Natl Acad Sci USA 102:491–496

Widnell KL, Self DW, Lane SB et al 1996 Regulation of CREB expression: in vivo evidence for a functional role in morphine action in the nucleus accumbens. J Pharmacol Exp Ther 276:306–315

Yakel JL 1997 Calcineurin regulation of synaptic function: from ion channels to transmitter release and gene transcription. Trends Pharmacol Sci 18:124–134

DISCUSSION

Chiamulera: Do you think that inhibition of calcineurin by cyslosporine could be a mechanism for smoking cessation in individuals already nicotine dependent?

Picciotto: This would be a big club to hit a problem that for many people is not important enough to suppress their immune system. It is more of a proof of concept. I have asked colleagues who do transplant studies whether their patients stop smoking. They tell me that their patients shouldn't be smoking if they have just received a new organ, so I doubt that the data are out there showing whether cyclosporine treatment would decrease the reinforcing properties of nicotine and smoking.

Chiamulera: Do you expect to see any brain regional differences in this effect on calcineurin?

Picciotto: I suspect that this will be more specific to neurons that rely on $\beta2$ rather than $\alpha7$ for signalling. We don't see much effect of $\alpha7$ antagonists on the calcineurin induction. Sue Wonnacott's group have shown that in a similar protocol in which they treat hippocampal neurons in culture with nicotine, they don't see a modulation of voltage-gated Ca^{2+} channels. Therefore there seems to be a difference between cortical and hippocampal neurons. In their hands most of their response to nicotine was through $\alpha7$ receptors; in our experiments while we see a contribution of both $\alpha7$ and $\beta2$ to the physiology, only the $\beta2$ receptors seem to recruit calcineurin.

Balfour: The sensitization of locomotory activity does not correlate with the sensitization of dopamine overflow. One of the mechanisms which I quite like as an explanation for the sensitization of locomotor activity is that there is post-synaptic sensitization of dopamine receptors. Do you have any evidence that some of your molecular mechanisms are altering the sensitivity of the post-synaptic dopamine receptors?

Picciotto: Not as far as we can tell. When we look at the responses to cyclosporine alone, we don't see effects in cortex or accumbens. This would suggest that the dopamine neurons are not getting access to the peripherally administered cyclosporine. The molecular evidence we have so far suggests that we are not modulating those downstream neurons. Dopamine itself could be altering the sensitivity of the downstream receptors, and mechanisms in the ventral tegmental area (VTA) could be those that are recruited by calcineurin. It's OK if it is not dopamine, because our original hypothesis was that it was glutamate, and that what we were really doing was modulating the response of this circuit to glutamatergic stimulation.

Balfour: There is evidence for a glutamate pathway that projects from the hippocampus that influences the responses to dopamine.

Bertrand: What was the concentration of nicotine that you used for the glutamate inhibition? It should be remembered that John Dani showed that nicotine will inhibit NMDA responses.

Picciotto: We didn't see any effect on NMDA responses in that study. We used $10\,\mu$M, which was optimal.

Bertrand: This is certainly a very high value, as it must be recalled that smokers experience concentrations in the hundreds of nanomoles.

Picciotto: It is very good at activating $\beta2$. If we use $1\,\mu$M we find similar effects but they are smaller. At 1 mM we don't see the effect.

Clarke: With regard to cyclosporine's effect on $\alpha7$ expression, are you perhaps thinking of work by Jim Patrick's group (i.e. Helekar et al 1994 and Helekar & Patrick 1997)?

Bertrand: Yes, the group of Jim Patrick reported that cyclosporine can modify the expression of $\alpha 7$.

Picciotto: I have searched cyclosporine and nicotine and haven't found it, but that doesn't mean it is not out there. We have looked for effects of $\alpha 7$ blockers. These had effects on nicotine-mediated neuroprotection, so clearly $\alpha 7$ had effects on these cortical neurons with respect to neuroprotection but not with respect to the glutamate-mediated Ca^{2+} entry.

Bertrand: Which $\alpha 7$ blocker have you tried to use?

Picciotto: Both α-bungaratoxin and MLA.

Clarke: Let's see whether we can arrive at a consensus on what would be an appropriate concentration of nicotine. In a moderate to heavy smoker between cigarettes, venous levels are 30–35 ng/ml. This puts the venous concentration at 0.2 μM. Animal data suggest that under steady-state conditions after a subcutaneous depot injection of nicotine, the brain maintains a gradient such that brain concentrations are about three- to fivefold greater than in plasma. Another complication is the boost in nicotine one gets from a cigarette puff. My estimation is that brain concentrations may at least transiently reach 1 μM.

Balfour: You need to be careful. The brain is a bowl of fat, effectively. When you measure nicotine in the brain you are not measuring free nicotine in the CSF; most of it is trapped in the fatty tissue. I would think that the concentration of nicotine in the CSF is much more relevant in terms of what is acting on the receptor.

Clarke: I largely agree. However, nicotinic receptors are surrounded by lipid and therefore I wonder if nicotine concentrations local to receptors could differ from the average concentration in CSF.

Corrigall: Presumably we should be looking at dose–effect studies, rather than comparing concentrations. The different species and paradigms might have very different dose ranges.

Bertrand: If we look at rat or human receptors we know their sensitivity. We know that even a low concentration of 100 nM causes detectable effects. Of course, the amplitude of the effect depends upon the concentration and will reach its maximal at much higher values.

Clarke: With respect to the notion that the exact dose doesn't matter, that is if rats are 10 times less sensitive to nicotine then let's increase the dose 10-fold, is this a real issue? Are there real species differences in terms of sensitivity to nicotine between rats and mice, and humans?

Picciotto: There are important species differences in clearance.

Bertrand: They are physiological and pharmacological differences in properties between rat and human receptors. But, the metabolism was reported to be six times higher in mice than human.

Clarke: Metabolism and clearance are going to be important for choosing an appropriate nicotine dose *in vivo*. But *in vitro*, where pharmacokinetics factors are largely absent, what are the issues we should be bearing in mind with respect to receptor differences between species?

Bertrand: My expectation is that differences in brain receptor distributions may cause larger differences than a small difference in sensitivity.

Caggiula: When trying to compare the effects of nicotine in rodents with those in humans, it doesn't just boil down to similarities and differences in drug metabolism, distribution or even receptor sensitivity although all three must be taken into account. I agree with Bill Corrigall, especially when we are dealing with *in vivo* preparations: we need to generate dose–response curves within a particular species for a particular function and use that as a basis for cross-species comparisons, rather than trying to directly equate drug dose or blood levels across species. Even if human nicotinic receptors had the same range of sensitivity to the drug as rat receptors, this doesn't mean that driving those receptors with nicotine will have the same downstream effects at each step along the way in the neural circuitry controlling a particular function in the two species. You can't stop at the receptor in looking for possible differences between species, even in slice preparations.

Tyndale: Julie Staley's imaging data suggest nicotine is hanging around in the brain for a long time occupying nicotinic receptors; this could mean theoretically that the concentrations of nicotine in the brain, or occupation of nicotinic receptors, may be irrelevant to some degree when we think about what triggers smoking every few hours. In addition, in models of chronic delivery of nicotine, in humans, monkeys and mice, it has been shown that chronic nicotine reduces the rates of nicotine metabolism. The effect of nicotine on day 1 could be substantially different from the effect of the same dose of nicotine on day 5, simply for metabolic reasons. We think that because rats use a different enzyme to metabolize nicotine than mice this regulation is going to be distinct across these two models. Mice look quite a lot like monkeys and humans from an enzymatic standpoint. If you are trying to look at a response to a drug when you are looking over time, there will be both species and a chronic component at the metabolic level. If nicotine is staying in various compartments of the brain for long periods, presumably this is in some manner/compartment that is not important to receptor function, otherwise you wouldn't see people smoke every two hours. There is some component that must be varying on a faster time, changes in receptor function if not binding.

Clarke: In these studies, how did they detect nicotine persisting in the brain?

Tyndale: In the monkeys treated with oral nicotine, and in the humans who smoked cigarettes, it was using imaging (Cosgrove et al 2004, Staley et al 2005). They also monitored plasma nicotine and showed that even after the plasma levels had dropped, the receptor was occupied for substantially longer (many hours to peak occupation).

Picciotto: Julie Staley and her collaborators are using a nicotinic ligand, A85380. They chronically treated the monkeys with nicotine and then looked for availability by A85380 binding. It took more than 10 d for the receptor to become available after they stopped chronic nicotine treatment.

Clarke: That is not necessarily evidence for nicotine physically persisting in brain matter. It could also be that the radioligand is binding less because nicotine has induced a prolonged internalization of its receptors, or has produced some other form of persistent receptor down-regulation.

Picciotto: If you are competing for a binding site then it suggests that whether or not you are active on your own, you are still going to have an effect on acetylcholine or nicotine signalling.

Brody: We haven't seen firm evidence for the same sequestration of nicotine/cotinine in our studies. We have smokers who are abstinent over night and we see very good binding of the receptors.

Balfour: The issue here is how nicotine is being delivered.

Shiffman: I have trouble buying the idea that we shouldn't care about absolute dose, and should just be looking at dose–response functions. We have heard that the dose–response function is often not linear. We have heard from Martin Jarvis' data that humans seem to regulate their nicotine levels within fairly narrow bounds. It seems to me that dose matters a lot.

Corrigall: At this stage we don't have a lot of models. We have none that have been validated for medication development for dependence. If we start throwing out models based on dose alone we will be in trouble. We need to look at the range of effective doses in each model. It seems unnecessary to say that self-administration of nicotine by a rat, examined over a full range of doses from where the animal doesn't do it to where it finds it aversive, needs to be over the same dose range as the self administration of nicotine by humans, by an inhalation route with a different vehicle, constrained by a different set of situations.

Shiffman: I agree. We shouldn't throw out something because it isn't the same dose, but it seems it would be fruitful to exercise some scepticism.

Picciotto: For $\beta 2$ nicotinic receptors we know a lot about the dose–response function for their opening. $10\,\mu M$ fits with the data we have for optimal doses that open $\beta 2$ receptors as opposed to optimal doses that open $\alpha 7$ receptors.

West: When I am talking to clinicians, one thing I try to say is that one of the core reasons that nicotine is addictive is that it rewards smoking and punishes abstinence. I also say that the mechanism underpinning this is something that evolved tens of millions of years ago before we got our 'crinkly cortex', and this is part of the problem: when smokers are thinking of stopping smoking this is the higher brain system that is doing this which is coming into conflict with what is primarily a midbrain system driving the behaviour and which is outside conscious awareness. There may be some hedonic value attached to this or not. This is a simple approach which probably isn't true. What I understand you to be saying is that from the animal data it isn't enough to postulate that nicotine is rewarding and that nicotine abstinence is punishing; we also have to take account of the fact that for some individuals there is neuroplasticity such that after exposure it is more rewarding and more punishing when it is taken away.

Picciotto: Yes. The CREB data are interesting in that they suggest that we could have an output that would do that kind of thing. That is, when the nicotine is on board we have a decrease in CREB phosphorylation. When the nicotine goes away not only is there a normalization, but there is an increase in CREB which has been shown by viral vector studies to be aversive on its own. These sorts of adaptations occur not only at the behavioural level but also at the molecular level.

West: Does this mean that the neural plasticity is what underpins dependence? Or is it just making a bad problem worse? This has implications for pharmacological targeting. If it is primarily a straightforward learning mechanism which has been reinforced endless times, that is one kind of neural plasticity.

Picciotto: I don't agree with the dichotomy. I am not sure that the learning you are talking about is distinguishable from systems level plasticity. The two are potentially the same.

References

Cosgrove K, Ellis S, Al-Tikriti M et al 2004 Assessment of the effects of chronic nicotine on b2-nicotinic acetylcholine receptors in nonhuman primate using [I-123]5-IA-85830 and SPECT. Sixty-Sixth Annual Scientific Meeting of the College on Problems of Drug Dependence. San Juan, Puerto Rico

Helekar SA, Char D, Neff S, Patrick J 1994 Prolyl isomerase requirement for the expression of functional homo-oligomeric ligand-gated ion channels. Neuron 12:179–189

Helekar SA, Patrick J 1997 Peptidyl prolyl cis-trans isomerase activity of cyclophilin A in functional homo-oligomeric receptor expression. Proc Natl Acad Sci USA 94:5432–5437

Staley JK, van Dyck CH, Weinzimmer D et al 2005 [123I]-5-IA-85380 SPECT measurement of nicotinic acetylcholine receptors in human brain by the constant infusion paradigm: feasibility and reproducibility. J Nuclear Med 46:1466–1472

Complementary roles for the accumbal shell and core in nicotine dependence

David Balfour

Section of Psychiatry, Division of Pathology & Neuroscience, University of Dundee Medical School, Ninewells Hospital, Dundee DD1 9SY, UK

Abstract. Recent studies suggest that the dopamine (DA) projections to the core and shell subdivisions of the nucleus accumbens play complementary roles in the neurobiology underlying nicotine dependence. This review focuses on the hypothesis that the increases in extracellular DA evoked in the accumbal shell by nicotine injections, are mediated by increased burst firing of the neurons which elicits a paracrine release of the monoamine. It is proposed that the primary consequence of this increased DA overflow is to enhance the pleasure derived from behaviours, such as smoking, that deliver nicotine. This increases the probability that the behaviour is repeated and learned efficiently. The working hypothesis predicts that the increased DA overflow in the accumbal core, evoked by repeated nicotine, also depends upon increased burst firing of the neurons and that its primary consequence is to increase the probability that drug-seeking behaviour is elicited by exposure to conditioned stimuli, such as sensory stimuli present in tobacco smoke, paired with delivery of the drug. Thus, the combined effects of nicotine on DA overflow in the shell and the core of the accumbens result in tobacco smoking becoming a highly pleasurable and compulsive behaviour that underpins the addiction to tobacco smoke.

2005 Understanding nicotine and tobacco addiction. Wiley, Chichester (Novartis Foundation Symposium 275) p 96–115

It is now widely accepted that the dopamine (DA) projections to the nucleus accumbens play an important role in the neurobiological mechanisms that underlie the development of nicotine dependence. Many of the microdialysis and behavioural studies, performed to explore the role of these neurons would seem to support the hypothesis that increased DA release in the nucleus accumbens mediates the rewarding properties of nicotine to which habitual users of the drug become addicted (Corrigall et al 1992, 1994, Di Chiara 2000). In recent years, however, this 'simple' explanation for the role of mesolimbic neurons has been challenged in a number of ways and this has resulted in some significant re-evaluation of the role of mesolimbic DA neurons in the dependence.

Our understanding of the mechanisms that mediate nicotine dependence gains much from comparing the neural and behavioural properties of the drug with those of other drugs of dependence, such as amphetamine and cocaine. These two illicit drugs of abuse exert their effects on DA overflow in the brain by acting as a substrate and an antagonist respectively at the neuronal DA transporter. However, when Rocha and colleagues (1998) investigated the reinforcing properties of cocaine in transgenic mice in which the DA transporter had been disabled, they found that the transgenic animals learned to self-administer cocaine in a similar way to wild-type animals. Thus, the reinforcing properties of cocaine cannot be explained entirely by its ability to inhibit the DA transporter. The data, therefore, cast some doubt on the role of increased DA overflow in the mechanisms underlying cocaine self-administration. Balfour et al (2000) noted that, in the transgenic animals, the extracellular levels of DA were elevated some six fold, to a concentration that was higher than that evoked by giving cocaine to wild-type animals. Thus, the data reported by Rocha et al (1998) did not exclude the possibility that raised extracellular DA was important to the development of cocaine self-administration although it, alone, does not fully explain the reinforcing properties of the drug. A more recent study, by Cannon & Palmiter (2003), however, has cast further doubt on the role of DA in rewarded behaviour by showing that mice, which have been genetically altered so that they cannot synthesize DA, nevertheless learn to respond for a sucrose reward. The data imply that increased DA overflow in the nucleus accumbens is not essential for the acquisition and maintenance of a rewarded behaviour. If this conclusion is correct, then why does stimulation of the mesolimbic DA systems seem to play a pivotal role in nicotine dependence? The hypothesis presented below will seek to address this paradox.

The effects of nicotine on dopamine release in the medial shell and core of the nucleus accumbens

The nucleus accumbens is composed of two principal subdivisions, the shell and the core, which are anatomically distinct and are thought to subserve different functions (Zahm & Brog 1992). Anatomically, the accumbal shell is limbic structure with major neural contacts with the amygdala, whereas the accumbal core sends major projections to areas of the brain concerned with the control of motor function (Heimer et al 1991). Acute injections of nicotine, like other psychostimulant drugs of abuse, preferentially stimulates DA overflow in the shell of the accumbens (Cadoni & Di Chiara 2000, Iyaniwura et al 2001). By contrast, increased DA overflow in the core subdivision is only observed in animals which have been sensitized to the drug by pretreatment with daily injections prior to the test day (Benwell & Balfour 1992, Cadoni & Di Chiara 2000, Iyaniwura et al 2001). This pretreatment regime also results in sensitization of the locomotor stimulant properties of nicotine and it was initially assumed that the sensitized locomotor response to the drug corresponded with the sensitization of the stimulatory effects of nicotine on DA overflow in the accumbal core (Benwell & Balfour 1992, Cadoni & Di Chiara 2000). However, a series of studies in our laboratory showed that it was possible to dissociate the effects of nicotine on DA overflow in the core of the accumbens and the development of sensitized locomotor responses to the drug (see Balfour et al 2000, Balfour 2004 for reviews). Thus, we suggested that the sensitized DA responses to nicotine may not be directly involved in sensitization of the effects of the drug on locomotor activity but mediate other psychopharmacological responses more directly involved with the neurobiology underlying dependence.

Rodd-Henricks et al (2002) have shown that rats can be trained to self-administer cocaine directly into the medial shell of the accumbens but will not learn to self-administer the drug into the accumbal core. Other studies by Sellings & Clarke (2003) have shown that the reinforcing properties of amphetamine are diminished by selective lesions of the DA projections to the medial shell whereas selective lesions of the DA projections to the core diminish the locomotor stimulant properties of the drug. These results support the hypothesis that the acquisition of psychostimulant-seeking behaviour depends upon increased DA overflow in the shell subdivision of the accumbens whereas the psychomotor stimulant properties of these drugs reflect increased DA overflow in the accumbal core. However, the latter conclusion must be treated with some caution since a more recent study by Ito et al (2004) suggests that the locomotor stimulant properties of cocaine may also be influenced by increased DA overflow in the shell, possibly as neurons from the core course through the shell subdivision as they project to motor areas of the brain.

In experimental models, the acquisition of a drug-seeking behaviour is often enhanced or facilitated by pairing delivery of the drug with a stimulus that signals delivery of the drug. Initially, this stimulus is neutral and has no predictable consequences. However, by being paired with delivery of a reinforcer, such as a drug of dependence, the stimulus acquires the properties of a conditioned stimulus (CS) or secondary reinforcer for which the animal will respond. A growing body of evidence now supports the conclusion that neural projections from the accumbal core play an important role in mediating the influence that conditioned reinforcers exert on drug-seeking behaviour. This conclusion is based on observations, such as those of Hall et al (2001), which have shown that selective lesions of the neurons in the accumbal core, but not the medial shell, attenuate the facilitatory effects of conditioned stimuli on responding for a food reward. Selective excitotoxic lesions of the accumbal core also attenuate the influence of a CS on cocaine-seeking behaviour whereas lesions of the shell have little effect on cocaine-seeking behaviour *per se* or responding in a second order schedule of reinforcement for the CS (Ito et al 2004).

Responding in a second order schedule to a CS is enhanced by the non-contingent microinjection of amphetamine in the nucleus accumbens (Taylor & Robbins 1984, Wyvell & Berridge 2000). More recently, Donny et al (2003) have shown that non-contingent nicotine also enhances responding for a visual reinforcer. These results suggest that simply increasing DA overflow in the accumbens enhances the effects of a CS on reward-seeking behaviour. Ito and colleagues (2000) used microdialysis to show that, in animals trained in a second order schedule of reinforcement for cocaine, responding when the drug was available caused increased DA overflow in both the medial shell and the core of the accumbens. This was an anticipated effect mediated by the effects of the cocaine the animals received. Drug-seeking behaviour, reinforced by the CS alone, had no effects of DA overflow in either subdivision of the accumbens. However, if the stimulus was presented non-contingently, it resulted in increased DA overflow in the core, but not the medial shell of the accumbens, and initiated drug-seeking behaviour.

Robinson & Berridge (1993, 2003) have long argued that the sensitization, evoked by repeated administration of psychostimulant drugs of abuse, plays a pivotal role in the development of dependence. They have proposed that a principal consequence of the sensitization is the attribution of incentive salience to conditioned stimuli that predict the availability of the drug. More recent studies have shown that the repetitive administration of nicotine, and other psychostimulant drugs of dependence, results in a selective sensitization of the DA projections to the accumbal core which is not observed in the medial shell of the accumbens (Cadoni et al 2000, Cadoni & Di Chiara 2000, Iyaniwura et al 2001). These results, when taken together, support the conclusion that the development of sensitized DA responses to these drugs influences the incentive salience of conditioned stimuli by acting on neurons within this subdivision of the accumbens that mediates the Pavlovian or compulsive drug-seeking behaviour evoked by these stimuli (Balfour 2004).

The putative role of extra-synaptic dopamine

Much of the evidence that nicotine, and other psychostimulant drugs of abuse, stimulate DA overflow in the nucleus accumbens is derived from microdialysis studies employing probes located in the medial shell or core of the structure. These probes are too large to directly sample the DA concentration in the synaptic cleft and, therefore, detect changes in neural activity by measuring changes in DA overflow into the interstitial space between the cells. A majority of the varicosities on the DA fibres that project to the nucleus accumbens do not appear to make tight synaptic contacts but form 'open synapses' that release DA directly into the interstitial space sampled by microdialysis probes (Nirenberg et al 1997). The neuronal transporters, which transport DA back into the neuron, are also arrayed along the fibre rather than the presynaptic membrane that faces into the synaptic cleft (Nirenberg et al 1997). Thus, it is thought that their primary role may be to regulate the DA concentration in the interstitial space between the cells. Significantly, these transporters represent the principal site of action for both cocaine and d-amphetamine and it seems reasonable to conclude that the primary effect of these drugs of abuse on DA release is to elicit a preferential increase in DA overflow into this extracellular space (Balfour et al 2000). By contrast, nicotine appears to increase DA release by acting on receptors on or close to the DA neurons in the ventral tegmental area and, thereby, influence impulse flow to the terminal fields (Balfour et al 2000, Nisell et al 1996). DA neurons in the midbrain can fire in two modes, as single irregular spikes or in bursts (Grace & Bunney 1984a,b). Increased DA over-flow into the interstitial space between the cells is enhanced preferentially by an increase in the proportion of the cells that exhibit burst firing rather than an increase in firing rate (Gonon 1988, Nissbrandt et al 1994). Nicotine injections increase burst firing of midbrain DA neurons (Nisell et al 1996). It seems reason-able to conclude, therefore, that the increases in DA overflow, elicited in the medial shell by acute and repeated nicotine and the core of the accumbens by repeated nicotine, are directly related to the increased burst firing evoked by the drug (Balfour et al 2000). Thus, the capacity to elicit substantial and sustained increases in the extra-synaptic DA concentration in the nucleus accumbens seems to be a property that is shared by psychostimulant drugs of dependence and may be pivotal to their ability to cause dependence (Balfour 2004).

From the data summarized earlier in this review, it is apparent that any hypoth-esis that is proposed to explain the role of mesolimbic DA neurons in nicotine dependence needs to take account of two, apparently conflicting, observations:

1. the acquisition and maintenance of responding for psychostimulant drugs of dependence is attenuated or abolished by lesions of the DA projections to the accumbens;
2. the acquisition of responding for the reinforcing properties of natural rewards is not absolutely dependent upon increased DA overflow in the accumbens.

We have suggested that this paradox can be addressed if it is assumed that the primary consequence of raised extracellular DA in the nucleus accumbens is the facilitation of both the acquisition and maintenance of reward-seeking behaviours (Balfour 2004). We have proposed that the data are consistent with the hypothesis that extra-synaptic DA in nucleus accumbens acts in a manner similar to a local hormone to enhance neural signals that emanate from, or project through the two principal subdivisions of the accumbens. Intravenous self-administration (IVSA) experiments with cocaine suggest that increased DA overflow in the medial shell of the accumbens facilitates the locomotor stimulant properties of the drug (Ito et al 2004) and the acquisition of cocaine-seeking behaviour (Rodd-Henricks et al 2002). Other studies suggest that increased in DA overflow in the accumbal shell promotes incentive or habit learning of behaviours associated with delivery of a reward (Di Chiara 2000, 2002). Di Chiara argues that the increase in DA overflow, evoked by drugs of dependence, is unphysiologically large and sustained and, as result, drug-seeking behaviour comes to dominate the behavioural repertoire of an addict. These observations are consistent with the working hypothesis that the primary role of increased DA overflow into the interstitial space of the accumbal shell maybe to confer increased hedonic value on the stimuli or behaviours experienced while the DA concentration remains elevated (Balfour 2004). As a result, the behaviour or stimulus itself becomes pleasurable. The putative psychophysiological value of this effect is to increase the probability that the animal will repeat a behaviour that delivers a reward. This, in turn, facilitates acquisition of the behaviour and associations between stimuli and the presentation of a reward. It is proposed that a natural reward, such as sucrose, exerts this effect by stimulating a circuit that results in stimulation of the DA fibres which project to the accumbal shell (Fig. 1A). Nicotine, and other psychostimulant drugs of abuse, however, stimulate the pathway directly. These drugs, therefore, have the potential to exert a substantial and sustained effect on the pathway and, thus, attribute a powerful hedonic impact on behaviours, such as lever-pressing in IVSA studies or cigarette smoking in humans, which deliver nicotine (Fig. 1B).

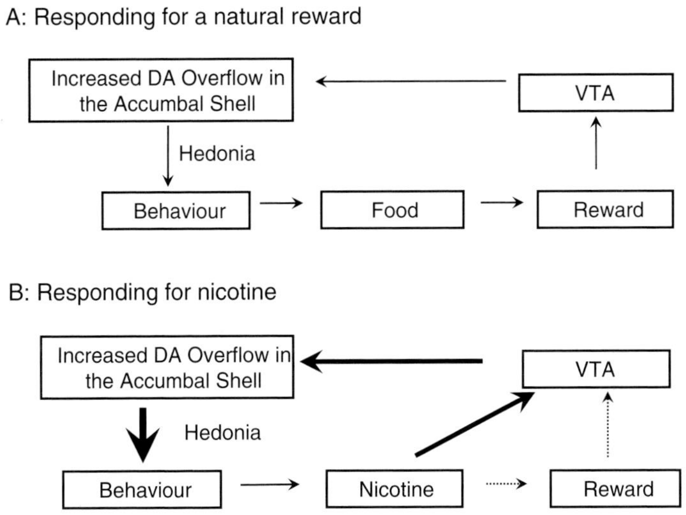

FIG. 1. The role of increased dopamine overflow in the accumbal medial shell on responding for a reward. (A) Outlines the proposed circuitry by which a natural reward, such as food, increases DA overflow in the accumbal medial shell. This increased DA overflow is hypothesized to confer hedonic characteristics on behaviour, such as a lever-pressing response, that results in presentation of the reward. (B) Illustrates the way in which nicotine may greatly enhance the hedonia associated with the behaviour by directly increasing extracellular DA in the accumbal medial shell, bypassing the need for the drug itself to exhibit 'rewarding' properties. (Reproduced with permission from Balfour 2004.)

The working hypothesis predicts that extracellular DA in the accumbal core also serves a paracrine role, but that in this subdivision of the accumbens, its primary role is to enhance the probability of Pavlovian responding to a CS (Balfour 2004). In the absence of drug, this effect serves to initiate drug-seeking behaviour and is thought to play an important role in the neurobiology underlying relapse. However, if the drug is also made available, IVSA results in increased DA overflow in both the core and the shell of the accumbens. In these circumstances, the hypothesis predicts that drug-seeking behaviour will be powerfully reinforced because (a) increased DA overflow in the shell confers powerful hedonic properties on the behaviour that results in IVSA and (b) Pavlovian or compulsive responding for a CS, paired with delivery of the drug, will be greatly magnified by the increase in DA overflow in the accumbal core (Fig. 2).

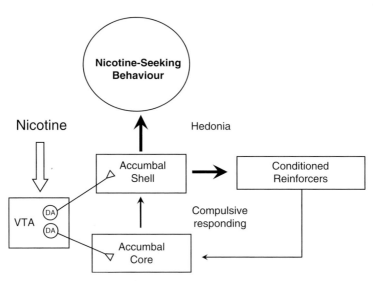

FIG. 2.   The putative roles of hedonia and conditioned reinforcers in nicotine-seeking behaviour. The figure summarizes the mechanisms that have been proposed in this review to explain how increased DA overflow in the medial shell and core of the nucleus accumbens, evoked by an injection of nicotine, play complementary roles in the expression of nicotine-seeking behaviour. The hypothesis posits that, in both subdivisions of the accumbens, extracellular DA serves to promote or amplify the signals that project from or through the structure. Stimulation of the projections to the medial shell of the accumbens enhances the hedonic value of the behaviour itself and of sensory and environmental stimuli associated with the delivery of nicotine. Stimulation of the projections to accumbal core promotes the effects of conditioned reinforcers or stimuli on nicotine-seeking behaviour. These conditioned responses can be amplified further by stimulation of the DA projections to medial shell, through which neurons from the core project. (Reproduced with permission from Balfour 2004.)

Dialysis experiments, similar to those performed by Ito et al (2000) with cocaine, have yet to be performed with animals self-administering nicotine. However, there is convincing evidence that the co-presentation of CS enhances nicotine-seeking behaviour in a manner similar to that seen for animals trained to respond for cocaine (Caggiula et al 2001). It seems reasonable to suggest, therefore, that the effects of nicotine on DA overflow in the shell and core of the accumbens also play an important complementary role in the neurobiology underlying nicotine reinforcement. These effects may be of particular importance to our understanding of the role of nicotine in tobacco dependence since nicotine, inhaled in tobacco smoke, is presented in the context of many complex sensory stimuli, present in the smoke, that could serve as conditioned stimuli. As a result, the tobacco vehicle, in which the nicotine is delivered, has the potential to greatly magnify the addictive properties of the nicotine contained within it. This conclusion is supported by the evidence that sensory cues within tobacco smoke play a fundamental role in the regulation of smoking behaviour and the craving to smoke (Rose et al 1993). Preclinical studies also support the conclusion that animals will continue to respond for a CS paired with the delivery of nicotine for a significant period of time following the withdrawal of the primary drug reinforcer (Caggiula et al 2001). This is likely to be fundamentally important to our understanding of the role of sensory stimuli, present in tobacco smoke, to the tobacco smoking habit because preclinical studies also suggest that many of the neuronal nicotinic receptors, which mediate the effects of nicotine on mesolimbic DA neurons are desensitized by sustained exposure to nicotine at concentrations commonly found in the blood of habitual smokers (Benwell et al 1995, Pidoplichko 1997). During periods when these receptors are desensitized, it seems likely that conditioned sensory stimuli present in the smoke continue to serve as secondary reinforcers that maintain the habit (Balfour et al 2000, Caggiula et al 2001, Balfour 2004). The salience of these conditioned stimuli are re-established at regular intervals when the smoker inhales tobacco smoke following a period of abstinence which allows the neuronal nicotinic receptors to re-sensitize and the nicotine present in the smoke again results in increased DA overflow in the accumbens.

Conclusion

This review has developed the hypothesis that nicotine shares with other psychostimulant drugs of dependence the ability to elicit a sustained and substantial increase in extracellular DA in the shell and core of the nucleus accumbens where it acts in a paracrine fashion to enhance drug-seeking behaviour. The hypothesis proposes that the role of extracellular DA in the shell subdivision confers hedonic properties upon behaviours that deliver the reward and, thus, facilitate acquisition of the behaviours. The primary role of increased extracellular DA in the accumbal core is to enhance compulsive or Pavlovian responding for CS associated with presentation of the drug. Thus, the co-incident increase of DA overflow in both subdivisions of the accumbens serves to render smoking the highly rewarding and compulsive behaviour that is characteristic of the addiction to tobacco.

Acknowledgements

Studies from the author's laboratory, discussed in this review, were performed with financial support from the Wellcome Trust.

References

Balfour DJK 2004 The neurobiology of nicotine dependence: a preclinical perspective on the role of the nucleus accumbens. Nic Tob Res 6:899–912

Balfour DJK, Wright AE, Benwell MEM, Birrell CE 2000 The putative role of extra-synaptic mesolimbic dopamine in the neurobiology of nicotine dependence. Behav Brain Res 113:73–83

Benwell MEM, Balfour DJK 1992 The effects of acute and repeated nicotine treatment on nucleus accumbens dopamine and locomotor activity. Br J Pharmacol 105:849–856

Benwell MEM, Balfour DJK, Birrell CE 1995 Desensitisation of nicotine-induced dopamine responses during constant infusion with nicotine. Br J Pharmacol 114:211–217

Cadoni C, Di Chiara G 2000 Differential changes in the accumbens medial shell and core dopamine in behavioural sensitization to nicotine. Eur J Pharmacol 387:R23–25

Cadoni C, Solinas M, Di Chiara G 2000 Psychostimulant sensitization: differential changes in accumbal medial shell and core dopamine. Eur J Pharmacol 388:69–76

Caggiula AR, Donny EC, White AR et al 2001 Cue dependency of nicotine self-administration and smoking. Pharmacol Biochem Behav 70:515–530

Cannon CM, Palmiter RD 2003 Reward without dopamine. J Neurosci 23:10827–10831

Corrigall WA, Franklin KJB, Coen KM, Clarke PBS 1992 The mesolimbic dopaminergic system is implicated in the reinforcing effects of nicotine. Psychopharmacology 107:285–289

Corrigall WA, Coen KM, Adamson KL 1994 Self-administered nicotine activates the mesolimbic dopamine system through the ventral tegmental area. Brain Res 653:278–284

Di Chiara G 2000 Behavioural pharmacology and neurobiology of nicotine reward and dependence. In: Clementi C, Fornasari D, Gotti C (eds) Handbook of experimental pharmacology. Springer, Berlin, vol 14:603–750

Di Chiara G 2002 Nucleus accumbens medial shell and core dopamine: differential role in behavior and addiction. Behav Brain Res 137:75–114

Donny EC, Chaudhri N, Caggiula AR et al 2003 Operant responding for a visual reinforcer in rats is enhanced by noncontingent nicotine: implications for nicotine self-administration and reinforcement. Psychopharmacology 169:68–76

Gonon FG 1988 Nonlinear relationship between impulse flow and dopamine released by rats midbrain dopaminergic neurons as studied by in vivo electrochemistry. Neuroscience 24:2419–2428

Grace AA, Bunney BS 1984a The control of firing pattern in nigral dopamine neurons: single spike firing. J Neurosci 4:2866–2876

Grace AA, Bunney BS 1984b The control of firing pattern in nigral dopamine neurons: burst firing. J Neurosci 4:2877–2890

Hall J, Parkinson JA, Connor TMF, Dickinson A, Everitt BJ 2001 Involvement of the central nucleus of the amygdala and nucleus accumbens core in mediating Pavlovian influences on instrumental behaviour. Eur J Neurosci 13:1984–1992

Heimer L, Zahm DS, Churchill L, Kalivas PW, Wohltman C 1991 Specificity in the projection patterns of accumbal core and medial shell in the rat. Neuroscience 41:89–125

Ito R, Dalley JW, Howes SR, Robbins TW, Everitt BJ 2000 Dissociation in conditioned dopamine release in the nucleus accumbens core and medial shell in response to cocaine cues and during cocaine-seeking behaviour in rats. J Neurosci 20:7489–7495

Ito R, Robbins TW, Everitt BJ 2004 Differential control over cocaine-seeking behaviour by nucleus accumbens core and shell. Nature Neurosci 7:389–397

Iyaniwura TT, Wright AE, Balfour DJK 2001 Evidence that mesoaccumbens dopamine and locomotor responses to nicotine in the rat are influenced by pre-treatment dose and strain. Psychopharmacology 158:73–79

Nirenberg NJ, Chan J, Pohorille A et al 1997 The dopamine transporter: comparative ultrastructure of dopaminergic axons in the limbic and motor components of the nucleus accumbens. J Neurosci 17:6988–6907

Nisell M, Nomikos GG, Hertel P, Panagis G, Svensson TH 1996 Condition-independent sensitization of locomotor stimulation and mesocortical dopamine release following chronic nicotine treatment in the rat. Synapse 22:369–381

Nissbrandt H, Elverfors A, Engberg G 1994 Pharmacologically induced cessation of burst activity in nigral dopamine neurons: significance for terminal dopamine efflux. Synapse 17:217–224

Pidoplichko V, De Biasi M, Williams JT, Dani J 1997 Nicotine activates and desensitizes midbrain dopamine neurones. Nature 390:401–404

Rocha BA, Fumagalli F, Gainetdinov RR et al 1998 Cocaine self-administration in dopamine-transporter knockout mice. Nature Neurosci 1:132–137

Robinson TE, Berridge KC 1993 The neural basis of drug craving: an incentive-sensitization theory of addiction. Brain Res Rev 18:247–291

Robinson TE, Berridge KC 2003 Addiction. Ann Rev Psychol 54:24–53

Rodd-Henricks ZA, McKenzie DL, Ting-Kai L, Murphy JM, McBride WJ 2002 Cocaine is self-administered into the medial shell but not the core of the nucleus accumbens of Wistar rats. J Pharmacol Exp Ther 303:1216–1226

Rose JE, Behm FM, Levin ED 1993 Role of nicotine dose and sensory cues in the regulation of smoke intake. Pharmacol Biochem Behav 44:891–900

Sellings LHL, Clarke PBS 2003 Segregation of amphetamine reward and locomotor stimulation between nucleus accumbens medial medial shell and core. J Neurosci 23:6295–6303

Taylor JR, Robbins TW 1984 Enhanced behavioural control by conditioned reinforcers following microinjections of d-amphetamine into the nucleus accumbens. Psychopharmacology 84:405–412

Wyvell CL, Berridge KC 2000 Intra-accumbens amphetamine increases the pure incentive salience of a Pavlovian cue for food reward: enhancement of 'wanting' without either 'liking' or reinforcement. J Neurosci 20:8122–8130

Zahm DS, Brog JS 1992 On the significance of subterritories in the 'accumbens' part of the rat ventral striatum. Neuroscience 50:751–767

DISCUSSION

Bertrand: You showed nice differences in sensitization. Can you cross-sensitize? Can you treat with cocaine and then infuse nicotine as a single pulse to see whether there is a larger response?

Balfour: We have not done it that way round yet. If we pretreat with nicotine and give amphetamine or cocaine, we don't see sensitization. There is cross-sensitization between amphetamine and cocaine.

Bertrand: Did you ever look at the histology of the core and the shell following nicotine treatment?

Balfour: No.

Corrigall: You used the term 'hedonia'. I'd like to make the point that what we are talking about here is reward and reinforcement, not hedonia.

Balfour: The reason why I used 'hedonia' is that smokers tend to say they like smoking. They don't say they like the effect of smoking.

Corrigall: The main point I am trying to make is that there is an issue of definition and its application. One can say 'I like chocolate', 'I like red wine' and so on. That is not hedonia. If you could tell me the definition of hedonia that would fit with the science, I would be happier. Then if you can tell me how that fits tobacco I would be happier still. But in an operational sense, I see this as reward and reinforcement, or approach and consummation.

Balfour: Why can an individual learn to do something which isn't in itself particularly rewarding? I am trying to come up with a hypothesis that addresses the issue that nicotine itself is not particularly pleasant to take.

Corrigall: The brain systems that subserve reward and reinforcement, or approach and consummation, or needing and wanting, are present for some survival reason. 'Wanting' or 'needing' is something that we have learned for survival, and 'liking' is the thing that gets us to what we want. The needing system could be co-opted by a drug of abuse, and in particular by nicotine, where the need may be strong but absent a lot of liking. Other drugs may have more of a balance. That's sort of an unfair answer because it falls back on non-science—this is the reason I asked that we don't use 'hedonia'.

Clarke: I still think your most interesting result is with the mini pumps, where you give a continuous subcutaneous infusion of nicotine and this abolishes the acute effect of nicotine on dopamine release. What is the implication of this for smokers? Perhaps half way through the day if you are a smoker you are not getting any dopamine response to nicotine: if this is the case, why are you still smoking? Is it instead because of the monoamine oxidase inhibition, or the history of reinforcement, or the acetaldehyde found in cigarette smoke? One way to test whether nicotinic receptor stimulation is still important half way through the day in a smoker would be to test smokers with mecamylamine at this time point. To date, have smokers only been tested with mecamylamine when they are abstinent?

Balfour: It would be a good experiment.

Shiffman: Jed Rose has done a study (Rose et al 1998) in which people were pretreated with mecamylamine during ad lib smoking and then progressed to quit. The result was largely unimpressive, with small reductions in smoking and modest effects on cessation.

Clarke: I thought the results were pretty good at 6 months and 1 year in his long-term study (Rose et al 1994).

Perkins: We did a mecamylamine study with nicotine spray discrimination and self-administration (Perkins et al 1999). Mecamylamine appeared to shift choice of nicotine versus placebo spray self-administration towards nicotine, which may be similar to compensation (due to blockade of nicotine receptors).

Clarke: This suggests that in your human subjects, there were still some working nicotinic receptors that were sensitive to mecamylamine. If all the receptors were desensitized, then an antagonist such as mecamylamine would have had no effect. However, your study used smokers that were overnight abstinent and hence their nicotinic receptors were presumably less desensitized than they would be during the daytime in a free-smoking context.

Balfour: One of the conditioned stimuli that I am arguing are present in tobacco smoke may be nicotine itself which we know irritates sensory receptors in the mouth and throat. The results reported by Jarvik & Assil (1988) and Rose et al (1989) suggest that mecamylamine blocks these effects, indicating that they are sensitive to blockade by nicotinic receptor antagonists. These results would tend to support that hypothesis.

Brody: From the human functional brain imaging literature there is a study correlating dopamine release with the hedonic response (Barrett et al 2004). They define this as 'pleasure'.

Corrigall: My discomfort with the term 'hedonic' is that it seems to be used loosely and is not defined.

Perkins: That is the problem of 'reward', also. I would define 'reward' as a hedonic characteristic of the drug.

Corrigall: Reward can be defined more precisely.

West: We have to. One of the things the incentive sensitization theory does is to claim that there is a dissociation between wanting and liking. This is a major conceptual advance. We can report how much we enjoy things and like things: there is a semi-quantitative scale we can use. We can also report how much we crave things and feel a need for them on a similar scale. When I first started working in this field what struck me was how strong the craving was compared with how much pleasure smokers experienced. One of the interesting things about this theory is that it seems to be the *smoking* that people are looking for. People aren't craving the effect of the cigarette, but the cigarette itself. Even if you get people to try to change from one cigarette to another that delivers the same nicotine level, they won't stick to that. There is something powerful about this notion that it is the set of stimuli associated with their cigarette that this captures. How would you characterize this sense of craving or urge to smoke within your model?

Balfour: Let me step back a little and say that my view is that the role of the shell is to increase the probability that the individual will repeat the behaviour that delivers the reward. The reason I argue it is hedonic is because that is the way you make the animal repeat the behaviour: if it enjoys doing it, it will do it again. When it takes its first injection of nicotine, the animal hasn't a clue why this is nice, but it repeats it. By association it learns that pressing the lever delivers something that is pleasurable. The role of the shell is to make particular behaviours pleasurable. When you switch to craving, that is driven by the core and is magnified by increased dopamine overflow in the core. When you smoke following a period of abstinence, you get an increase in dopamine overflow in the core and this magnifies the value of the conditioned stimuli.

Shiffman: In your theory you are focusing not on the wanting but on the liking. I have data which suggest that how much people like smoking is not very relevant. The way you have just said this, it is suggesting that developing hedonic sensations is natural selection's way of getting us to repeat the behaviour. But once this circuit has been drawn, it is easy to imagine bypassing it: that is, in the normal course of things we tend to develop likings. Might it not be possible for that circuit to generate repetition of that behaviour bypassing the circuit that generates liking? Might you end up wanting something you don't actually like?

Balfour: I think the wanting is a core activity; liking is a shell activity. I focused on increasing dopamine overflow in the shell and core. Extracellular dopamine in the shell and core set the level of liking and the level of wanting. In the absence of the drug, there a basal tone that maintains some extracellular dopamine which influences liking and wanting. However, when dopamine overflow in the shell and the core are 'driven' pharmacologically by a drug, this relationship begins to be disturbed and addiction may result.

Markou: There is no way to define experimentally the liking and wanting, in either humans or animals. I subscribe to more of an incentive motivational approach, where a stimulus becomes more attractive if an individual is in a withdrawal state. After dependence develops, you may not reach this hedonic state that you used to when you started using the drug, but you might bring levels back up to the euthymic baseline state. There is reinforcement, but this reinforcement is of a different quality, in the sense that is negative reinforcement, that is alleviation of a negative affective state and return to the baseline euthymic state.

Shiffman: This is a fundamental issue whenever researchers working on humans and animals get together. There is a tendency to say that any data obtained by self report are somehow less scientific. It may be that these constructs are softer than we would like, but we can get semi-quantitative ratings. Craving is not that special in this respect: pain is something we have to get by self-report. We can operationalize it in the lab by putting a rat's tail on a hot plate, for example, but this is not pain: it is a pain-producing stimulus.

Corrigall: My objection was to the terms 'hedonia' and 'euphoria'. We seem to have shifted to an objection to self-report and other associated data. I do not have a problem with data of this kind, given well-defined terms that can be operationalized. I am arguing none of this has much to do with hedonia.

Markou: Craving may have to do with hedonia. Either from self-reports or hard-core experimentation, we cannot readily differentiate the two: the wanting/liking and hedonia. We define these two the same way in the animal based on the animal's behaviour. The same can be done in humans, where self-reports can be complemented by behavioural data.

Corrigall: Animals will do a number of things that we would not describe as hedonia or euphoria, as will humans. I suspect that many of them might have a dopamine component, because it is a motivational system.

Balfour: You are equating hedonia with euphoria. For me hedonia is simply pleasure or enjoyment.

Jarvis: You described a pattern of dopamine release in the nucleus accumbens related to nicotine. To what extent do you see similar or different patterns with other drugs of abuse? Is this potentially another way through to drawing inferences about some of these knotty problems?

Balfour: First of all the sensitization in the core only happens following repetitive administration of drugs that are abused. We also know that natural rewards, when presented, stimulate dopamine overflow in the shell. If you give water to a rat, you get a modest increase in dopamine overflow. If you give water to a thirsty rat you get quite a big increase in dopamine overflow in the shell.

Jarvis: Can you differentiate nicotine from other drugs in terms of these dopamine responses?

Balfour: In the sense of what they do to the core and the shell, not particularly. The mechanism by which nicotine elicits its effects is different. Cocaine and amphetamine act at the level of the transporter. The opiates remove inhibitory inputs in the ventral tegmental area (VTA), and nicotine stimulates the dopamine neurons directly. The mechanism is different but the outcome in the core and the shell is the same.

Jarvis: It comes down to this question of to what extent these things are the same phenomenon. In terms of what influences nicotine addiction and treatment, it is entirely specific. One doesn't see treatments that work for nicotine and other dependencies.

Corrigall: Arguments are made for them however, for example, naltrexone?

Jarvis: I thought the evidence for this was mixed.

Stolerman: The distinctions attempted between hedonic and motivational states are hard to express in operational terms and are driving me back towards my more radical-behavioural roots. Reinforcing effects of drugs are defined by behavioural changes and they may have little or nothing to do with changes in subjective state and mood. Cocaine is the drug par excellence for euphoria, yet human subjects in cocaine self-administration experiments have been shown to self-administer doses that are too small for them to be able to report a subjective effect. This is just one illustration of the danger of assuming there is a primacy of feelings, moods and sensations over actual behaviour. It may be the other way round. We don't know of a neural mechanism through which a mood change actually influences behaviour.

West: What is fascinating about this research is that it takes us beyond a simple common-sense analysis of what the phenomena are. The rather crude measures of subjective states that we have are sufficient to enable us to refute certain common-sense hypotheses about what is involved in nicotine dependence. We can measure liking and wanting and demonstrate that the two aren't terribly well correlated. I reported in my presentation that enjoyment showed no correlation with ability to remain abstinent. The relationship with craving is there, but it is very weak. The subjective measures are potentially important in linking this more scientific research with the clinical experience. How does your model account for the objective reduction in the hazard function in relation to relapse, which is also accompanied by the reduction in craving that occurs as a result of time since last cigarette when you are trying to achieve abstinence? So your probability of relapse starts high and decreases sort of exponentially, as a result of simply being abstinent. What changes are taking place in your system that would account for that phenomenon?

Balfour: I can only speculate. If a conditioned stimulus is presented non-contingently, this results in a burst of dopamine release in the core which magnifies the influence that stimulus exerts on behaviour. My argument is that the behaviour is being driven. As you become abstinent, unless that stimulus is presented, the factors driving the craving become diminished. Under these circumstances, there is nothing driving the dopamine system to magnify the Pavlovian response. If an addicted individual then experiences a conditioned stimulus this craving may be re-established and be exacerbated by an increase in dopamine overflow in the accumbal core.

West: You would predict that if we were to take someone who has been abstinent from cigarettes for a week and give them nicotine, they would crave again.

Balfour: You are assuming that nicotine is the stimulus.

West: What if we give them a de-nicotinized cigarette?

Balfour: I think their craving would go back up again.

Shiffman: Would their hedonic response to that stimulus be important? You are putting a good deal of focus on that.

Balfour: I am still arguing that what smokers find most pleasurable is the behaviour of smoking. But the conditioned stimuli themselves do not have to be particularly pleasurable, although I believe they probably do acquire some hedonic characteristics.

Changeux: I am interested by the discussion about subjective states. I agree that we can ask the subject to rate their experience on a subjective scale, but in humans there is an enormous difficulty here. I gave a course on neuroaesthetics this year at the Collège de France on the neuronal bases of music perception. There exists a broad diversity of lesions or congenital diseases that create a selective dissociation of music perception. They are called amusias.

As far as craving is concerned, there are mutants such as the αCGRP (α-calcitonin gene-related peptide) knockout mouse that show an altered craving without modified dependence and/or tolerance (Salmon et al 2001, 2004).

Shiffman: How do you know this?

Changeux: Behavioural analysis offers clues to dissect craving from tolerance and dependence. Why not use the mutant animals to carry out this kind of analysis? Perhaps there are also pharmacological tools other than those of glutamate and/or dopamine pharmacology which might help to dissect these different subjective states. Also there is neurology. What about a study of genetic disease in humans where there are alterations of addictive or craving abilities? In schizophrenic patients there is indeed a tendency for chain smoking. We could use these new tools to look at these issues.

Balfour: One of the factors that we need to remember about the mesolimbic dopamine system is that it is a phylogenetically old system. Rats and mice are using it, but I suspect they don't experience 'euphoria' or 'pleasure' in quite the sense that humans do. They simply do things they like and don't do things they don't like. As animals evolve this evolves into what we interpret as pleasure and so on. The other issue is that as we learn that the projections to different parts of the brain play different roles, it is very difficult to selectively lesion these. The toxin-based techniques that I have used can't differentiate between them. The attraction of using transgenic methodologies may lie in the discovery that certain types of nicotinic receptor are expressed selectively in the neurons that project to the core and the shell and frontal cortex and so on. I don't think we can do this any other way.

Stolerman: Others have reported selective lesions of core and shell. Do you not think that has been achieved?

Balfour: They are destroying neurons within the core and the shell. This is the evidence that the core is necessary for a conditioned stimulus.

Bertrand: Do we know of cerebral vascular accidents that will cause people to quit smoking? Some of the vascular accidents are very localized and may be informative to understand the anatomical determinants involved in addiction.

Powell: I have worked with a neurological population, exploring whether commonly observed deficits of motivation might reflect disruption to brain reward pathways. We found that treatment with bromocriptine, a D2 agonist, was effective in promoting not only locomotor activity but also reward-motivated behaviour assessed both in daily life and on a laboratory task of response to financial incentives. Likewise, when we tested brain-injured patients before and after smoking we found that smoking produced a similar increase in their response to incentives on this experimental task.

Corrigall: I have a more general question. Which are the receptors that we do need to pay attention to, and which ones can we forget about? Do we have a short list?

Changeux: The only thing I can say is that all those that we have tested seem to have effects. I may add that those where effects were not seen may have to be further investigated! For example, the role the $\alpha7$ subunit is still an open question. $\beta2$ and $\alpha4$ subunits are widespread in the brain and there is good evidence that they make a strong contribution to nicotine addiction and cognitive functions. The so-called nAChR 'minor' subunits need to be further investigated. We have constructed an $\alpha6$-subunit knockout which we are presently studying. The $\alpha6$ subunit seems to be preferentially expressed in the dopaminergic axon terminals (Champtiaux et al 2003). These are fine topologies that might be critical for some aspects of nicotine effects on physiology and behaviour.

Corrigall: Such as nicotine affecting release in the terminal region?

Changeux: There is a major difference between acetylcholine and nicotine: acetylcholine is released at the level of endings of cholinergic terminals whereas nicotine is acting everywhere it has access. There is a fundamental difference between an artificial reinforcer like nicotine and the physiological neurotransmitter. There might be receptors which are accessible to nicotine but not to acetylcholine. Whether all the receptors that are present in the brain are involved in a physiological response is an open question still. It is not just the type of receptor and its localization, but also its accessibility to the physiological reward and/or nicotine. Nicotine stimulates processes which bypass, alter or modify physiological reward processes, for instance at the level of the minor subunits present in the dopaminergic neuron of the VTA whose complex subunit composition is still not fully understood. Continuing on this issue of receptors, 'non-conventional' pathways of receptor activation and propagation of signals may exist, for instance at the level of the prefrontal cortex. Indeed we have been concerned by the effect of nicotine on 'states of consciousness' (we should not be afraid of using this word that qualifies subjective states) and I would like to throw into the discussion the observation we made that there are nicotinic receptors on axons that we referred to as 'preterminal' and that are possibly located at the nodes of Ranvier (Lena et al 1993). Whole-cell recordings performed on rat interpeduncular nucleus neurons using the thin-slice technique showed that nicotine dramatically increased the frequency of postsynaptic GABAergic currents. This presynaptic action was suppressed in the presence of TTX. A comparable effect of nicotine was found using a preparation of acutely isolated neurons that had retained synaptic terminals attached to their cell body as evidenced by immunoreactivity to synaptophysin and presence of spontaneous GABAergic and glutamatergic synaptic activity. This action was also suppressed in the presence of TTX. This means that receptors sensitive to nicotine are present on axons, and that their activation can elicit an action potential which is abolished by TTX. Since one may correlate the abundance of white matter with the development of prefrontal cortex and thus of consciousness (there is a dramatic increase in white matter from mice to humans; Sherwood et al 2005, Schenker et al 2005), nicotine may act at this level and modify states of consciousness. The first morning cigarette changes the way the smoker is able to read a newspaper, speak and interact. In other words, nicotine may affect the state of attentive wakefulness. Is this taking place at the level of the prefrontal white matter?

Picciotto: There are clearly a number of models of nicotine's pharmacological effect in mice. We have to remember that the absence of a subunit throughout development is not the same as showing that it doesn't have an acute role when an animal that grows up with a normal complement of receptors is treated. Jean-Pierre's experiments with the rescue will help us to find out whether there is a developmental or long-term change in these animals, or whether there is an acute role for the receptors during a particular behaviour. There is compartmentalization of effects of different receptor subtypes. This is just emerging from the knockout receptor field. There are some hints that the $\beta4$ and $\alpha3$ receptors may have effects on anxiety-like behaviours. They may be important for withdrawal (Salas et al 2004). There is evidence from double receptor knockouts that $\alpha7$ and $\beta2$ together may be important for some cognitive behaviours such as passive avoidance (Marubio & Paylor 2004). The complement of receptors are not simply redundant. They don't all do the same thing, and when we limit ourselves to examining models of drug reinforcement you are going to pull out particular subtypes. It is not sufficient to say that these are the subtypes that are important for smoking when we know that the attentional effects and effects on mood and even pain sensation are contributing to an ongoing complex behaviour. Without the drive of the motivational system, perhaps all the rest is not enough. You need some initial strong drive, but tobacco smoking is different from other drugs, in part because nicotine is good at doing so many different things that help us function at optimum levels. It is a good homeostatic molecule. So the doors are still open for other subunits in modifications of behaviours that are important to smoking.

Bertrand: The fact that nicotinic receptors have been kept through evolution suggest that they are important. Interestingly, treatments that are used for elderly people such as tacrine, have to be given for weeks before any effect is detected. However, we do not know if such treatment modifies the pattern of receptor expression and receptor distribution is likely to be very important.

Corrigall: I have a question for the receptor people here. What are the tools that would advance our understanding of these questions?

Bertrand: For me, there are two tools needed: (i) a better genetic approach to human populations of smokers and non-smokers, and (ii) a selective modulator of the different nicotine receptor subtypes.

Tyndale: We have found differences in the frequency of genetic polymorphisms in the nicotinic receptor between smoker and non-smoker schizophrenics (De Luca et al 2004). Caryn Lerman has shown that variation in the opiate receptors affects treatment with nicotine. I am not aware of anyone doing specific experimental studies of smoking behaviours between people with various genetic variants however there is some of this type of work being done by Paul Cinciripini.

Balfour: When we think about human genetics, nicotinic receptors are one issue, but there are also roles for all kinds of receptors and transporters.

Changeux: The technology we developed (Maskos et al 2005) was used with knockout mice, but it can also be used to inactivate genes in normal mice, rats and even monkeys. An interesting alternative to lesion or stimulation studies might be to locally change the subunit composition of receptors *in situ*.

Walton: From the genetic point of view we have looked at various different targets, but I have always steered clear of the nicotinic receptor because it is so complex. There's a differing composition of subunits and there's a change in shape. One polymorphism in a particular part of a protein could stabilize or destabilize a particular form of receptor. This could be anywhere in the protein, and not just in the active site.

Tyndale: That would also be true for the dopamine receptors.

Stolerman: Desensitization is the big difference between nicotinic sites and many of the others that we are interested in. One of our fundamental difficulties remains not knowing to what extent desensitization of receptors is the primary mechanism for the effects of nicotine even when it is given acutely. Or is desensitization something that becomes important upon chronic exposure? The latter position doesn't fit well with the findings of the very rapid desensitization seen in studies at the cellular level. And we have to account for the fact that tolerance develops to many effects of nicotine; this is difficult to understand if desensitization is the main mechanism for acute effects; if its acute effect is desensitization of the receptors and then tolerance develops, then there is a rather implausible implication that there is less desensitization as the nicotine is given repeatedly.

Clarke: We need to be very careful about desensitization and the pharmacokinetics of nicotine. If we give the nicotine too fast and too infrequently, we may be biasing things towards a dopaminergic mechanism which may not be the case in humans. Speaking more generally, we have to recognize that the answer we get may depend critically on the animal model used. For example, there are probably multiple reward systems in the brain; we know this from the opiate system, where the reward can be dependent on or independent of dopamine, depending on how much exposure the animal has had to the drug (Nader et al 1997). Hence, depending on how fast we give nicotine and for how long, we could quite conceivably tap into different brain systems.

Chiamulera: I am surprised that there is no research to investigate the mechanism of action of nicotine-replacement therapy (NRT). Different NRTs have different pharmacokinetic profiles. We could speculate that the different forms of NRT would have different dynamic patterns of binding to nicotinic receptors and therefore of activation and desensitization allosteric states of the receptor.

References

Barrett SP, Boileau I, Okker J, Pihl RO, Dagher A 2004 The hedonic response to cigarette smoking is proportional to dopamine release in the human striatum as measured by positron emission tomography and [^{11}C]raclopride. Synapse 54:65–71

Champtiaux N, Gotti C, Cordero-Erausquin M et al 2003 Subunit composition of functional nicotinic receptors in dopaminergic neurons investigated with knock-out mice. J Neurosci 23:7820–7829

De Luca V, Wong AH, Muller DJ, Wong GW, Tyndale RF, Kennedy JL 2004 Evidence of association between smoking and alpha7 nicotinic receptor subunit gene in schizophrenia patients. Neuropsychopharmacology 29:1522–1526

Jarvik ME, Assil KM 1988 Mecamylamine blocks the burning sensation of nicotine on the tongue. Chem Senses 13:213–217

Lena C, Changeux JP, Mulle C 1993 Evidence for 'preterminal' nicotinic receptors on GABAergic axons in the rat interpeduncular nucleus. J Neurosci 13:2680–2688

Marubio LM, Paylor R 2004 Impaired passive avoidance learning in mice lacking central neuronal nicotinic acetylcholine receptors. Neuroscience 129:575–582

Maskos U, Molles BE, Pons S et al 2005 Nicotine reinforcement and cognition restored by targeted expression of nicotinic receptors. Nature 436:103–107

Nader K, Bechara A, van der Kooy D 1997 Neurobiological constraints on behavioral models of motivation. Annu Rev Psychol 48:85–114

Perkins KA, Sanders M, Fonte C et al 1999 Effects of central and peripheral nicotinic blockade on human nicotine discrimination. Psychopharmacology 142:158–164

Rose JE, Behm FM, Westman EC, Levin ED, Stein RM, Ripka GV 1994 Mecamylamine combined with nicotine skin patch facilitates smoking cessation beyond nicotine patch treatment alone. Clin Pharmacol Ther 56:86–99

Rose JE, Sampson A, Levin ED, Henningfield JE 1989 Mecamylamine increases nicotine preference and attenuates nicotine discrimination. Pharmacol Biochem Behav 32:933–938

Rose JE, Behm FM, Westman EC 1998 Nicotine-mecamylamine treatment for smoking cessation: the role of pre-cessation therapy. Exp Clin Psychopharmacol 6:331–343

Salas R, Pieri F, DeBiasi M 2004 Decreased signs of nicotine withdrawal in mice null for the beta4 nicotinic acetylcholine receptor subunit. J Neurosci 24:10035–10039

Salmon AM, Damaj MI, Marubio LM, Epping-Jordan MP, Merlo-Pich E, Changeux JP 2001 Altered neuroadaptation in opiate dependence and neurogenic inflammatory nociception in alpha CGRP-deficient mice. Nat Neurosci 4:357–358

Salmon AM, Evrard A, Damaj I, Changeux JP 2004 Reduction of withdrawal signs after chronic nicotine exposure of alpha-calcitonin gene-related peptide knock-out mice. Neurosci Lett 360:73–76

Schenker NM, Desgouttes AM, Semendeferi K 2005 Neural connectivity and cortical substrates of cognition in hominoids. J Hum Evol 49:547–569

Sherwood CC, Holloway RL, Semendeferi K, Hof PR 2005 Is prefrontal white matter enlargement a human evolutionary specialization? Nat Neurosci 8:537–538

The dopamine D₃ system: new opportunities for dopamine-based reward

Christian Heidbreder

Department of Neuropsychopharmacology, Centre of Excellence for Drug Discovery in Psychiatry, GlaxoSmithKline Pharmaceuticals, Via A. Fleming 4, 37135 Verona, Italy

Abstract. The mesolimbic dopamine (DA) system has been the framework for theories exploring the chemoarchitectural substrates of reward and motivation, including aspects of drug addiction. Recent findings support the idea that mesolimbic DA neurotransmission is implicated in the learning of the motivational significance of a stimulus rather than in the mediation of the hedonic or aversive valence of the stimulus *per se*. As such, enhanced mesolimbic DA activity would facilitate incentive learning or the attribution of incentive salience to cues. In this context, the high binding affinity of the DA D₃ receptor to endogenous DA, its high expression in the so-called brain reward regions, as well as its up-regulation in the ventral striatum of cocaine overdose victims and in rodents after cocaine self-administration or behavioural sensitization to cocaine- or nicotine-associated cues make the DA D₃ receptor an attractive new opportunity for the pharmacotherapeutic management of drug addiction. The present paper will introduce the concept that selective antagonism at the DA D₃ receptor might be a new strategy to prevent environmental and pharmacological stimuli from triggering and maintaining drug-seeking behaviour.

2005 Understanding nicotine and tobacco addiction. Wiley, Chichester (Novartis Foundation Symposium 275) p 116–131

Drug addiction refers to compulsive drug use despite physical, psychological or social harm, and is characterized by loss of control over amount and frequency of drug use, irresistible cravings and urges, denial of indisputable negative consequences, and the emergence of a negative emotional state when the drug is absent. Thus, from a psychiatric perspective, drug addiction has aspects of impulse control and compulsive disorders, which may lead to relapse or reinstatement of drug-seeking behaviours even after relatively long periods of abstinence. It is this late relapse that makes the therapeutic management of drug addiction a major challenge for current research and drug development.

Recent surveys confirm that there are about 200 million users of illegal drugs worldwide, which represent 3.4% of the world population. Alcohol dependence

116

impacts 32 million adults in the top seven markets whereas about 1.2 billion smokers are estimated worldwide, comprising approximately one-third of the global population aged 15 or older. The World Health Organization (WHO) estimates that the worldwide number of smokers will continue to increase to 1.6 billion by 2025. Among other neuropsychiatric diseases, alcohol and drug abuse *per se* costs the American economy an estimated overall $544.11 billion per year in lost productivity, health care expenditures, crime and other conditions (Uhl & Grow 2004).

Despite the societal burden of drug addiction and related psychiatric comorbidities, efficacious pharmacotherapeutic strategies promoting long-lasting drug abstinence and long-term recovery, and ensuring satisfactory patient compliance are still lacking. Significant room for improvement exists in both the efficacy (acute cessation, reduction in the number of cessation attempts, reduction in craving, prevention of relapse, long-term maintenance of abstinence, and compliance to treatment) and safety (improved side-effect profile) domains. As such, the continued elucidation of the neurobiological and neurochemical underpinnings of withdrawal symptoms, drug intake, craving, relapse and co-morbid psychiatric associations is critical for the development of new pharmacotherapeutic approaches for the treatment of drug addiction.

Mesolimbic dopamine and attentional processing of environmental stimuli

Virtually all drugs of abuse, but also natural rewards such as food and sexual interaction, elicit a significant increase in extracellular dopamine (DA) in the mesolimbic system that originates in the ventral tegmental area (VTA) and projects toward limbic forebrain regions including the nucleus accumbens (NAc) (Wise 2004). Substantial data sets correlating DA with the hedonic value of rewarding stimuli contributed to the practice of referring to the mesolimbic DA system as the 'brain reward circuit'. Recently, however, the concept that mesolimbic DA simply encodes hedonic tone has been called into question. First, enhanced dopaminergic activity in the NAc is not only elicited by reward-related stimuli, but can also be triggered by aversive stimuli or exposure to a novel environment that has no obvious rewarding property (Gray et al 1997). Second, rats with extensive neurotoxic lesions of the DA neurons in the NAc show normal hedonic response patterns to sucrose (Berridge & Robinson 1998). Third, a drug like cocaine is still rewarding in mutant mice lacking the DA transporter (e.g. Rocha et al 1998) suggesting that additional transporters and/or mechanisms contribute to the reinforcing properties of the drug. Fourth, DA-deficient (DD) mice provided with both sucrose and water still demonstrate significant preference for sucrose (Cannon & Palmiter 2003). Fifth, analysis of response patterns of single DA neurons to reward presentation has led to the suggestion that mesolimbic DA may be more involved in prediction of reward and the use of such information to strengthen behaviours and increase their future likelihood (Schultz 2002).

These findings clearly support the idea that the mesolimbic DA system is implicated in the learning of the *motivational significance* of a stimulus rather than in the mediation of the hedonic/aversive value of the stimulus *per se*. As such, DA would play a rheostatic role modifying synaptic weights depending on the valence (better-than-expected *vs.* worse-than-expected) of the environmental stimuli. In order to apply this hypothesis to drug addiction, one must assume that any response to the drug that occurs during the period of raised extracellular DA may have the potential of acquiring incentive salience and contribute to increased attentional processing of drug-related cues. A corollary hypothesis is that this attentional bias toward drug-related cues elicits drug craving and contributes to compulsive drug use and relapse to drug-seeking behaviour.

Mesolimbic dopamine and regulation of drug-seeking behaviour

The neurocircuitry underlying reinstatement of drug seeking behaviour remains largely unknown. However, recent studies have shown that presentation of a drug-associated conditioned stimulus (CS) to animals can induce large conditioned increases in extracellular DA levels in the NAc (Di Ciano et al 1998, Ito et al 2000), suggesting that DA neurotransmission in the NAc is involved in cue-controlled drug-seeking behaviour (Wyvell & Berridge 2000). In addition, the amygdala has been reported to play an important role in drug-enhanced stimulus–reward associations (Harmer & Phillips 1999), which may underlie drug craving and compulsive drug-taking in humans (O'Brien et al 1998). Enhanced monoaminergic tone in the basolateral subregion of the amygdala (BLA) appears to increase the motivational properties or salience of cocaine-associated cues during reinstatement of cocaine-seeking behaviour, whereas inactivation of the BLA produces the reverse effect (Ledford et al 2003). The central amygdala (CeA) may mediate conditioned increases in DA measured in the NAc following the non-contingent presentation of a CS (Ledford et al 2003), and seems to also play a key role in stress-triggered relapse to cocaine-seeking behaviour (Erb et al 2001, Leri et al 2002). Finally, the anterior cingulate cortex (ACC) seems to serve as a common link in the neural circuitry underlying reinstatement of drug-seeking behaviours (Heidbreder & Groenewegen 2003).

Functional magnetic resonance imaging (fMRI) and positron emission tomography (PET) scan studies provide evidence for overlapping between regions activated during drug craving and those activated during a working memory (e.g. Grant et al 1996) suggesting that both craving and attentional processes may involve similar neural circuits. The ACC is activated both in selective attention and response competition processes (Tamminga 1999), as well as in cue-induced cocaine craving (e.g. Childress et al 1999). Importantly, the ACC has reciprocal connections with both the BLA/CeA and NAc (for a comprehensive review, see Heidbreder & Groe-newegen 2003). Thus, one may suggest that the ACC, in concert with the NAc and the BLA/CeA, contributes to discriminate between multiple stimuli on the basis of their association with reward. This notion further supports the idea that sustained increase of the DA signal following exposure to drugs of abuse or stress might result in an attentional narrowing toward drug-related stimuli, which would lead to craving and ultimately relapse.

Mesolimbic dopamine and the dopamine D$_3$ receptor

The role of DA in the attentional processing of drug-related cues together with drug-induced increase in DA in the mesolimbic system as a key factor for the expression of drug-seeking behaviour clearly point toward the potential use of DA receptor antagonists as candidate medications to reduce drug seeking and craving. However, non-selective DA receptor antagonists, which have been shown to increase abstinence and/or attenuate measures of drug- and cue-induced craving in humans (Modell et al 1993, Shaw et al 1994) have the potential to induce long-term neurological side effects and are not suitable as anti-craving medications.

A growing body of evidence is increasing the likelihood that DA D$_3$ receptors are significantly involved in the control of drug-seeking behaviour. There are four main arguments in support of a key role of the DA D$_3$ receptor in drug addiction. First, DA D$_3$ receptors show highest density in limbic regions such as the ventral striatum and amygdala, brain areas that seem to play a key role in behaviours controlled by the presentation of drug-associated cues. Although inter-species differences have been reported in the distribution of the DA D$_3$ receptor, its expression in the human brain follows a similar pattern as the one observed in the rodent brain. Second, studies show that DA D$_3$ receptors are up-regulated in the NAc of cocaine overdose fatalities. Third, DA D$_3$ mRNA and receptors are increased in cocaine cue conditioned hyperlocomotion, and termination of a cocaine self-administration regimen increases DA D$_3$ binding over time in the NAc core and ventral caudate-putamen. In addition, nicotine-induced conditioned locomotion and nicotine behavioural sensitization are both associated with a significant increase in D$_3$ receptor binding and mRNA levels in the NAc shell. Sub-chronic administration of morphine also produces a significant increase in D$_3$ receptor mRNA in the caudate-putamen and ventral midbrain. Fourth, selective blockade of DA D$_3$ receptors by SB-277011A (trans-N-[4-[2-(6-cyano-1,2,3,4-tetrahydroisoquinolin-2yl)ethyl]cyclo-hexyl]-4-quinolininecarbo-xamide), a highly-potent and highly-selective DA D$_3$ receptor antagonist, is efficacious in models of cocaine-, nicotine-, alcohol-, and heroin-seeking behaviours in the rat (for a comprehensive review in support of these four arguments, see Heidbreder et al 2005).

Selective DA D_3 receptor antagonists and rewarding efficacy of drugs of abuse

A commonality shared by selective DA D_3 receptor antagonists is that they significantly reduce drug self-administration only when the self-administration workload imposed upon the animal is increased either in terms of progressive-ratio [PR] break-point or in the transition from low fixed-ratio [FR] (e.g. FR1-FR2) to high FR (e.g. FR10) schedules of reinforcement, or when the unit dose of reinforcing drug is lowered. This is an important observation because low FR schedules of reinforcement measure the pattern of rate of drug intake, but not the degree of reinforcing efficacy (Wise & Gardner 2004). Since the PR break-point is an index of the relative strength of a reinforcer independent of response rate, the shift in PR break-point produced by selective DA D_3 receptor antagonists indicates that these agents decrease the reinforcing value of drugs in rats. Although such a conclusion is warranted, interpretation of the effects of new selective DA D_3 receptor antagonists on drug self-administration under different schedules of reinforcement can always be confounded by a number of factors. Thus, one may argue that selective DA D_3 receptor antagonists may produce non-specific effects, such as sedation, memory impairment, motor dysfunctions, or rewarding/aversive actions *per se*. However, it has already been demonstrated that selective DA D_3 receptor antagonists (a) do not have abuse liability as evidenced by the observation that they do not maintain drug self-administration (Xi et al 2005); (b) do not produce conditioned preference or aversion (Vorel et al 2002, Gyertyán & Gál 2003), and (c) do not alter intracranial self-stimulation thresholds (Vorel et al 2002). In addition, selective DA D_3 receptor antagonists do not alter the reinforcing action of natural rewards such as sucrose (Di Ciano et al 2003) or food (Vorel et al 2002). Furthermore, selective DA D_3 receptor antagonists significantly improve the learning deficit produced by the non-selective muscarinic antagonist scopolamine and the anxiogenic benzodiazepine inverse agonist FG-7142 without altering the normal learning process in non-impaired rats (Laszy et al 2005), and produce an increase in extracellular levels of acetylcholine in the anterior cingulate cortex (Lacroix et al 2003). These latter effects would be expected to improve rather than interfere with memory.

One may also argue that the efficacy of selective DA D_3 receptor antagonists in reducing drug-seeking behaviour may be partly related to their action at DA D_2 receptors. This, however, is unlikely as evidenced by the functional difference between selective D_3 vs. D_1/D_2 antagonism in animal models commonly used to assess drug-induced reward processes. First, DA D_1- and D_2-preferring antagonists typically produce a right-shift along the pulse frequency axis in the rate-frequency curve paradigm (Miliaressis et al 1986). Furthermore, the efficacy of DA receptor antagonists in producing right shifts is correlated with their relative efficacy in displacing DA D$_2$ binding (Gallistel & Davis 1983). In contrast, selective DA D$_3$ receptor antagonists do not alter electrical brain-reward thresholds (Vorel et al 2002). Second, whereas DA D$_1$-preferring and mixed D$_1$/D$_2$ antagonists produce conditioned aversion (for a review, see Tzschentke 1998), DA D$_3$ receptor antagonists produce neither reward nor aversion (Vorel et al 2002, Ashby et al 2003, Gyertyán & Gál 2003). Third, DA D$_1$- and D$_2$-preferring antagonists are negative reinforcers (Kandel & Schuster 1977) while highly-selective DA D$_3$ receptor antagonists do not support self-administration, and thus appear devoid of reward efficacy (Xi et al 2005).

Finally, selective antagonism at DA D$_3$ receptors does not produce functional antagonism at DA D$_2$ receptors in laboratory rodents *in vivo*. In contrast to DA D$_2$ receptor antagonists, selective antagonism at DA D$_3$ receptors (a) does not elicit catalepsy; (b) does not affect spontaneous or stimulant-induced locomotion; (c) does not increase serum prolactin levels; and (d) does not increase DA levels in the striatum (Reavill et al 2000). Furthermore, the motor coordination and psychomotor activity profile of selective antagonism at DA D$_3$ receptors is significantly different from that of haloperidol, a mixed DA D$_2$/D$_3$ receptor antagonist, which significantly reduces locomotor activity and rearing behaviour, increases catalepsy, and impairs motor coordination. Conversely, selective DA D$_3$ receptor antagonists do not alter locomotor activity or motor coordination (Xi et al 2005).

Conclusions

Addiction at the human level is characterized by an increase in motivation to self-administer drug(s) despite adverse consequences. Although the proof of efficacy of pharmacotherapeutic agents is to be derived ultimately from clinical trials, the preclinical findings that selective antagonism at DA D$_3$ receptors reduces such motivation and reduces the reinforcing efficacy of drugs such as nicotine, alcohol, cocaine, heroin, and marijuana adds to an accumulating body of evidence that selective DA D$_3$ receptor antagonists may hold highest promise in the treatment of drug addiction.

References

Ashby CR Jr, Paul M, Gardner EL, Heidbreder CA, Hagan JJ 2003 Acute administration of the selective D$_3$ receptor antagonist SB-277011-A blocks the acquisition and expression of the conditioned place preference response to heroin in male rats. Synapse 48:154–156

Berridge KC, Robinson TE 1998 What is the role of dopamine in reward: hedonic impact, reward learning, or incentive salience? Brain Res Brain Res Rev 28:309–369

Cannon CM, Palmiter RD 2003 Reward without dopamine. J Neurosci 23:10827–10831

Childress AR, Mozley PD, McElgin W, Fitzgerald J, Reivich M, O'Brien CP 1999 Limbic activation during cue-induced cocaine craving. Am J Psychiatry 156:11–18

Di Ciano P, Blaha CD, Phillips AG 1998 Conditioned changes in dopamine oxidation currents in the nucleus accumbens of rats by stimuli paired with self-administration or yoked administration of d-amphetamine. Eur J Neurosci 10:1121–1127

Di Ciano P, Underwood RJ, Hagan JJ, Everitt BJ 2003 Attenuation of cue-controlled cocaine-seeking by a selective D$_3$ dopamine receptor antagonist SB-277011-A. Neuropsychopharmacology 28:329–338

Erb S, Salmaso N, Rodaros D, Stewart J 2001 A role for the CRF-containing pathway from central nucleus of the amygdala to bed nucleus of the stria terminalis in the stress-induced reinstatement of cocaine seeking in rats. Psychopharmacology (Berl) 158:360–365

Gallistel CR, Davis AJ 1983 Affinity for the dopamine D2 receptor predicts neuroleptic potency in blocking the reinforcing effect of MFB stimulation. Pharmacol Biochem Behav 19:867–872

Gray JA, Moran PM, Grigoryan G, Peters SL, Young AM, Joseph MH 1997 Latent inhibition: the nucleus accumbens connection revisited. Behav Brain Res 88:27–34

Grant S, London ED, Newlin DB et al 1996 Activation of memory circuits during cue-elicited cocaine craving. Proc Natl Acad Sci USA 93:12040–12045

Gyertyán I, Gál K 2003 Dopamine D$_3$ receptor ligands show place conditioning effect but do not influence cocaine-induced place preference. Neuroreport 14:93–98

Harmer CJ, Phillips GD 1999 Enhanced dopamine efflux in the amygdala by a predictive, but not a non-predictive, stimulus: facilitation by prior repeated d-amphetamine. Neuroscience 90:119–130

Heidbreder CA, Groenewegen HJ 2003 The medial prefrontal cortex in the rat: evidence for a dorso-ventral distinction based upon functional and anatomical characteristics. Neurosci Biobehav Rev 27:555–579

Heidbreder CA, Gardner EL, Xi Z-X et al 2005 The role of central dopamine D$_3$ receptors in drug addiction: a review of pharmacological evidence. Brain Res Rev 49:77–105

Ito R, Dalley JW, Howes SR, Robbins TW, Everitt BJ 2000 Dissociation in conditioned dopamine release in the nucleus accumbens core and shell in response to cocaine cues and during cocaine-seeking behavior in rats. J Neurosci 20:7489–7495

Kandel DA, Schuster CR 1977 An investigation of nalorphine and perphenazine as negative reinforcers in an escape paradigm. Pharmacol Biochem Behav 6:61–71

Lacroix LP, Hows MEP, Shah AJ, Hagan JJ, Heidbreder CA 2003 Selective antagonism at dopamine D$_3$ receptors enhances monoaminergic and cholinergic neurotransmission in the rat anterior cingulate cortex. Neuropsychopharmacology 28:839–849

Laszy J, Laszlovszky I, Gyertyán I 2005 Dopamine D$_3$ receptor antagonists improve the learning performance in memory-impaired rats. Psychopharmacology 179:567–575

Ledford CC, Fuchs RA, See RE 2003 Potentiated reinstatement of cocaine-seeking behavior following D-amphetamine infusion into the basolateral amygdala. Neuropsychopharmacology 28:1721–1729

Leri F, Flores J, Rodaros D, Stewart J 2002 Blockade of stress-induced but not cocaine-induced reinstatement by infusion of noradrenergic antagonists into the bed nucleus of the stria terminalis or the central nucleus of the amygdala. J Neurosci 22:5713–5718

Miliaressis E, Rompre PP, Laviolette P Philippe L, Coulombe D 1986 The curve-shift paradigm in self-administration. Physiol Behav 37:85–93

Modell JG, Mountz JM, Glaser FB, Lee JY 1993 Effect of haloperidol on measures of craving and impaired control in alcoholic subjects. Alcohol Clin Exp Res 17:234–240

O'Brien CP, Childress AR, Ehrman RN, Robbins SJ 1998 Conditioning factors in drug abuse: can they explain compulsion? J Psychopharmacology 12:15–22

Reavill C, Taylor SG, Wood MD et al 2000 Pharmacological actions of a novel, high-affinity, and selective human dopamine D$_3$ receptor antagonist, SB-277011-A. J Pharmacol Exp Ther 294:1154–1165

Rocha BA, Fumagalli F, Gainetdinov RR et al 1998 Cocaine self-administration in dopamine-transporter knockout mice. Nat Neurosci 1:132–137

Schultz W 2002 Getting formal with dopamine and reward. Neuron 36:241–263

Shaw GK, Waller S, Majumdar SK, Latham CJ, Dunn G 1994 Tiapride in the prevention of relapse in recently detoxified alcoholics. Br J Psychiatry 165:515–523

Tamminga CA 1999 The anterior cingulate and response conflict. Am J Psychiatry 156:1849

Tzschentke TM 1998 Measuring reward with the conditioned place preference paradigm: a comprehensive review of drug effects, recent progress and new issues. Prog Neurobiol 56:613–672

Uhl GR, Grow RW 2004 The burden of complex genetics in brain disorders. Arch Gen Psychiatry 61:223–229

Vorel SR, Ashby CR Jr, Paul M et al 2002 Dopamine D$_3$ receptor antagonism inhibits cocaine-seeking and cocaine-enhanced brain reward in rats. J Neurosci 22:9595–9603

Wise RA 2004 Dopamine, learning and motivation. Nat Rev Neurosci 5:483–494

Wise RA, Gardner EL 2004 Animal models of addiction. In: Charney DS, Nestler EJ (eds), Neurobiology of mental illness, 2nd edn. Oxford Univ Press, p 683–697

Wyvell CL, Berridge KC 2000 Intra-accumbens amphetamine increases the conditioned incentive salience of sucrose reward: enhancement of reward 'wanting' without enhanced 'liking' or response reinforcement. J Neurosci 20:8122–8130

Xi Z-X, Gilbert JG, Pak AC, Ashby CR Jr, Heidbreder CA, Gardner EL 2005 Selective dopamine D3 receptor antagonism by SB-277011A attenuates cocaine reinforcement as assessed by progressive-ratio and variable-cost/variable-payoff fixed-ratio cocaine self-administration in rats. Eur J Neurosci 21:3427–3438

DISCUSSION

Markou: I would like to raise a topic we haven't discussed yet but which is relevant here. A lot of schizophrenia patients smoke. Dopamine D$_3$ receptor antagonists have been suggested as antipsychotic medications. Do you see D$_3$ receptors antagonists being useful in schizophrenia, and if yes, what aspects of schizophrenia will these medications be treating that may currently be being self-medicated by smoking?

Heidbreder: This is an interesting question. Our D$_3$ receptor antagonist programme was originally developed for schizophrenia, not drug addiction. There are several arguments in support of a role of D$_3$ receptors in schizophrenia. For example, levels of D$_3$ receptors are elevated in schizophrenics that are off antipsychotics, which might reflect a hyperdopaminergic state of the mesolimbic dopamine system (Gurevitch et al 1997). Dopamine D$_3$ receptors could also be regulated by extrinsic non-dopaminergic signals, such as brain-derived neurotrophic factor, which is controlled by dopamine tone. In actuality, elevated dopamine may result in enhanced release of brain-derived neurotrophic factor (BDNF) from cortico-striatal fibres and an increase in D$_3$ receptor levels in the nucleus accumbens (Guillin et al 2001). Interestingly, antipsychotic treatment leads to a reduction in levels of BDNF (Dawson et al 2001). We also know that a Ser9Gly polymorphism in the D$_3$ receptor could be associated with a higher risk of developing schizophrenia in some subgroups of patients (Dubertret et al 1998, Jonsson et al 2003). In my opinion selective dopamine D_3 receptor antagonists might be very useful in treating the negative symptoms of schizophrenia, particularly cognitive dysfunction. Importantly, selective dopamine D_3 antagonists are not expected to elicit a marked extrapyramidal syndrome, which is important with regards to the treatment of these negative symptoms. We know, for example, that administration of selective dopamine D_3 receptor antagonists consistently reduces the electrical activity of ventral tegmental area-derived mesolimbic dopamine neurons (Ashby et al 2000). Like clozapine, this action is selective, compared with substantia nigra-derived nigrostriatal neurons, which is in accordance with a low extra-pyramidal syndrome potential of selective D_3 receptor antagonists. Finally, recent studies demonstrated that the acute administration of selective dopamine D_3 receptor antagonists significantly improves the learning deficit produced by the non-selective muscarinic antagonist scopolamine and the anxiogenic benzodiazepine inverse agonist FG-7142 without altering the normal learning process in non-impaired rats (Laszy et al 2005). We have also recently shown that selective dopamine D_3 receptor antagonists produce an increase in extracellular levels of acetylcholine in the anterior cingulate cortex (Lacroix et al 2003). Together these effects would be expected to improve cognitive functions.

Caggiula: You showed that the antagonist attenuated cocaine and nicotine conditioned place preference (CPP). It also attenuated nicotine- or cocaine-induced reinstatement after extinction, and cocaine cue-induced reinstatement. Did you also do nicotine cue-induced reinstatement?

Heidbreder: This experiment is currently ongoing.

Caggiula: Could you speculate on the possible functional significance of the time-dependent increase in D_3 binding that occurs after the termination of cocaine self administration?

Heidbreder: The study I was referring to was published by Neisewander's group last year (Neisewander et al 2004). In this elegant series of experiments, Neisewander and colleagues showed that termination of a cocaine self-administration regimen progressively increases dopamine D_3 binding up to 32 days. This effect may occur through regulatory responses to an increase in phasic dopamine levels associated with cocaine-taking and -seeking behaviour. The extent to which this effect is maintained over longer periods of time and how it relates to craving is currently unknown, but it seems that these alterations are long-lasting.

Changeux: You used only one drug throughout these studies. What is the range of specificity of this compound, and how does it compare with other compounds in the same series? Have you clearly demonstrated that the compound is acting only on the target that you are assuming the drug is acting on?

Heidbreder: The compound I referred to is SB-277011A (trans-N-[4-[2-(6-cyano-1,2,3,4-tetrahydroisoquinolin-2yl)ethyl]cyclo-hexyl]-4-quinolininecarbo-xamide). This compound was one of the first selective brain-penetrant dopamine D_3 receptor antagonists with high affinity for the human and rat cloned dopamine D$_3$ receptor and greater than 100-fold selectivity for about 60 additional receptors, enzymes, and ion channels (Reavill et al 2000; for a comprehensive review, see Heidbreder et al 2005). Similar results have now been observed with other selective dopamine D$_3$ receptor antagonists (Campiani et al 2003, Macdonald et al 2003). We have so far tested a range of compounds from three different chemical series.

Changeux: The knockout has been done: why didn't you talk about it?

Heidbreder: Yes, it is true that studies have been performed using dopamine D$_3$-deficient mice. The behavioural phenotype of D$_3$ knockout mice, however, is rather unclear. Some studies reported that in D$_3$ receptor knockout mice, physical dependence to ethanol is increased (Narita et al 2002), although other studies indicated that deleting the D$_3$ receptor in C57BL/6j mice does not significantly alter the rewarding effects of ethanol as assessed by operant ethanol self-administration (Boyce-Rustay & Risinger 2003). These findings are in direct contrast with our pharmacological data indicating that selective antagonism at D$_3$ receptors by SB-277011A significantly decreases the intake of ethanol by rats and mice (for comprehensive reviews, see Heidbreder et al 2004, 2005). I am sceptical about some of these constitutive knockout studies because we don't know what counter-adaptations may have taken place. In fact, the discrepancies between findings from pharmacological studies and dopamine D$_3$ receptor knockout studies might be explained by changes during the development of the genetically modified animal to compensate for the absence of the D$_3$ receptor. In support of this suggestion are findings that haloperidol-treated animals acquire ethanol conditioned place preference normally (Risinger et al 1992) whereas dopamine D$_2$ receptor knockout mice fail to acquire the conditioned place preference response (Cunningham et al 2000). These findings demonstrate that the behavioural effects produced by a selective receptor antagonist are not always compatible with those produced by genetically deleting the receptor at which the antagonist acts. The technology you have presented earlier today (Maskos et al 2005), however, by stereotaxically injecting a lentiviral vector directed toward a specific target into a specific brain region of mice carrying selective deletions at the target, would be an extremely elegant way to address this issue.

Chiamulera: What was the rationale for testing the compound on the learning and memory test? How do you put this in the context of nicotine addiction in general? And how can you explain the reversal of learning impairment with the effects with the CPP paradigm?

Heidbreder: As mentioned previously, our initial aim was to profile selective dopamine D$_3$ receptor antagonists for the treatment of schizophrenia as a primary therapeutic indication. In this context, we characterized the neurochemical fingerprints of clozapine, olanzapine, risperidone, haloperidol vs. our selective dopamine D$_3$ receptor antagonists. It became clear that D2 receptor antagonists do not alter cholinergic function in the medial prefrontal cortex. However selective dopamine D_3 antagonists do enhance extracellular levels of acetylcholine in the anterior cingulate cortex in the same line as the effects observed following acute clozapine or olanzapine treatment (Lacroix et al 2003). Furthermore, there is growing evidence suggesting that selective dopamine D_3 receptor antagonists can reverse learning deficits produced by either scopolamine or the anxiogenic drug FG-7142 without altering the normal learning process in non-impaired rats (Laszy et al 2005). We currently do not have a clear explanation as to the mechanisms involved in these potential cognitive enhancing effects. I was previously referring to compulsive drug use as a result of attentional narrowing toward drugs and drug-related stimuli. We also know that chronic drug use hampers frontal cortex function (Volkow & Fowler 2000), and that such deficits may contribute to impaired impulse control, as well as lack of judgement and risk assessment (Bechara et al 1994). As such, I think that having a compound that increases cholinergic function in such a key brain region as the anterior cingulate cortex holds highest promise in counteracting these cognitive deficits.

Shiffman: You speculated that the increased binding over time might be a substrate for craving. The puzzle is that both in cocaine and nicotine addiction, craving decreases over time and abstinence, yet you are seeing progressively increased binding. In terms of the time course this would seem like a substrate for the *diminution* of craving.

Picciotto: There are some nice studies by Yavin Shaham and his group suggesting that craving for cocaine decreases over time with withdrawal, but the liability to cue- or drug-induced relapse incubates (Grimm et al 2001). As the withdrawal time gets longer relapse to cocaine seeking grows. He has shown for cocaine that the behaviour after extinction can be triggered potently and there is a neurochemical substrate. He has looked at BDNF, in particular in the amygdala as well as the accumbens (Lu et al 2005). The D_3 receptor up-regulation may parallel the BDNF increase. It may also parallel increases in CREB. Is there a cAMP response element in the D_3 promoter?

Heidbreder: As mentioned earlier, the relationship between D_3 and BDNF is quite well established, and sustained increase in extracellular dopamine levels may result in enhanced release of BDNF from corticostriatal fibres and an increase in D_3 receptor levels in the nucleus accumbens.

West: That couldn't be the case for humans, because the profile for humans is exactly the opposite.

Shiffman: There is a shift in the profile: more cue-induced relapse is seen later on in smokers, particularly with alcohol, whereas there is more affect and stress triggering is seen early on.

West: Is this seen in absolute terms, or relative to other sources of relapse? The early stages of abstinence have everything going on.

Shiffman: And that is damping out. You showed data primarily on reinstatement paradigms. Have you looked at self-administration itself?

Heidbreder: We did look at nicotine or cocaine self-administration under low fixed ratio schedules of reinforcement. There is something very interesting to point out at this stage. A commonality shared by selective DA D$_3$ receptor antagonists is that they significantly reduce drug self-administration only when the self-administration workload imposed upon the animal is increased either in terms of progressive-ratio [PR] break-point or in the transition from low fixed-ratio [FR] (e.g. FR1–FR2) to high FR (e.g. FR10) schedules of reinforcement, or when the unit dose of reinforcing drug is lowered. This is an important observation because low FR schedules of reinforcement measure the pattern of rate of drug intake, but not the degree of reinforcing efficacy. Since the PR break-point is an index of the relative strength of a reinforcer independent of response rate, the shift in PR break-point produced by selective DA D$_3$ receptor antagonists indicates that these agents decrease the reinforcing value of drugs in rats.

Balfour: What does cocaine administration *per se* and chronic administration of your antagonist do to the expression of D$_3$ receptors?

Heidbreder: I am not aware of any studies looking at the expression of D$_3$ following acute injection of cocaine. The only chronic study is the Neisewander et al (2004) paper with different time points following cessation of cocaine self-administration. We have never looked at the effect of chronic treatment with our selective D$_3$ receptor antagonists on expression of D$_3$ mRNA or proteins.

Balfour: Could the increase simply be recovery to normal levels?

Heidbreder: It is possible, but we don't have any evidence of this. However, similar increases in D$_3$ binding have been observed in post-mortem studies on the brains of cocaine overdose fatalities (Staley & Mash 1996).

Balfour: Given the work in Barry Everitt's laboratory in Cambridge (Ito et al 2004) which suggests that excitotoxic lesions of accumbal core diminish responding for a conditioned stimulus paired with cocaine whereas lesions of the shell have very little effect on responding for either the drug or the conditioned stimulus. Where do you think the D$_3$ receptors are located in the shell?

Heidbreder: This is an interesting question if we are to focus on the nucleus accumbens. Most of expression studies are performed using autoradiography with 7-OH-DPAT or 7-OH-PIPAT. What these studies typically and reliably report is that dopamine D$_3$ receptors are expressed in highest densities in the islands of Calleja, olfactory bulb, nucleus accumbens, and intermediate lobe of the pituitary. However, we also see a low signal in other regions such as the amygdala, possibly the basolateral amygdala. When one considers the important role of the basolateral amygdala in rheostating the motivational properties or salience of cocaine-associated cues during reinstatement of cocaine-seeking behaviour, one may be tempted to hypothesize that D_3 receptors in that brain region may play a key role in our behavioural findings.

Balfour: Your microinfusion studies showed reduced responding as well.

Heidbreder: That is correct in the case of stress-triggered relapse to cocaine seeking behaviour, but this is just one study that we did in the shell subregion of the nucleus accumbens. We now need to investigate other brain regions in additional paradigms.

Gasparini: I have a more general question related to the probability of success of D_3 antagonists. You mentioned that there are a number of projects, involving a variety of targets, for treating addiction states. You also pointed out a couple of elements which might explain why they haven't been successful. What makes you so confident that the D_3 antagonist will have a high chance of success in humans? Is it the results in animal models? For which sub-syndrome of addiction will D_3 antagonists likely prove most successful?

Heidbreder: You are working in drug discovery as well. You know that drug discovery people must remain very optimistic! There are limitations with animal models, but in the drug addiction field the models have a reasonable construct validity, and for some paradigms such as self-administration, a good face validity as well. Predictive validity is more problematic as we have very few gold standards for comparative purposes, even though some of our behavioural paradigms have been used successfully to profile compounds such as acamprosate, naltrexone, baclofen, bupropion, and more recently rimonabant or varenicline, which all showed signs of efficacy in clinical trials for alcohol and/or nicotine dependence. We have used the best animal models currently available to test our dopamine D_3 receptor antagonists. Based on the results we got so far I am optimistic. I believe that there is also scope for these selective antagonists beyond drug addiction. Relapse prevention looks like a very interesting target for these selective D_3 receptor antagonists. We also need to reconsider schizophrenia and further investigate compulsive/impulsive disorders. In fact, there is a *Bal1* polymorphism of the DA D_3 receptor gene that is associated with measures of impulsiveness and novelty seeking, and the personality trait of novelty seeking, of which impulsiveness is one component, is linked to DA function and addictive propensity, and predicts later alcoholism and relapse rate in detoxified alcoholics (for a comprehensive review, see Heidbreder et al 2004).

Bizarro: Did you say that this compound does not affect alcohol oral self-administration?

Heidbreder: No, alcohol is affected as well. We performed different studies on alcohol self-administration and prevention of relapse, and saw a similar pattern as for nicotine and cocaine.

Bizarro: You mentioned a clinical trial on alcohol-addicted patients. 85% of them might be dependent on nicotine as well. What is the expectation for this, taking into account nicotine as well as alcohol?

Heidbreder: It is a difficult question. There are now some clinical trials trying to take advantage of the comorbidity between alcohol and nicotine addiction. For example, a recent paper (Johnson et al 2003) revealed that patients who received topiramate, compared with placebo, were significantly less likely to have positive serum cotinine levels, and that drinking reductions were accompanied by smoking decreases in the topiramate group, but not the placebo group. Further studies are now warranted to assess whether or not topiramate may be useful to treat both nicotine and alcohol dependencies (Johnson 2004).

West: I wasn't sure of the rationale for why D_3 antagonism would work with drugs of abuse but not with naturally occurring reinforcers.

Heidbreder: We need to make a distinction here between natural reinforcers, as assessed in operant procedures, and food intake or binge eating. When I was talking about lack of efficacy of selective dopamine D_3 receptor antagonists on natural reinforcers this was strictly in the context of operant conditioning procedures under similar schedules of reinforcement.

West: I still can't quite see how, if you set up the same kinds of parameters but with nicotine or food reward, why antagonizing the D_3 receptors would have a profound effect in one case and no detectable effect in the other.

Heidbreder: One potential explanation is that the neurocircuitries underlying natural reinforcement and drug-induced reinforcement are partly different.

West: I find that implausible. I don't think we would have evolved special circuitries for getting reward out of nicotine or alcohol. Most of our theorizing on this subject is based on the idea that drugs of abuse tap into existing reward pathways. The midbrain dopamine pathway has been posited as a final pathway in that sense.

Corrigall: But many of us can drink alcohol for example without abusing it or using other drugs. There can be differences in degree.

West: Is it differences in degree? This is an important question.

Heidbreder: We are dealing with a receptor that has a very focal distribution in the so-called mesolimbic systems. We are not talking about the entire mesolimbic system. In addition, whereas both dopamine and glutamate have been clearly involved in mediating the reinforcing properties of most drugs of abuse—and in particular psychostimulants—the evidence is not as clear for food-seeking and taking behaviours.

References

Grimm JW, Hope BT, Wise RA, Shaham Y 2001 Neuroadaptation. Incubation of cocaine craving after withdrawal. Nature 412:141–142

Lu L, Hope BT, Dempsey J, Liu SY, Bossert JM, Shaham Y 2005 Central amygdala ERK signaling pathway is critical to incubation of cocaine craving. Nat Neurosci 8:212–219

Ashby CR Jr, Minabe Y, Stemp G, Hagan JJ, Middlemiss DN 2000 Acute and chronic adminis-tration of the selective D_3 receptor antagonist SB-277011-A alters activity of midbrain dopamine neurons in rats: An in vivo electrophysiological study. J Pharmacol Exp Ther 294:1166–1174

Bechara A, Damasio AR, Damasio H, Anderson SW 1994 Insensitivity to future consequences following damage to human prefrontal cortex. Cognition 50:7–15

Boyce-Rustay JM, Risinger FO 2003 Dopamine D3 receptor knockout mice and the motivational effect of ethanol. Pharmacol Biochem Behav 75:373–379

Campiani G, Butini S, Trotta F et al 2003 Synthesis and pharmacological evaluation of potent and highly selective D3 receptor ligands: inihibition of cocaine-seeking behavior and the role of dopamine D3/D2 receptors. J Med Chem 46:3822–3839

Cunningham CL, Howard MA, Gill SJ, Rubinstein M, Low MJ, Grandy DK 2000 Ethanol-conditioned place preference is reduced in dopamine D2 receptor-deficient mice. Pharmacol Biochem Behav 67:693–699

Dawson NM, Hamid EH, Egan MF, Meredith GE 2001 Changes in the pattern of brain-derived neurotrophic factor immunoreactivity in the rat brain after acute and subchronic haloperidol treatment. Synapse 39:70–81

Dubertret C, Gorwood P, Ades J, Feingold J, Schwartz JC, Sokoloff P 1998 Meta-analysis of Drd3 gene and schizophrenia: ethnic heterogeneity and significant association in Caucasians. Am J Med Genet 81:318–322

Guillin O, Diaz J, Carroll P, Griffon N, Schwartz JC, Sokoloff P 2001 BDNF controls dopamine D3 receptor expression and triggers behavioural sensitization. Nature 411:86–89

Gurevich EV, Bordelon Y, Shapiro RM, Arnold SE, Gur RE, Joyce JN 1997 Mesolimbic dopamine D3 receptors and use of antipsychotics in patients with schizophrenia. A postmortem study. Arch Gen Psychiatry 54:225–232

Heidbreder CA, Andreoli M, Marcon C, Thanos PK, Ashby CR Jr, Gardner EL 2004 Role of dopamine D3 receptors in the addictive properties of ethanol. Drugs Today 40:355–365

Heidbreder CA, Gardner EL, Xi Z-X et al 2005 The role of central dopamine D3 receptors in drug addiction: a review of pharmacological evidence. Brain Res Rev 49:77–105

Ito R, Robbins TW, Everitt BJ 2004 Differential control over cocaine-seeking behavior by nucleus accumbens core and shell. Nat Neurosci 7:389–397

Johnson BA 2004 Topiramate-induced neuromodulation of cortico-mesolimbic dopamine func-tion: a new vista for the treatment of comorbid alcohol and nicotine dependence? Addict Behav 29:1465–1479

Johnson BA, Ait-Daoud N, Bowden CL et al 2003 Oral topiramate for treatment of alcohol dependence: a randomised controlled trial. Lancet 361:1677–1685

Jonsson EG, Flyckt L, Burgert E et al 2003 Dopamine D3 receptor gene Ser9Gly variant and schizophrenia: association study and meta-analysis. Psychiatr Genet 13:1–12

Lacroix LP, Hows MEP, Shah AJ, Hagan JJ, Heidbreder CA 2003 Selective antagonism at dopamine D3 receptors enhances monoaminergic and cholinergic neurotransmission in the rat anterior cingulate cortex. Neuropsychopharmacology 28:839–849

Laszy J, Laszlovszky I, Gyertyán I 2005 Dopamine D3 receptor antagonists improve the learn-ing performance of memory-impaired rats. Psychopharmacology 179:567–575

Macdonald GJ, Branch CL, Hadley MS et al 2003 Design and synthesis of trans-3-(2-(4-((3-(3-(5-methyl-1,2,4-oxadiazolyl)) phenyl)carboxamido)cyclohexyl)ethyl)-7-methylsulfonyl-2,3,4,5-tetrahydro-1H-3-benzazepine (SB-414796): a potent and selective dopamine D3 receptor antagonist. J Med Chem 46:4952–4964.

Maskos U, Molles BE, Pons S et al 2005 Nicotine reinforcement and cognition restored by targeted expression of nicotinic receptors. Nature 436:103–107

Narita M, Soma M, Tamaki H, Suzuki T 2002 Intensification of the development of ethanol dependence in mice lacking dopamine D3 receptor. Neurosci Lett 324:129–132

Neisewander JL, Fuchs RA, Tran-Nguyen LT, Weber SM, Coffey GP, Joyce JN 2004 Increases in dopamine D₃ receptor binding in rats receiving a cocaine challenge at various time points after cocaine self-administration: implications for cocaine-seeking behavior. Neuropsychopharmacology 29:1479–1487

Reavill C, Taylor SG, Wood MD et al 2000 Pharmacological actions of a novel, high-affinity, and selective human dopamine D3 receptor antagonist, SB-277011-A. J Pharmacol Exp Ther 294:1154–1165

Risinger FO, Dickinson SD, Cunningham CL 1992 Haloperidol reduces ethanol-induced motor activity stimulation but not conditioned place preference. Psychopharmacology (Berl) 107:453–456

Staley JK, Mash DC 1996 Adaptive increase in D3 dopamine receptors in the brain reward circuits of human cocaine fatalities. J Neurosci 16:6100–6106

Volkow ND, Fowler JS 2000 Addiction, a disease of compulsion and drive: involvement of the orbitofrontal cortex. Cereb Cortex 10:318–325

Pathways and systems involved in nicotine dependence

Athina Markou

Molecular and Integrative Neuroscience Department, SP2400 The Scripps Research Institute, 10550 North Torrey Pines Rd., La Jolla, CA 92037, USA

Abstract. Nicotine dependence is defined by the persistence of drug-taking and the withdrawal symptoms observed upon cessation of nicotine administration. Interactions between cholinergic, glutamatergic, γ-aminobutyric acid (GABA) and dopaminergic neurotransmitter systems in limbic brain sites mediate nicotine's rewarding effects. Administration of antagonists at nicotinic acetylcholine, dopaminergic, metabotropic glutamate or $GABA_B$ receptors decreases nicotine self-administration in rats. Further, microinjections of nicotinic antagonists or $GABA_B$ receptor agonists into the ventral tegmental area (VTA) or the pedunculopontine nucleus, that projects to the VTA, decrease self-administration. The critical role of the VTA to the nucleus accumbens dopaminergic projection is indicated by lesion and microdialyis studies. With the development of dependence, neuroadaptations occur in components of these systems to counteract chronic nicotine exposure. Nicotine withdrawal is associated with elevations in brain reward thresholds reflecting an anhedonic effect. Similar threshold elevations are induced in nicotine-dependent rats after systemic or intra-VTA administration of nicotinic antagonists or a metabotropic glutamate 2/3 receptor ($mGluR_{2/3}$) agonist, but not after $GABA_B$ agonist administration. Thus, with nicotine dependence there is decreased activity of nicotinic receptors, increased activity of $mGluR_{2/3}$, and no change in $GABA_B$ receptor activity in the VTA. The net outcome is decreased dopamine output in the nucleus accumbens during nicotine withdrawal.

2005 Understanding nicotine and tobacco addiction. Wiley, Chichester (Novartis Foundation Symposium 275) p 132–152

It is widely recognized that tobacco products are among the most addictive of all dependence-producing substances. Although there are over 4000 chemicals in tobacco products that could contribute to dependence, there is little debate that nicotine is a major component in tobacco responsible for addiction. Thus, research to promote our understanding of the neurobiology of tobacco dependence focuses on the mechanisms mediating nicotine dependence.

Dependence on drugs of abuse, including nicotine, is often defined by both the persistence of drug-taking behaviour despite adverse consequences, and the emergence of withdrawal symptoms upon abrupt cessation of drug administration (American Psychiatric Association 1994). Therefore, both the neurosubstrates mediating the reinforcing effects of acute nicotine and those mediating the withdrawal syndrome are relevant to drug dependence. The systems that develop neuroadaptations with the development of nicotine dependence and lead to the emergence of the withdrawal signs upon cessation of drug administration are likely to be the same or interacting with the systems mediating the acute nicotine effects (Markou et al 1998). That is, drug dependence develops as an adaptation to chronic drug exposure. In this review, the systems and pathways mediating the reinforcing effects of nicotine will be reviewed. Then, the neurobiological mechanisms exhibiting adaptations with chronic nicotine exposure will be discussed as the substrates for nicotine dependence.

Neurosubstrates of nicotine reinforcement

In humans, acute nicotine administration produces positive effects including mild euphoria. Such subjective positive effects support reliable intravenous nicotine self-administration behaviour in a variety of species, such as rats, mice, non-human primates and humans (e.g. Markou & Paterson 2001, Picciotto & Corrigall 2002).

The mesolimbic dopaminergic system and nicotinic acetylcholine receptors (nAchRs) within that system are critically involved in the reinforcing properties of nicotine (for reviews, Picciotto & Corrigall 2002, Balfour 2004; Fig. 1 for anatomy diagram). Acute nicotine administration increased the firing rate of ventral tegmental area (VTA) dopaminergic neurons, and elevated dialysate dopamine levels in the shell of the nucleus accumbens (Balfour 2004), possibly through excitatory actions at nAchRs on mesolimbic dopaminergic neurons in both the VTA and the nucleus accumbens (Nisell et al 1997). Interestingly, nAChRs in the VTA were shown to play a more important role than those in the nucleus accumbens in the effects of nicotine on nucleus accumbens dopamine release (Nisell et al 1997).

Other mechanisms by which nicotine may elevate striatal dopamine levels are by increasing frontal cortex glutamatergic stimulation of ventral striatum dopamine release, and/or glutamatergic stimulation of VTA dopaminergic neurons projecting to the striatum. Nicotine increases glutamate release by agonist actions at excitatory presynaptic nAchRs on glutamatergic terminals in various brain sites, including the VTA, nucleus accumbens, prefrontal cortex and hippocampus (Mansvelder & McGehee 2000, Kenny & Markou 2004). In the VTA, nicotine acts at presynaptic $\alpha 7$ nAChRs located upon glutamate afferents to increase glutamate release in the VTA which in turn stimulates dopamine release in the nucleus accumbens (Schilstrom et al 1998, Mansvelder & McGehee 2000, Kenny & Markou 2004). This increased glutamate release then acts at metabotropic and ionotropic glutamate receptors on postsynaptic dopamine neurons and increases their bursting activity and neurotransmitter release.

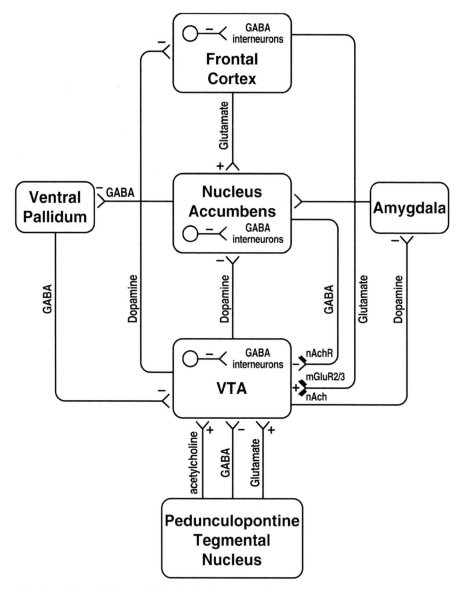

FIG. 1.   Schematic diagram depicting brain circuits and neurotransmitter interactions hypothesized to be involved in mediating nicotine reinforcement, and nicotine dependence and withdrawal. The diagram is limited to the projections and brain sites discussed here.

Accordingly, blockade of postsynaptic metabotropic glutamate 5 receptors (mGluR$_5$) with MPEP [2-methyl-6-(phenylethynyl)-pyridine] decreased intravenous nicotine self-administration in rats and mice (Paterson et al 2003; Fig. 2) and the motivation to self-administer nicotine (Paterson & Markou 2005), possibly by decreasing nicotine-stimulated dopamine release in the mesolimbic system. Similar decreases in nicotine self-administration are also seen after administration of dopaminergic and nAchR antagonists (Watkins et al 1999, Picciotto & Corrigall 2002). It is important to emphasize that MPEP, at doses that blocked nicotine self-administration, had no effect on responding for food (Paterson et al 2003), while in the progressive ratio schedule the effects on breaking points for nicotine were larger than those for food (Paterson & Markou 2005). The selectivity of the effects of MPEP for nicotine versus food reinforcement suggests that MPEP selectively blocks the reinforcing effects of nicotine without affecting motor performance or food reinforcement.

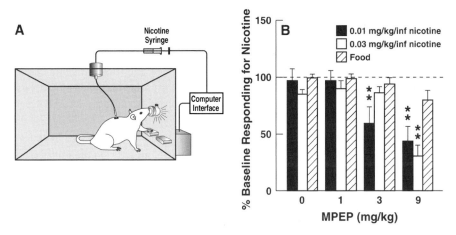

FIG. 2.   (A) The intravenous nicotine self-administration procedure is a method for evaluating the positive euphoric effects of nicotine and the effects of pharmacological treatments on nicotine intake. Rats or mice are prepared with catheters into the jugular vein. Usually two levers are present in the testing chamber. Responses on one lever result in an intravenous nicotine infusion, and responses on the other lever have no consequences. A light above the active lever is illuminated during the nicotine infusion and remains on for a few seconds afterward to signal the nicotine delivery. (Reproduced from Cryan et al 2003b, with permission from Elsevier) (B) Administration of the mGlu$_5$ receptor antagonist MPEP decreased self-administration of either of two nicotine doses available to the animals, while not affecting responding for food. These results suggest that the mGlu$_5$ receptor antagonist selectively blocked the reinforcing effects of nicotine without affecting the reinforcing effects of food or the subjects' ability to perform the task. (Reproduced with permission from Paterson et al 2003, copyright 2003 Springer-Verlag.)

The role of nAchRs on VTA dopaminergic neurons in nicotine reinforcement is supported by findings indicating that injections of the competitive nAchR antagonist dihydro-β-erythroidine (DHβE) into the VTA, but not into the nucleus accumbens, or lesions of the mesolimbic dopaminergic projections, or cholinergic lesions of the pedunculopontine nucleus or systemic administration of dopamine receptor antagonists decreased nicotine self-administration in rats (Picciotto & Corrigall 2002). In terms of nAchRs subtypes, studies suggest an involvement of the $\alpha4\beta2$ and $\alpha7$ nAchR subtypes in both nicotine-induced dopamine release and nicotine reinforcement (Schilstrom et al 1998, Watkins et al 1999, Markou & Paterson 2001, Picciotto & Corrigall 2002). Further, mutant mice with hypersensitive $\alpha4$-containing nAchRs show a 50-fold increased sensitivity to the reinforcing effects of nicotine, as measured by a place preference procedure (Tapper et al 2004), further indicating a critical role of $\alpha4$-containing nAchRs in nicotine reinforcement.

In addition to dopamine and glutamate, another neurotransmitter system critically involved in the reinforcing effects of acute nicotine is γ-aminobutyric acid (GABA). The dopaminergic neurons projecting from the VTA to the nucleus accumbens receive descending GABAergic input from the ventral pallidum and the nucleus accumbens, and ascending GABAergic input from the tegmental pedunculopontine nucleus. These GABAergic neurons, and intra-VTA GABA interneurons, have an inhibitory effect on dopaminergic tone at both the VTA and the nucleus accumbens. There are GABA inhibitory afferents to dopaminergic VTA neurons, inhibitory GABA interneurons within the VTA, and medium spiny GABA neurons in the nucleus accumbens that also inhibit mesolimbic dopamine release (for review, Mansvelder & McGehee 2000). Accordingly, increased GABAergic transmission abolished both dopamine increases in the nucleus accumbens and the reinforcing effects of nicotine (Brebner et al 2002). Specifically, systemic injections of γ-vinyl GABA (GVG, also referred to as vigabatrin, an irreversible inhibitor of GABA transaminase, the primary enzyme involved in GABA metabolism) that leads to increased GABA levels decreased nicotine self-administration in rats (Paterson & Markou 2002), and abolished the expression and acquisition of nicotine-induced conditioned place preference (Brebner et al 2002). Further, GVG administration dose- and time-dependently lowered nicotine-induced increases in nucleus accumbens dopamine in both naïve and chronically nicotine-treated rats measured by *in vivo* microdialysis, and abolished nicotine-induced increases in dopamine in the striatum of primates measured by positron emission tomography (Brebner et al 2002).

The use of receptor-selective agonists suggested the involvement of GABA$_B$ receptors in these effects. Systemic or microinjections of baclofen or CGP44532 [(3-amino-2[S]-hydroxypropyl)-methylphosphinic acid], two GABA$_B$ receptor agonists, into the nucleus accumbens shell, the VTA or the tegmental pedunculopontine nucleus that sends cholinergic, GABAergic and glutamatergic projections to the

VTA, but not injections into the caudate-putamen, decreased the reinforcing effects of nicotine (Paterson et al 2004, Picciotto & Corrigall 2002). These decreases in nicotine self-administration persisted even after chronic administration of CGP44532 for 14 days, indicating little tolerance to this effect of the $GABA_B$ receptor agonist with this length of treatment (Paterson et al 2005b). The issue of tolerance is important because drug therapies have to be administered chronically to humans for smoking cessation. However, GVG and $GABA_B$ receptor agonists also decreased responding for food, although at higher doses than the threshold doses for inducing decreases in nicotine self-administration (Paterson & Markou 2002, Paterson et al 2004, 2005b). These effects on responding for food may reflect non-specific performance effects of the GABAergic compounds or specific effects on food intake. The latter possibility is intriguing as abstinence-associated weight gain is often a concern for smokers, especially women, who wish to quit smoking.

Thus, increased GABA transmission through activation of $GABA_B$ receptors blocks the reinforcing effects of nicotine. Interestingly, however, a human clinical study showed that a single acute dose of baclofen had no effect on either the number of cigarettes smoked or craving for nicotine (Cousins et al 2001). Nevertheless, other clinical studies showed that chronic baclofen reduced cocaine and alcohol abuse, and cue-induced brain activation (e.g. Addolorato et al 2002). Therefore, chronic treatment with these GABAergic drugs may be required before tobacco smoking is decreased in humans.

Neurosubstrates of nicotine dependence and withdrawal

Smoking cessation leads to an aversive withdrawal syndrome in humans, components of which are exhibited for 1–10 weeks post-smoking. This withdrawal syndrome is comprised of affective, somatic and cognitive components. Affective symptoms are primarily depressed mood and anhedonia, dysphoria, craving, anxiety and irritability. The most common somatic symptoms include bradycardia and gastrointestinal discomfort. A cognitive symptom of withdrawal is difficulty concentrating (American Psychiatric Association 1994). This nicotine withdrawal syndrome is hypothesized to be an important motivational factor that contributes to the perpetuation of nicotine dependence and the tobacco smoking habit (Markou et al 1998). It is our working hypothesis that the withdrawal signs are mediated by the neuroadaptations that occur as a result of chronic nicotine exposure, and which are left unopposed when nicotine administration is stopped. Accordingly, withdrawal signs are often opposite in direction to the acute drug effects.

Several rodent models were developed to investigate the neurobiology of the nicotine withdrawal syndrome and dependence. One of the first and most widely used measures is the frequency of somatic signs that are reliably seen in rats, but are less reliably observed in mice (Hildebrand et al 1999, Epping-Jordan et al 1998,

Isola et al 1999, Carboni et al 2000, Semenova et al 2003, Salas et al 2004, Malin 2001). The most prominent somatic signs in the rat are abdominal constrictions (writhes), gasps, ptosis, facial fasciculation and eyeblinks. These somatic signs are both centrally and peripherally mediated (Malin 2001, Hildebrand et al 1999, Watkins et al 2000, Carboni et al 2000, Cryan et al 2003a).

Although the somatic components of nicotine withdrawal are certainly unpleasant, avoidance of the negative affective depression-like components of withdrawal is hypothesized to play a more important role in the maintenance of nicotine dependence than the somatic aspects of withdrawal (Markou et al 1998). A valid and reliable measure of the affective and motivational aspects of drug withdrawal is elevation of brain reward thresholds observed after cessation of chronic nicotine administration (Epping-Jordan et al 1998, Harrison et al 2001, Semenova & Markou 2003, Cryan et al 2003a, Fig. 3). Elevations of reward thresholds are an operational measure of 'diminished interest or pleasure' in rewarding stimuli (i.e. anhedonia) that is a symptom of nicotine withdrawal, and a core symptom of depression (American Psychiatric Association 1994). Similar threshold elevations are seen during withdrawal from all major drugs of abuse (Markou et al 1998). Interestingly, several dissociations have been identified between the threshold elevations and the somatic signs associated with nicotine withdrawal, suggesting that the various aspects of withdrawal are mediated by different substrates (Epping-Jordan et al 1998, Watkins et al 2000, Harrison et al 2001, Semenova & Markou 2003).

There are two experimental approaches used to investigate the neuronal substrates of nicotine dependence and withdrawal. In one of these approaches, nicotine-dependent and control rats are injected with drugs that probe various neurotransmitter systems and receptors. Precipitation of nicotine withdrawal signs in nicotine-treated, but not control saline-treated, rats suggests that chronic nicotine exposure induces adaptations in the specific system/receptor. Using this approach, not surprisingly, it was found that administration of a variety of nAchR antagonists precipitated nicotine withdrawal signs in nicotine-treated rats. Specifically, systemic or intra-VTA administration of mecamylamine, or systemic or intraventricular administration of chlorisondamine induced somatic signs and/or reward threshold elevations in nicotine-dependent rats only (Hildebrand et al 1999, Watkins et al 2000). Administration of the nAchR antagonist DHβE, that is relatively selective for the α4-containing high-affinity nAChRs, induced threshold elevations but no increases in somatic signs in dependent rats, demonstrating that the threshold elevations are not due to non-specific performance effects of the antagonists (Epping-Jordan et al 1998). Further, intra-VTA administration of the nAchR antagonists mecamylamine (Hildebrand et al 1999) or DHβE (Bruijnzeel & Markou 2004; Fig. 4) was sufficient to induce the somatic signs or threshold elevations, respectively, in nicotine-dependent rats, demonstrating the involvement of nAchRs in the VTA in both the somatic and affective aspects of withdrawal. In addition, work in

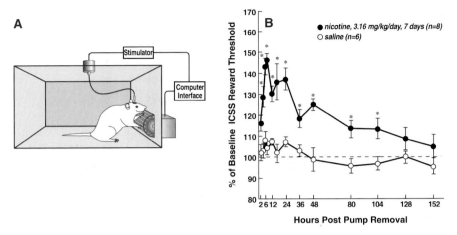

FIG. 3.   (A) The intracranial self-stimulation procedure is a method for assessing the function of the brain's reward pathways, and provides a unique measure of the affective depression-like aspects of nicotine withdrawal. Rats are prepared with electrodes into a specific brain site that is part of the brain's reward circuit. The functioning of the reward circuit is assessed by measuring the minimal electrical current intensity for which the animals will perform an easy response, such as turning a wheel, to receive the stimulation. The minimal current intensity that the subject is willing to self-deliver is the reward threshold. Subjects can detect current intensities significantly lower than the ones for which they are willing to work, indicating that these current-intensity thresholds are indeed reward thresholds. Usually a discrete-trial procedure is used that allows the assessment of reward thresholds that are not affected by non-specific motor effects of the drug treatments. (Reproduced from Cryan et al 2003b, with permission from Elsevier.) (B) Nicotine withdrawal is associated with elevations in brain reward thresholds in rats, reflecting a depression-like anhedonic state. Rats trained on the intracranial self-stimulation procedure were prepared with subcutaneous osmotic minipumps delivering either nicotine (3.16 mg/kg/day, free base) or saline. After seven days, the minipumps were removed and the rats' thresholds were assessed at regular intervals. Rats pre-treated with nicotine exhibited significant elevations in brain reward thresholds during nicotine withdrawal that gradually returned to baseline threshold levels. The thresholds of the rats pretreated with saline remained stable during the assessment period. (Reproduced with permission from Nature, Epping-Jordan et al 1998.)

knockout mice demonstrated a critical role of the β4-containing, but not β2-containing, nAchRs in the somatic signs of withdrawal (Salas et al 2004). It is of interest to mention here that, by contrast, β2-containing nAchRs are critical for the reinforcing effects of nicotine (Picciotto & Corrigall, 2002), while α4-containing receptors appear to be critical in both the reinforcing effects of nicotine (Tapper et al 2004) and nicotine dependence (see above). Finally, administration of the α7-containing nAchR antagonist methyllycaconitine did not precipitate either somatic signs or threshold elevations in nicotine-dependent rats suggesting that these receptors may not be involved in the development of nicotine dependence, despite the

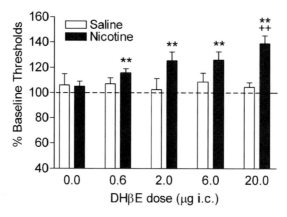

FIG. 4. Injection of the nAchR antagonist DHβE into the VTA of nicotine-dependent rats resulted in reward threshold elevations similar to those seen during spontaneous nicotine withdrawal. Rats were treated chronically with either nicotine or saline administered by subcutaneous osmotic minipumps. Nicotine-dependent rats exhibited elevations in brain reward thresholds when the nAchR antagonist DHβE was injected into the VTA, but not dorsal to the VTA. There were no effects of DHβE injections in rats chronically treated with saline. This pattern of results indicates that blockade of nAchRs in the VTA is sufficient to precipitate the depression-like aspects of nicotine withdrawal. (Reprinted from Bruijnzeel & Markou 2004, with permission from Elsevier.)

fact that α7-containing receptors undergo rapid desensitization in the presence of concentrations of nicotine achieved in the brains of smokers and appear to be involved in the reinforcing effects of nicotine (Markou & Paterson 2001). Overall, the observation that nAchR antagonists precipitate symptoms of withdrawal in nicotine-dependent but not control rats suggests that chronic nicotine exposure induces compensatory decreases in the overall activity of the cholinergic system that contributes to the nicotine withdrawal syndrome.

During nicotine withdrawal precipitated by systemic or intra-VTA administration of the nAchR antagonist mecamylamine in nicotine-treated rats, or after cessation of nicotine self-administration dopamine dialysate levels decreased in the nucleus accumbens and the central nucleus of the amygdale (e.g. Hildebrand et al 1999, Rahman et al 2004). Similar dopamine decreases in the nucleus accumbens are also associated with withdrawal from other drugs of abuse. It is noteworthy that the smoking cessation aid bupropion (an atypical antidepressant; trade name Zyban or Wellbutrin) acts partly by inhibiting neuronal uptake of dopamine and thereby increasing dopamine transmission. Consistent with the above, bupropion reversed both the threshold elevations and the somatic signs of nicotine withdrawal in rats (Cryan et al 2003a). Interestingly, the effects of bupropion on nicotine self-administration are inconsistent (for review, Bruijnzeel & Markou 2003). Taken together, the above data suggest that decreased mesolimbic dopamine transmission mediates aspects of nicotine withdrawal.

In terms of the glutamate system, based on the stimulatory actions of glutamate on dopamine release (Mansvelder & McGehee 2000, Schilstrom et al 1998), it is hypothesized that decreased glutamate transmission mediates nicotine withdrawal. Indeed, systemic or intra-VTA administration of the metabotropic glutamate 2/3 ($mGlu_{2/3}$) receptor agonist LY314582 precipitated withdrawal-like threshold elevations in nicotine-dependent but not control rats (Kenny et al 2003; Fig. 5). These $mGlu_{2/3}$ receptors are found primarily presynaptically where they negatively regu-

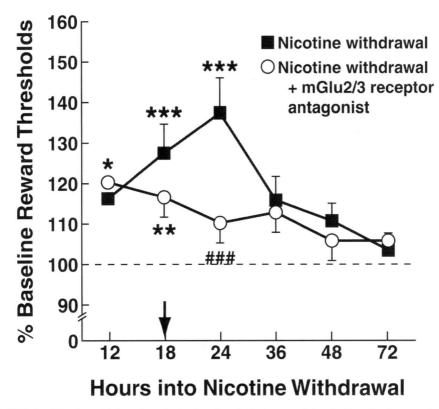

FIG. 5.   Nicotine withdrawal results in elevations in brain reward thresholds reflecting an anhedonic state. Administration of the $mGlu_{2/3}$ receptor antagonist LY341495 reversed this depression-like state seen during nicotine withdrawal. The top line shows the elevated thresholds of nicotine withdrawing rats, similar to what is seen in Fig. 3B. The bottom line shows that after administration of the $mGlu_{2/3}$ receptor antagonist, reward thresholds were restored to baseline (100% of pre-nicotine values). The arrow shows the time-point at which the $mGlu_{2/3}$ receptor antagonist was administered. (Reproduced with permission from Kenny et al 2003.)

late glutamate transmission (Kenny & Markou 2004). Thus, it appears that with the development of nicotine dependence there is increased negative regulation of glutamate transmission through $mGluR_{2/3}$ receptors that results in decreases in glutamate release when nicotine is no longer present. Consistent with this hypothesis, the $mGlu_{2/3}$ receptor antagonist LY341495 reversed the threshold elevations observed in rats undergoing spontaneous nicotine withdrawal (Kenny et al 2003). Similarly, it was found that there was decreased activity of postsynaptic AMPA/kainate receptors, while there did not appear to be adaptations in $mGlu_5$ receptors in nicotine-dependent rats (Kenny et al 2003; Fig. 5), despite the important role that this receptor has in the reinforcing effects of nicotine (Paterson et al 2003, Paterson & Markou 2005). In conclusion, decreased glutamate transmission, resulting from adaptations in both pre- and post-synaptic receptors, may contribute to the affective aspects of nicotine withdrawal.

The above data about the lack of adaptations in $mGlu_5$ receptor activity highlight the fact that not all systems involved in the reinforcing effects of nicotine will necessarily develop changes when chronically exposed to nicotine. This notion is also supported by data demonstrating that there are no changes in GABA transmission, $GABA_B$ receptor activity or $\alpha 7$ nAchR receptor activity in nicotine-dependent rats, despite the important role of these receptors in the reinforcing effects of nicotine (Markou & Paterson 2001, Paterson & Markou 2002, Paterson et al 2004, 2005a, 2005b). Finally, despite the demonstrated roles of the $\beta 2$-containing and $\alpha 7$ nAchR in the reinforcing effects of nicotine, this receptor does not appear involved in withdrawal (Markou & Paterson 2001, Picciotto & Corrigall 2002, Salas et al 2004).

Commonalities in neurosubstrates mediating depression and the depression-like aspects of nicotine withdrawal

The second experimental approach used to identify the systems mediating nicotine withdrawal and dependence is the study of the pharmacological manipulations that reverse spontaneous nicotine withdrawal, and thus infer the underlying abnormality from the treatment. Based on the phenomenological similarities between depression, the depression-like aspects of nicotine withdrawal and the negative symptoms of schizophrenia, it was hypothesized that overlapping neurobiological substrates may mediate these depressive symptoms. Accordingly, we predicted that clinically used antidepressant treatments would alleviate the depression-like aspects of nicotine withdrawal. Consistent with this hypothesis, the co-administration of the selective serotonin reuptake inhibitor fluoxetine and the serotonin 1A ($5-HT_{1A}$) receptor antagonist p-MPPI reversed the threshold elevations seen in nicotine withdrawing rats, while having no effect on the somatic signs of withdrawal (Harrison et al 2001). Thus, similarly to depression, reversal of decreased serotonergic transmission ameliorates the depression-like aspects of nicotine withdrawal. Further, the antidepressant bupropion that acts primarily by inhibiting the dopamine transporter reversed both the affective and somatic signs of nicotine withdrawal in rats (Cryan et al 2003a), suggesting that decreased dopamine transmission also characterizes nicotine withdrawal. Finally, chronic pretreatment with the atypical antipsychotic clozapine, that is the most effective antipsychotic against the negative depression-like aspects of schizophrenia, attenuated the severity of the nicotine withdrawal syndrome in rats (Semenova & Markou 2003). Taken together, these data support the hypothesis of commonalities in the substrates mediating depressive symptoms of nicotine withdrawal and those seen in psychiatric populations. Such common substrates may contribute to the high rates of tobacco smoking among psychiatric populations.

Acknowledgements

This work was supported by National Institutes of Health (NIH) of the USA grants R01 DA11946, U01 MH69062 and Tobacco Related Disease Research Program from the State of California grant 12RT-0231. The author would like to thank Mr Mike Arends for outstanding editorial assistance, and Drs Neil Paterson, Paul Kenny, Svetlana Semenova, Adrie Bruijnzeel, Mark Epping-Jordan, Shelly Watkins, John Cryan, Amanda Harrison and Karin Sandoval for their contributions to the experimental and conceptual work from my laboratory discussed in this document. This is publication 17392-NP of The Scripps Research Institute.

References

Addolorato G, Caputo F, Capristo E et al 2002 Baclofen efficacy in reducing alcohol craving and intake: a preliminary double-blind randomized controlled study. Alcohol 37:504–508

American Psychiatric Association 1994 Diagnostic and statistical manual of mental disorders. 4th edn, American Psychiatric Press, Washington, DC

Balfour DJK 2004 The neurobiology of tobacco dependence: a preclinical perspective on the role of the dopamine projections to the nucleus. Nicotine Tob Res 6:899–912

Brebner K, Childress AR, Roberts DCS 2002 A potential role for GABA$_B$ agonists in the treatment of psychostimulant addiction. Alcohol Alcohol 5:478–484

Bruijnzeel AW, Markou A 2003 Characterization of the effects of bupropion on the reinforcing properties of nicotine and food in rats. Synapse 50:20–28

Bruijnzeel AW, Markou A 2004 Adaptations in cholinergic transmission in the ventral tegmental area associated with the affective signs of nicotine withdrawal in rats. Neuropharmacology 47:572–579

Carboni E, Bortone L, Giua C, Di Chiara G 2000 Dissociation of physical abstinence signs from changes in extracellular dopamine in the nucleus accumbens and in the prefrontal cortex of nicotine dependent rats. Drug Alcohol Depend 58:93–102

Cousins MS, Stamat HM, de Wit H 2001 Effects of a single dose of baclofen on self-reported subjective effects and tobacco smoking. Nicotine Tob Res 3:123–129

Cryan JF, Bruijnzeel AW, Skjei KL, Markou A 2003a Bupropion enhances brain reward function and reverses the affective and somatic aspects of nicotine withdrawal in the rat. Psychopharmacology 168:347–358

Cryan JF, Gasparini F, van Heeke G, Markou A 2003b Non-nicotinic neuropharmacological strategies for nicotine dependence: beyond bupropion. Drug Discov Today 22:1025–1034

Epping-Jordan MP, Watkins SS, Koob GF, Markou A 1998 Dramatic decreases in brain reward function during nicotine withdrawal. Nature 393:76–79

Harrison AA, Liem YT, Markou A 2001 Fluoxetine combined with a serotonin-1A receptor antagonist reversed reward deficits observed during nicotine and amphetamine withdrawal in rats. Neuropsychopharmacology 25:55–71

Hildebrand BE, Panagis G, Svensson TH, Nomikos GG 1999 Behavioral and biochemical manifestations of mecamylamine-precipitated nicotine withdrawal in the rat: role of nicotinic receptors in the ventral tegmental area. Neurosychopharmacology 21:560–574

Isola R, Vogelsberg V, Wemlinger TA, Neff NH, Hadjiconstantinou M 1999 Nicotine abstinence in the mouse. Brain Res 850:189–196

Kenny PJ, Markou A 2004 The ups and downs of addiction: Role of metabotropic glutamate receptors. Trends Pharmacol Sci 25:265–272

Kenny PJ, Gasparini F, Markou A 2003 Group II metabotropic and α-amino-3-hydroxy-5-methyl-4-isoxazole propionate (AMPA)/kainate glutamate receptors regulate the deficit in brain reward function associated with nicotine withdrawal in rats. J Pharmacol Exp Ther 306:1068–1076

Malin DH 2001 Nicotine dependence: studies with a laboratory model. Pharmacol Biochem Behav 70:551–559

Mansvelder HD, McGehee DS 2000 Long-term potentiation of excitatory inputs to brain reward areas by nicotine. Neuron 27:349–357

Markou A, Paterson NE 2001 The nicotinic antagonist methyllycaconitine has differential effects on nicotine self-administration and nicotine withdrawal in the rat. Nicotine Tob Res 3:361–373

Markou A, Kosten TR, Koob GF 1998 Neurobiological similarities in depression and drug dependence: A self-medication hypothesis. Neuropsychopharmacology 18: 135–174

Nisell M, Marcus M, Nomikos GG, Svensson TH 1997 Differential effects of acute and chronic nicotine on dopamine output in the core and shell of the rat nucleus accumbens. J Neural Transm 104:1–10

Paterson NE, Markou A 2002 Increased GABA neurotransmission via administration of γ-vinyl GABA decreased nicotine self-administration in the rat. Synapse 44:252–253

Paterson NE, Markou A 2005 The mGluR5 antagonist MPEP selectively decreased break points for nicotine and cocaine but not food. Psychopharmacology 1:255–261

Paterson NE, Semenova S, Gasparini F, Markou A 2003 The mGluR5 antagonist MPEP decreased nicotine self-administration in rats and mice. Psychopharmacology 167:257–264

Paterson NE, Froestl W, Markou A 2004 The GABA$_B$ receptor agonists baclofen and CGP44532 decreased nicotine self-administration in the rat. Psychopharmacology 172:179–186

Paterson NE, Bruijnzeel AW, Kenny PJ, Wright CD, Froestl W, Markou A 2005a Prolonged nicotine exposure does not alter GABA$_B$ receptor-mediated regulation of brain reward function. Neuropharmacology 49:953–962

Paterson NE, Froestl W, Markou A 2005b Repeated administration of the GABA$_B$ receptor agonist CGP44532 decreased nicotine self-administration, and acute administration decreased cue-reinstatement of nicotine- seeking in rats. Neuropsychopharmacology 30:119–128

Picciotto MR, Corrigall WA 2002 Neuronal systems underlying behaviors related to nicotine addiction: Neural circuits and molecular genetics. J Neurosci 22:3338–3341

Rahman S, Zhang J, Engleman EA, Corrigall WA 2004 Neuroadaptive changes in the mesoaccumbens dopamine system after chronic nicotine self-administration: A microdialysis study. Neuroscience 129:415–424

Salas R, Pieri F, De Biasi M 2004 Decreased signs of nicotine withdrawal in mice null for the b4 nicotinic acetylcholine receptor subunit. J Neurosci 24:10035–10039

Schilstrom B, Svensson HM, Svensson TH, Nomikos GG 1998 Nicotine and food induced dopamine release in the nucleus accumbens of the rat: Putative role of alpha7 nicotinic receptors in the ventral tegmental area. Neuroscience 85:1005–1009

Semenova S, Bespalov A, Markou A 2003 Decreased prepulse inhibition during nicotine withdrawal in DBA/2J mice is reversed by nicotine self-administration. Eur J Pharmacol 472:99–110

Semenova S, Markou A 2003 Clozapine treatment attenuated somatic and affective signs of nicotine and amphetamine withdrawal in subsets of rats that exhibited hyposensitivity to the initial effects of clozapine. Biol Psychiatry 54:1249–1264

Tapper AR, McKinney SL, Nashmi R et al 2004 Nicotine activation of alpha4 receptors: sufficient for reward, tolerance, and sensitization. Science 3061029–1032

Watkins SS, Epping-Jordan MP, Koob GF, Markou A 1999 Blockade of nicotine self-administration with nicotinic antagonists in rats. Pharmacol Biochem Behav 62: 743–751

Watkins SS, Stinus L, Koob GF, Markou A 2000 Reward and somatic changes during precipitated nicotine withdrawal in rats: Centrally and peripherally mediated effects. J Pharmacol Exp Ther 292:1053–1064

DISCUSSION

Changeux: You said that there is no adaptation in the GABAergic system. Do you mean the metabotropic glutamate receptor, or in the GABA receptor system in general, including the ligand-gated ion channel?

Markou: As you may know, vigabatrin inhibits the enzyme that breaks down GABA. When this compound is administered, levels of GABA in the synapse are increased. When we injected this compound to nicotine-dependent rats, we did see GABAergic modulation of reward at the higher doses used, but no differential effects between control animals and nicotine-dependent animals. This result indicates that globally there doesn't seem to be a change in the way that the GABA system is functioning in nicotine dependence. Nevertheless, we thought that some adaptations that may occur in the GABA system function might be masked by opposing changes in different brain sites or receptors, so we administered an agonist for the metabotropic glutamate receptor $GABA_B$ receptor systemically or directly into the VTA. We thought that the different sites might counteract each other, but again there were no differential effects between control and nicotine-dependent rats on reward when the $GABA_B$ receptor agonist was administered. On the basis of these data, taking everything together, I would say that there are no changes in the way in which the GABA system functions globally with the development of nicotine dependence.

Changeux: With all the drugs you used, you didn't mention the benzodiazepines. Why not? Are they effective in tobacco smoking?

Markou: I haven't looked at these. Perhaps benzodiazepines would be effective considering that nicotine withdrawal is characterized by anxiety and irritability, and benzodiazepines are anxiolytics.

Shiffman: That has been well studied and they are not.

Changeux: Benzodiazepines are highly addictive drugs.

Shiffman: No, they are only mildly addictive.

West: A problem is that most of the people for whom it is stated that there is strong dependence on benzodiazepines were prescribed these drugs as an anxiolytic. When anxiety occurs when people stop taking an anxiolytic, this is a functional dependence but not dependence in the sense we are discussing at this meeting.

Stolerman: There is clear tolerance to main effects of benzodiazepines, clearly demonstrated withdrawal syndromes in animals and humans, and animal self-administration behaviour. And there is a tremendous amount of illicit benzodiazepine use. To my eyes, this all adds up to a serious degree of dependence.

West: There is. It is complex: it often accompanies other forms of dependence, and is frequently part of polydrug use syndrome.

Changeux: There is pressure here from companies who want to sell benzodiazepines to talk down the addictive properties of these drugs, but as scientists we may be concerned by this. An important issue is whether the inhibitory networks adapt through the mechanism of addiction or not. Since there is an indication that benzodiazepines create dependence, they may have an effect on synaptic plasticity.

Stolerman: I think it would be useful to dissect a bit further the dissociation that Markou described between the effects of a particular compound on the withdrawal measure and on self-administration. I think you said that you hadn't found any effect on self-administration and there was an effect on withdrawal. But this is a measure of withdrawal that you argue is motivationally relevant. The implication is that the self-administration procedure is not tapping into the withdrawal relief as a sort of reward/reinforcement mechanism. Do we not need a model of nicotine self-administration where withdrawal is an important motivating factor? Is there any reason why we don't have this? Given that the animals are intravenously cannulated, they could be dosed 24 h round the clock for a period, and then you could look at the effect of terminating that on self-administration? Is this too complicated?

Markou: Yes, it is very complicated. We tried this with 6 h daily, 12 h daily and 23 h daily nicotine self-administration in rats. Animals do develop dependence as defined by somatic signs of withdrawal, but we have not got the animals to self-administer enough nicotine that upon cessation they would show elevations in brain reward thresholds. We have some intriguing recent findings suggesting that if anything, after prolonged periods of nicotine self-administration, rats exhibit lower reward thresholds than baseline, as thought these subjects have a permanent resetting of their reward system (Kenny & Markou 2005). This finding is consistent with what David Balfour argues, that nicotine may reset the system where other stimuli in the environment are perceived as very rewarding. It is puzzling and different to what is seen with cocaine self-administration.

Balfour: In our hands it takes 24–48 h to resensitize all receptors once the dopamine system has been desensitized. If the drug is withdrawn and you look for self-administration, it is possible that if you do it too quickly the critical receptors are still desensitized.

Stolerman: In time-consuming experiments like this it is difficult to hit the right time. Did you say that this is different for cocaine?

Markou: If we let animals self-administer a lot of cocaine, then during the self-administration process if we assess the threshold just before they have access to cocaine or after they stop the cocaine self-administration, they show elevations in reward threshold. This is exactly what I was alluding to: we can do this with cocaine with passive or active administration, but with nicotine we don't know how to get the animals to the same conditions of dependence. It is possible that it might take a much longer exposure to nicotine for the subjects to reach that stage of dependence.

Shiffman: Forgetting the drug probes, the data you show on intercranial self stimulation suggest that the thresholds return to baseline in about 5 or 6 days. Can you interpret time the same way for this species as one would for humans? What do you think this says about the time course of at least this aspect of nicotine withdrawal?

Markou: Typically in our experiments, we expose rats to nicotine for just one week, while in humans tobacco smoking goes on for years or even decades before the person attempts abstinence. I think the duration of the withdrawal is a function of how long the experimental animal or the human has been exposed to nicotine. We have actually showed experimentally that the longer the exposure to nicotine and the higher the nicotine dose, the longer the reward threshold elevation. In these experiments, we exposed animals for three or four weeks to nicotine. In these animals, after the cessation of nicotine administration, the elevation in reward thresholds was only 10–15%, but it was there for the entire duration of testing which was more than one month (Skjei & Markou 2003). Although 10–15% does not sound much, 10–15% depression in mood over a period of month could be clinically significant in humans.

Shiffman: Would you speculate that under conditions of prolonged self-administration that it might never return to baseline?

Markou: Yes.

Shiffman: Part of my interest is that there clearly is an acute phase of withdrawal, but this resolves more rapidly than we have thought in humans. On the over hand, we certainly see relapse and reinstatement still being very likely long after that. We may need a two-factor model to explain this.

Markou: With our most recent data that I described above, I started to think also that there are two withdrawal phases. One acute phase that resolves within a few days and possibly weeks in humans, and a more protracted withdrawal phase that can last for months and even years. The majority of the data that I presented are mostly relevant to this acute early phase. However, the few data that we have with prolonged exposure to nicotine may be relevant to the protracted withdrawal phase.

Shiffman: In some human data, we see return to baseline within 5–6 days. I have another question. For some drugs you showed a clear interaction where the probe drug only eliminated the change in threshold in the nicotine-pretreated animals. For buproprion it seems more ambiguous. On this model, should we care whether a drug is specific? Isn't the implication that any drug that lowers the threshold, even if it is not specific to nicotine pre-treated organisms, would be a treatment for this aspect of withdrawal?

Markou: That is a good point. We did a dose–response study examining the effects of various doses of bupropion on nicotine withdrawal and found exactly what you describe: even without nicotine withdrawal, bupropion lowers thresholds indicating an intrinsic reward enhancing effect of bupropion. If we were to use a subthreshold dose of bupropion that would have no effect in control rats, we still would not know whether we have an additive effect. In the case of buproprion it is clear that we might be substituting one mild psychostimulant drug, nicotine, with another mild psychostimulant drug, bupropion.

Shiffman: In humans the clinical trials suggest that subthreshold doses of buproprion actually *increase* the severity of withdrawal. Let me ask my question another way: are there drugs that are known to decrease the threshold, which should be tested as treatments for that phase of withdrawal? They needn't be nicotine specific. You have set this up as a final common pathway for hedonia.

Markou: It is possible that every drug that lowers reward thresholds may alleviate nicotine withdrawal in terms of the anhedonic depression-like aspects of nicotine withdrawal. I am confident, for example, that amphetamine would alleviate nicotine withdrawal. I should clarify though that elevations in brain reward thresholds reflect the anhedonic depression-like aspects of nicotine withdrawal, and these are the aspects of nicotine withdrawal that one would predict would get alleviated by treatments that lower reward thresholds under baseline conditions.

Picciotto: There is a confound here. Of the antidepressants that have been tested, buproprion works pretty well for smoking cessation, but most of the other antidepressants have been modest at best. There are some effects that come out in the literature but overall there is a huge gap between the ability of general antidepressants to get people through acute withdrawal and the ability of buproprion to do the same. If it is the common ability to decrease brain reward thresholds, wouldn't you expect that they would all be equally affected?

West: That's not quite true. Monoamine oxidase A (MAOA) inhibitors do the same. Your point is right, though: why doesn't fluoxetine work? It is a big contradiction in the literature.

Shiffman: When Niaura analysed for blood levels (Hitsman et al 2001), there was an effect in people with high blood levels. It may be the heterogeneity of pharmacokinetics that is responsible for this uncertainty.

Walton: You said that you could ameliorate withdrawal with a specific serotonin reuptake inhibitor (SSRI), but you had also manipulated the serotonin 1A (5-HT$_{1A}$) receptor at the same time. Is this a useful therapeutic strategy?

Markou: The reason I used the 5-HT$_{1A}$ receptor antagonist in combination with the SRRI was because the acute withdrawal phase, as we discussed previously, is not long enough to allow us to administer the SSRI chronically to see the therapeutic effect. The 5-HT$_{1A}$ receptor antagonist combined with SSRI strategy is used in the clinic to elevate rapidly the serotonin level. It has been suggested that this rapid increase in serotonin levels also accelerates the action of the therapeutic effect. I had to combine fluoxetine with the 5-HT$_{1A}$ receptor antagonist so I could get a rapid elevation in serotonin levels which would hopefully would also lead to a rapid therapeutic effect that I could detect during the early acute withdrawal phase. And indeed it worked. We also examined the effects of the exact same therapeutic drug combination, SSRI combined with a 5-HT$_{1A}$ receptor antagonist, on amphetamine withdrawal, and again we saw reversal of amphetamine withdrawal with this drug combination (Harrison et al 2001, Markou et al 2005). Taken together, these data suggest that increases in serotonin transmission reverse the depression-like aspects of nicotine or amphetamine withdrawal. Further, these data indicate that elevations in brain reward thresholds reflect an anhedonic depression-like state that is reversible by clinical antidepressant medications.

Walton: In human treatment for depression, augmentation with 5-HT$_{1A}$ antagonists works quite well.

Markou: It is my understanding of the clinical literature that antidepressants worked for smoking cessation if one pre-selected the patients who exhibited depressive symptamatology. Not every person who stops smoking necessarily exhibits depressive symptoms. But if one were to pre-select the people that do show depression, then I think the success rates of antidepressant treatments for smoking cessation would increase.

Shiffman: The literature is very mixed. At that point you have a mechanistic question about whether you are treating depression and having a knock-on effect on smoking, or whether you are really treating smoking addiction. Conversely, buproprion has been specifically shown to work if you exclude anyone with depression.

Stolerman: On the question of bupropion compared with the other antidepressants, I'd like to mention the hypothesis that it acts as a nicotine antagonist. While I am not convinced that the antagonist action is the main mode of action, it might be a property that bupropion has and other antidepressants lack?

Balfour: Many of the ones that have been tested also have some nicotinic receptor antagonist properties.

Picciotto: There is a broad ability of different antidepressant classes to block nicotinic receptors non-competitively. The affinity changes across classes and it is not clear that buproprion has the highest affinity, but potentially this is a common aspect of antidepressants.

Stolerman: So it doesn't correlate with their efficacy in smoking cessation.

Picciotto: That hasn't been done. If buproprion is a really good nicotinic antagonist, in brain stimulation reward threshold experiments you would expect it to have some effect in the opposite direction.

Markou: In fact, it appears that at high doses bupropion reverses the acute effects of nicotine in reward threshold, perhaps reflecting the nicotinic antagonist properties of bupropion (Cryan et al 2003). However, this gets complicated with the issue of receptor desensitization and up-regulation that is seen in the *in vitro* work, while our *in vivo* data in behaving rats clearly indicate that overall there is decreased activity of nicotinic acetylcholine receptors in nicotine dependence What would be very important for the field would be to explain how the well established phenomenon of receptor desensitization and up-regulation relates or does not relate to the behavioural data that I presented indicating decreased activity of nicotinic receptors in nicotine dependence.

Clarke: I have a question concerning the validity of animal models. With your ICSS threshold model it seems to me that you have a predictive model. This is sufficient to make it useful. I am a little troubled, though, because I remember the early papers by Malin (2001) showing that the nicotine withdrawal signs had some commonality with opiate withdrawal. There were also some pharmacological similarities.

Markou: Malin finds that opiate receptor antagonists precipitate nicotine withdrawal in nicotine-dependent animals. We could not replicate his findings (Watkins et al 2000). In terms of the somatic signs, those of the nicotine withdrawal syndrome are not as overt as those of the opiate-withdrawal syndrome: it takes more of a trained eye to see them. Further, it is interesting to note that we see many dissociation between the somatic signs of nicotine withdrawal and the elevations in brain reward thresholds. That is, some nicotinic receptor antagonists will induce one or not the other, for example, while some pharmacological treatments would reverse the threshold elevations but not the somatic signs and vice versa. Further, we see elevations in thresholds even when there are no somatic signs, indicating that elevation of thresholds is not because the animal is feeling malaise.

Clarke: To what extent do you think the somatic signs of withdrawal are a reflection of some adaptation in the periphery?

Markou: That is what they are, I think. This is another point where I do not confirm Malin's findings. Malin finds that the somatic signs of nicotine withdrawal are centrally mediated. Using chlorisondamine, the nicotinic receptor antagonist that does not readily cross the blood–brain barrier, we found that the somatic signs are peripherally mediated (Watkins et al 2000).

Clarke: Would it help if we could somehow reverse the somatic signs in smokers?

Markou: They might be clinically relevant, but I hypothesize that the treatment of the affective aspects of withdrawal are most relevant to the prevention of relapse.

Clarke: You talk about this ICSS threshold test as a test of hedonia. We really want to know whether the electrical stimulation is pleasant in humans.

Markou: The only thing I can say is that there is an anthropomorphic indication of pleasure: if you see an animal having its first access to ICSS, it seems clear that this is extremely hedonic.

Clarke: I have seen the same thing and regarded it as a compulsive behaviour. In the human ICSS literature, the stimulation doesn't produce unalloyed pleasure. When R.G. Heath asked his patients why they were self stimulating, it wasn't as if they were having an orgasm.

Markou: Some were. There was a woman who had her first one!

Picciotto: Why do you think it would be a problem with the model if there are some commonalities between nicotine withdrawal and the opiate system?

Clarke: I believe it is possible to give too much nicotine to an animal. You could give a large dose that could induce a kind of withdrawal that may not be relevant to the human condition. I think the ultimate test is predictive validity, and Athina Markou shows evidence that she has that.

Picciotto: I agree that you can give too much nicotine to an animal and then the model wouldn't be relevant to humans. However, if you give naltrexone to a smoker you get signs that resemble strongly the anhedonia related to nicotine withdrawal. There is some human validity to the idea that there is an opiate component to the nicotine experience even in humans.

Clarke: That isn't good news for Athina.

Corrigall: Just as a point for the record about opiate antagonists and smoking, I would like to note that there is a history of human lab studies that show very diverse results, including an absence of effects on tobacco smoking as well as small effects. The opiate system is not a good exemplar for neurochemical manipulations related to tobacco addiction.

Bertrand: Let me add a comment. We have published that dihydro-β-erytroidine (DHβE) is a competitive antagonist of the nicotine receptor. This compound is, however, a very broad antagonist which, depending upon the concentration, inhibits all the known receptors. We have also shown that DHβE causes up-regulation of the $\alpha 4\beta 2$ receptor. I therefore have problems with experiments carried out with DHβE. In your experiments with DHβE, were the doses specific for $\alpha 4\beta 2$ or were they general doses and for how long did you apply the compound?

Markou: The doses of DHβE that we used were up to 6 mg/kg given systemically, and what is relevant here is the comparison between DHβE and mechamelamine. When we injected mechamelamine to nicotine-dependent animals, mechamelamine induced both the somatic signs of nicotine withdrawal and the threshold elevations. Interestingly, DHβE administration induced only the threshold elevations. Thus, I would argue that mechamelamine is a broader nicotine receptor antagonist than DHβE.

Bertrand: I think that we should consider the difference in mechanisms of blockade. Mechamelamine is an open channel blocker that will act only when the agonist is present. Instead, DHβE is a competitive inhibitor which, as I mentioned earlier causes multiple effects. Therefore, you are not starting from equal points and I would predict that in terms of neuronal network the effects will be different.

Markou: I didn't make any arguments about specific nicotinic receptors, in terms of the selectivity of the antagonist for the nicotine receptor subtypes. I am only arguing that the behavioural output after the development of nicotine dependence clearly indicates an overall balance of the nicotinic receptor that reflects decreased activity in general.

Brody: What is the status of giving these drugs to humans? I have been hearing about GABA$_B$ agonism for years, and baclofen is on the market.

Markou: Baclofen has been used in some small clinical trials for alcohol and cocaine, and has shown some efficacy. But as far as I know the effects of baclofen or other GABA$_B$ receptor agonists have not been tested for smoking cessation yet.

References

Cryan JF, Bruijnzeel AW, Skjei KL, Markou A 2003 Bupropion enhances brain reward function and reverses the affective and somatic aspects of nicotine withdrawal in the rat. Psychopharmacology 168:347–358

Harrison AA, Liem YT, Markou A 2001 Fluoxetine combined with a serotonin-1A receptor antagonist reversed reward deficits observed during nicotine and amphetamine withdrawal in rats. Neuropsychopharmacology 25:55–71

Hitsman B, Spring B, Borrelli B, Niaura R, Papandonatos GD 2001 Influence of antidepressant pharmacotherapy on behavioral treatment adherence and smoking cessation outcome in a combined treatment involving fluoxetine. Exp Clin Psychopharmacol 9:355–362

Kenny PJ, Markou A 2005 Nicotine may permanently increase the sensitivity of brain reward systems. Neuropsychopharmacology, in press

Malin DH 2001 Nicotine dependence: studies with a laboratory model. Pharmacol Biochem Behav 70:551–559

Markou A, Harrison AA, Chevrette J, Hoyer D 2005 Paroxetine combined with a 5-HT1A receptor antagonist reversed reward deficits observed during amphetamine withdrawal in rats. Psychopharmacology 178:133–142

Skjei KL, Markou A 2003 Effects of repeated withdrawal episodes, nicotine dose, and duration of nicotine exposure on the severity and duration of nicotine withdrawal in rats. Psychopharmacology 168:280–292

Watkins SS, Stinus L, Koob GF, Markou A 2000 Reward and somatic changes during precipitated nicotine withdrawal in rats: centrally and peripherally mediated effects. J Pharmacol Exp Therap 292:1053–1064

Localizing tobacco dependence pathways with functional brain imaging

Arthur L. Brody

UCLA Department of Psychiatry & Biobehavioral Sciences, 300 UCLA Medical Plaza, Suite 2200, Los Angeles, CA 90095, USA

Abstract. Localizing tobacco dependence pathways with functional brain imaging may (in conjunction with other lines of research) lead to improved treatments for this condition. Mediation of cigarette craving and responses to acute and chronic nicotine administration/smoking have been reported. Cigarette craving is associated with activation of limbic and paralimbic brain structures. Acute administration of nicotine/smoking results in: reduced global brain activity; activation of the prefrontal cortex, thalamus, and visual system; activation of the thalamus and visual cortex during visual cognitive tasks; and increased dopamine (DA) concentration in the ventral striatum. Chronic nicotine/cigarette exposure results in decreased monoamine oxidase (MAO) A and B activity and a reduction in $\alpha_4\beta_2$ nicotinic acetylcholine receptor (nAChR) availability. This group of findings demonstrates a number of ways in which smoking might enhance neurotransmission through cortico-basal ganglia-thalamic circuits originating in the lateral prefrontal and/or paralimbic cortex. This enhancement may result from direct stimulation by nicotine of nAChRs on cortical or paralimbic structures, or perhaps more potently through subcortical stimulation of nAChRs in the thalamus or via DA release and MAO inhibition in the basal ganglia. Brain circuit activation may explain the effects of smoking (such as heightened attention and withdrawal symptom alleviation) in tobacco-dependent subjects.

2005 Understanding nicotine and tobacco addiction. Wiley, Chichester (Novartis Foundation Symposium 275) p 153–170

Functional brain imaging (in conjunction with cellular and molecular research) holds great promise for elucidating both brain circuits and molecular targets that mediate the acute effects of cigarette smoking and chronic effects of tobacco dependence. A greater understanding of brain function associated with smoking may result in improved treatments for tobacco dependence.

In this paper, studies using four primary imaging modalities will be reviewed, namely (1) functional magnetic resonance imaging (fMRI), (2) positron emission tomography (PET), (3) single photon emission computed tomography (SPECT), and (4) autoradiography. These imaging modalities have been used to determine relationships between brain function and effects of acute and chronic cigarette smoking and of smoking-related behaviours. In order to build a cohesive model of brain activity responses to acute and chronic smoking, nicotine and cigarette studies will be reviewed together, while recognizing that cigarette smoke has many constituents other than nicotine (Baker et al 2004). The purpose of this paper is to synthesize findings from functional brain imaging studies of tobacco use and dependence, and present a coherent model of brain function in smokers. Cigarette craving responses will be reviewed first, followed by acute brain responses to nicotine/smoking, followed by chronic responses to nicotine/smoking, and concluding with a discussion of these imaging findings in the context of neuroanatomical work and the effects of smoking in tobacco-dependent subjects.

Functional brain imaging studies of cigarette craving

In tobacco-dependent smokers, craving (urge to smoke) begins within minutes after the last cigarette, and the intensity of craving rises over the next 3–6 h (Schuh & Stitzer 1995). Cigarette-related cues reliably enhance craving during this period, when compared to neutral cues (Carter & Tiffany 1999).

Two recent studies used a cigarette versus neutral cue paradigm paired with functional imaging to evaluate brain mediation of cigarette craving. In one study (Due et al 2002), 6 smokers and 6 non-smokers underwent event-related fMRI when presented with smoking images (colour photographs) compared with neutral images, for 4 s each. For the smoker group, craving increased during the testing session and exposure to smoking images resulted in activation of mesolimbic (right posterior amygdala, posterior hippocampus, ventral tegmental area and medial thalamus) and visuospatial cortical attention (bilateral prefrontal and parietal cortex and right fusiform gyrus) circuitry, while the non-smoker group did not have these changes. In the second study (Brody et al 2002), 20 smokers and 20 non-smokers underwent two [^{18}F]fluorodeoxyglucose-PET (FDG-PET) sessions. For one PET session, subjects held a cigarette and watched a cigarette-related video, while for the other, subjects held a pen and watched a nature video (randomized order) during the 30 min uptake period of FDG. When presented with smoking-related (compared to neutral) cues, smokers had higher regional metabolism in the bilateral anterior cingulate cortex (ACC), left orbitofrontal cortex (OFC), and left anterior temporal lobe. Change in craving scores was also positively correlated with change in metabolism in the OFC, dorsolateral prefrontal cortex and anterior insula bilaterally.

These studies of cigarette craving indicate that immediate responses to visual smoking-related cues (fMRI study) activate the brain reward system, limbic regions, and the visual processing system, while longer exposure to cues (FDG-PET study) leads to activation of the ACC, which mediates anxiety, alertness, and arousal (Kimbrell et al 1999, Naito et al 2000) and the OFC, which functions in part as a secondary processing centre for sensory information (Rolls et al 1998).

In a study examining effects of treatment on brain mediation of craving, 17 smokers underwent the same FDG-PET craving versus neutral cue protocol as in the second study of craving listed above (Brody et al 2002) after a standard course of treatment with bupropion HCl. Bupropion-treated smokers had reduced cigarette cue-induced craving and diminished ACC activation when presented with cigarette-related cues, compared to untreated smokers (Brody et al 2004a). This diminished ACC activation was due to elevated baseline normalized ACC activity in treated smokers, giving an indication that bupropion treatment of smokers increases resting ACC metabolism.

Acute nicotine administration and cigarette smoking

Brain activity responses to nicotine/cigarette administration

The effects of administration of nicotine or cigarette smoking compared with a placebo or control state has been examined many times with functional brain imaging (Table 1). Though a wide range of brain regions have been reported to have altered activity in response to nicotine or cigarette smoking, several global and regional findings have been replicated, leading to general conclusions about the acute effects of nicotine or smoking on brain activity.

One common finding is that administration of nicotine (Stapleton et al 2003, Domino et al 2000b) or cigarette smoking (Yamamoto et al 2003) during scanning results in decreased global brain activity. Similarly, smokers who smoke ad lib prior to SPECT scanning (including the morning of the scan) have decreased global brain activity compared to former smokers and non-smokers (Rourke et al 1997). A large recent study (Fallon et al 2004) further characterized this decreased global activity with nicotine administration. FDG-PET was performed while smokers and ex-smokers performed the Bushman aggression task (designed to elicit an aggressive state). Subjects had nicotine administered via a 0, 3.5 or 21 mg nicotine patch. Smokers who were rated high on the personality trait 'hostility' had widespread cerebral metabolic decreases while wearing the 21 mg patch and performing the aggression task. Low hostility smokers did not have these changes during PET, suggesting that personality profile may determine which smokers have global metabolic decreases in response to nicotine.

In studies examining regional brain responses to nicotine or smoking, the most common findings are relative increases in activity in the prefrontal cortex (including the dorsolateral prefrontal cortex, and inferior frontal, medial frontal, and orbitofrontal gyri) (Stein et al 1998, Domino et al 2000b, Rose et al 2003), thalamus (Domino et al 2000a, Stein et al 1998, Domino et al 2000b, Zubieta et al 2001, London et al 1988), and visual system (Domino et al 2000a, 2000b, London et al 1988, Zubieta et al 2005). Additionally, a ^{133}Xe inhalation study reported increases

TABLE 1 Human brain imaging studies of nicotine or cigarette administration

Authors	Subjects	Method	Intervention	Results
Rourke et al (1997)	8 smokers; 8 former smokers; 17 non-smokers	iodine-123 iodoamphetamine (IMP) SPECT	Smokers smoked the morning of the scan; other groups did not	↓ cortical uptake of IMP (a measure of blood flow) in current smokers compared to other groups
Stein et al (1998)	16 smokers	fMRI	IV nic (0.75–2.25 mg/70 kg wt) vs. placebo	↑ R NAc and bilateral amyg, cingulate, frontal lobes, thal, others
Domino et al (2000a)	18 smokers	^{15}O-PET	Nic nasal spray vs. pepper spray	↑ thal, pons, visual cortex, cereb
Domino et al (2000b)	11 smokers	FDG-PET	Nic nasal spray vs. pepper spray	Small ↓ global; ↑ L IFG, L PC, R thal, visual cortex; ↓ normalized L ins and R inf occ ctx
Zubieta et al (2001)	18 smokers	^{15}O-PET	Nic nasal spray vs. pepper spray	↑ anterior thal; ↓ L ant temp and R amyg
Rose et al (2003)	34 smokers	^{15}O-PET	Cigarette vs. no nic control conditions	↑ L frontal factor (incl prefrontal and ACC), ↓ L amyg rCBF
Yamamoto et al (2003)	10 smokers	^{99m}Tc-ECD SPECT	Cigarette vs. abstinence	↓ global blood flow
Stapleton et al (2003)	4 smokers; 2 non-smokers	2 FDG-PETs (Fully quantified)	IV nic (1.5 mg) vs. placebo	↓ global and most regions studied
Zubieta et al (2005)	19 smokers	^{15}O-PET	Cigarette vs. denicotinized cigarette vs. baseline	↑ visual cortex and cerebellum, ↓ ACC and NAc

All regional changes represent normalized activity, unless otherwise stated. Nic, nicotine; thal, thalamus; cereb, cerebellum; SPECT, single photon emission computed tomography; fMRI, functional magnetic resonance imaging; IV, intravenous; R, right; L, left; NAc, nucleus accumbens; amyg, amygdala; FDG, ^{18}F-fluorodeoxyglucose; PET, positron emission tomography; IFG, inferior frontal gyrus; PC, posterior cingulate; ins, insula; inf occ ctx, inferior occipital cortex; ant, anterior; temp, temporal lobe; ACC, anterior cingulate cortex.

in frontal lobe and thalamic blood flow in smokers who smoked a cigarette (Nakamura et al 2000). While this group of studies demonstrate specific regional activation with nicotine or smoking, they also imply activation of cortico-basal ganglia-thalamic brain circuits (Alexander et al 1990) that may mediate the subjective effects of smoking (see below).

Since regional activity was normalized to whole brain activity in at least some of these studies, and whole brain activity has been found to decrease with nicotine or cigarette administration (cited above), the regional findings presented here may represent either increased regional activity, or possibly, less of a decrease in regional activity than in other brain areas. Regional decreases in activity are generally not seen with nicotine or cigarette administration, though at least two studies found relatively decreased activity in the left (Rose et al 2003) and right (Zubieta et al 2001) amygdala.

Effect of nicotine on brain activation during cognitive tasks

The most commonly replicated cognitive effect of nicotine administration is improved performance on tasks that require vigilant attention in nicotine-dependent smokers (Newhouse et al 2004). Nicotine administration also has been reported to improve reaction time (regardless of smoking status) as well. Consistent with these findings are studies which demonstrate that acute abstinence from smoking (within 12 h) results in slowed response times (Thompson et al 2002).

In examining brain mediation of the cognitive effects of smoking, several groups have performed functional imaging studies in subjects performing cognitive tasks during administration of nicotine compared to a control condition. For most of these studies, subjects performed a cognitive task that involved visual recognition and working memory, such as the n-back task. Results of these studies have been somewhat mixed, showing both decreased (Ghatan et al 1998, Ernst et al 2001) and increased (Kumari et al 2003, Jacobsen et al 2004) ACC activation in response to nicotine administration while performing the task. Brain activation responses to nicotine during cognitive tasks have been more consistent in other brain areas such as the thalamus (Jacobsen et al 2004, Lawrence et al 2002) and visual cortex (Ghatan et al 1998, Lawrence et al 2002).

Brain dopamine responses to nicotine and smoking

A common pathway for the rewarding effects of most, if not all, addictive drugs is the brain dopamine (DA) system (Koob 1992). Laboratory animal studies demonstrate that DA release in the ventral striatum (VST)/nucleus accumbens (NAc) underlies the reinforcing properties of nicotine (Koob 1992). Microdialysis (Di Chiara & Imperato 1988, Pontieri et al 1996) and lesion (Corrigall et al 1992) studies in rats indicate that nicotine-induced DA release is strongest in this region, and is more robust than the DA release found in associated structures receiving dopaminergic input, such as the dorsal striatum (Di Chiara & Imperato 1988). These studies generally used nicotine dosages that simulated human cigarette smoking. Additionally, many *in vitro* studies of the VST have reported DA release in response to nicotine (e.g. Rowell et al 1987).

Human brain imaging studies of the DA system (Table 2) corroborate and expand upon these laboratory studies. Striatal DA release in response to a nicotine or cigarette challenge has been demonstrated repeatedly in both non-human primates and humans (Dewey et al 1999, Marenco et al 2004, Brody et al 2004, Tsukada et al 2002), with the majority of these studies using PET and the radiotracer [^{11}C]raclopride (a relatively specific D_2 receptor binder) to demonstrate DA release through radiotracer displacement. These studies have reported a wide range of DA concentration changes. In two studies that examined the question directly (Tsukada et al 2002, Marenco et al 2004), nicotine was found to result in less radiotracer displacement than amphetamine, while it has also been reported that nicotine-induced DA release is comparable in magnitude to that induced by other addictive drugs (Pontieri et al 1996). Also, an association between [^{11}C]raclopride displacement and the hedonic effects of smoking (defined as elation and euphoria) has been demonstrated (Barrett et al 2004), though this study did not find an overall difference between the smoking and non-smoking conditions. Thus, while the majority of studies do provide evidence for nicotine/smoking-induced DA release, there are disparities between studies as to the extent of human smoking-induced DA release. Disparities between these studies may be due to differences in methodology (e.g. nicotine administration versus cigarette smoking) and/or technical complexities in performing such studies.

Nicotine-induced DA release in the NAc has been reported to be mediated by stimulation of nicotinic acetylcholine receptors (nAChRs) on cells of the ventral tegmental area (VTA) that project to the NAc rather than by nicotinic receptors within the NAc itself (Nisell et al 1994). Lesioning of mesolimbic VTA neurons projecting to the NAc leads to decreased nicotine self-administration (Corrigall et al 1992). Additionally, the effects of nicotine on the dopaminergic system appear to be modulated by glutamatergic and GABAergic neurons (Picciotto & Corrigall 2002), with nicotine stimulation of glutamatergic tracts from the prefrontal cortex to the VTA leading to increased DA neuron firing and GABA agonism leading to a dampening of DA neuron responses.

Glutamatergic (and other) effects of nicotine/cigarette smoking

Recent autoradiography studies of rodents are determining effects of nicotine/smoking in other brain systems that may be activated by nicotine

TABLE 2 Functional imaging studies of dopaminergic (DA) effects of nicotine administration or smoking

Authors	Subjects	Method	Intervention	Results/conclusions
Dewey et al (1999)	16 baboons	^{11}C-raclopride PET (double bolus)	IV nic (0.3 mg)	↓ DV tracer (indicating ↑ DA concentration) in NAc
Dagher et al (2001)	11 smokers; 18 non-smokers	^{11}C-SCH 23390 PET		↓ BP in smokers (indicating ↓ D1 receptor density) in ventral striatum
Tsukada et al (2002)	4 Macada mulatto monkeys	^{11}C-raclopride PET (B/I)	IV nic (B/I)	Slight ↓ BP (indicating ↑ DA concentration) in anesthetized, but not conscious monkeys, in dorsal striatum
Salokangas et al (2000)	9 smokers; 10 non-smokers	^{18}F-DOPA PET		↑ uptake (indicating ↑ DA activity) in cd and Put of smokers
Marenco et al (2004)	5 rhesus monkeys	^{11}C-raclopride PET (double bolus & B/I)	IV nic (0.01 to 0.06 mg/kg)	↓ BP (indicating ↑ DA concentration) in basal ganglia with nic administration
Brody et al (2004)	20 smokers	^{11}C-raclopride PET (B/I)	Single cigarette versus no smoking	↓ BP (indicating ↑ DA concentration) in smoking, but not no smoking, condition in L ventral cd and put
Barrett et al (2004)	10 smokers	^{11}C-raclopride PET (double bolus)	Smoking every 12 minutes versus no smoking	↓ BP correlated with hedonic response to smoking in cd and posterior put

PET, positron emission tomography; IV, intravenous; nic, nicotine; DV, volume of distribution; DA, dopamine; BP, binding potential; B/I, bolus-plus-infusion; cd, caudate; put, putamen; SPECT, single photon emission computed tomography; DAT, dopamine transporter; ADHD, attention deficit hyperactivity disorder; beta-CIT, 2β-carbomethoxy-3 beta-(4-iodophenyl)-tropane; 5-HT, serotonin.

stimulation of nAChRs. For example, in response to nicotine, glutamate is released in the prelimbic prefrontal cortex (Gioanni et al 1999), and glutamate and aspartate are released in the VTA (Schilstrom et al 2000). Importantly, one of these studies (Gioanni et al 1999) also demonstrated that nicotine administration facilitates thalamo-cortical neurotransmission through stimulation of nAChRs on glutamatergic neurons.

Brain function responses to chronic nicotine administration and cigarette smoking

Monoamine oxidase (MAO) function in smokers

Fowler and colleagues have performed a series of studies demonstrating decreases in MAO A and B activity in cigarette smokers using the PET tracers [^{11}C]clorgyline and [^{11}C]L-deprenyl-D2, respectively (Fowler et al 2003). When compared to former smokers and non-smokers, average reductions for current smokers are 30 and 40% for MAO A and B (Fowler et al 2003). These reductions are the result of chronic smoking behaviour rather than a single administration of intravenous nicotine or smoking a single cigarette, and are less than those seen with antidepressant MAO inhibitors. Additionally, a human post-mortem study of chronic smokers demonstrated a modest reduction in MAO A binding that did not reach statistical significance (Klimek et al 2001).

MAO participates in the catabolism of dopamine, norepinephrine and serotonin (Fowler et al 2003), and it has been postulated that some of the clinical effects of smoking are due to MAO inhibition, leading to decreases in monoamine breakdown with a subsequent increase in monoamine availability. Thus, the rewarding properties of smoking may be due to DA release (as described above) and/or MAO inhibition. Smoking may also alter mood and anxiety through MAO inhibition effects on norepinephrine and serotonin availability and turnover.

Functional imaging of nicotinic acetylcholine receptors (nAChRs)

Because stimulation of nicotinic acetylcholine receptors (nAChRs) is intimately linked with effects of smoking, a longstanding and still developing area of research is the labelling of nAChRs during functional brain imaging. Nicotine binds to nAChRs in the brain to mediate a variety of behavioural states (Lukas 1998), such as heightened arousal and improved reaction time and psychomotor function (Paterson & Nordberg 2000). Nicotine administration also produces reward through DA release in the NAc, at least in part through stimulation of nAChRs in the ventral tegmental area (e.g. Corrigall et al 1994, Nisell et al 1994) as discussed above. Nicotinic acetylcholine receptors are widespread throughout the brain, with a rank order distribution of nAChR density being: thalamus >basal ganglia >cerebral cortex >hippocampus >cerebellum (e.g. London et al 1985, Davila-Garcia et al 1999).

Radiotracers for the nAChR have been developed in recent years, with labelled A-85380 (3-(2(S)-azetidinylmethoxy) pyridine) (Koren et al 1998) compounds having the most widespread use. Studies of non-human primates and humans have examined distributions of nAChRs with these new radiotracers, and found regional densities of these receptors similar to those in the animal work cited above (e.g.

Kimes et al 2003, Fujita et al 2003). In initial human studies, no subjective or cardiovascular effects of 2-FA have been reported; however, studies of tobacco dependent subjects have not yet been published. In two recent studies of baboons, the effects of nicotine or tobacco smoke on nAChR availability were examined. In a PET study using the radiotracer 2-FA (Valette et al 2003), IV nicotine (0.6 mg), inhalation of tobacco smoke from one cigarette (0.9 mg nicotine), and IV nornicotine were all found to reduce the volume of distribution of the radiotracer by roughly 30–60% in the thalamus and putamen at 80 minutes, and this reduction of 2-FA binding was relatively long-lived (up to 6 hours). Similarly, a 50% reduction in nAChR availability was found with IV nicotine administration to baboons using an epibatidine analogue and PET scanning (Ding et al 2000). Taken together, these studies demonstrate that radiotracers for nAChRs can be administered safely to measure nAChR densities, and that administration of nicotine and smoking substantially decrease $\alpha_4\beta_2$ nAChR availability.

Discussion: localizing tobacco dependence pathways

Functional brain imaging has been used to determine both acute and chronic effects of nicotine/cigarette exposure. Responses to acute administration of nicotine/ smoking include: a reduction in global brain activity; activation of the prefrontal cortex, thalamus, and visual system; activation of the thalamus and visual cortex (and possibly ACC) during visual cognitive tasks; and increased DA concentration in the ventral striatum/NAc. Responses to chronic nicotine/cigarette administration include decreased MAO A and B activity and a substantial reduction in $\alpha_4\beta_2$ nAChR availability in the thalamus and putamen (accompanied by an overall up-regulation of these receptors).

This group of findings demonstrates a number of ways in which smoking might enhance neurotransmission through cortico-basal ganglia-thalamic circuits (Alexander et al 1990) (in addition to demonstrating direct effects of chronic nicotine exposure on nAChR availability) (Fig. 1). Given that the thalamus and ventral striatum/NAc function as relay centres for information and for paralimbic and motor processing in the brain, the net effect of smoking may be to enhance neurotransmission along cortico-basal ganglia-thalamic loops originating in paralimbic cortex. Neurotransmission through these circuits may be stimulated directly by the interconnected nAChR-rich thalamus and visual systems, and/or indirectly through effects on MAO inhibition and DA release in the ventral striatum/NAc. In the thalamus, for example, nicotine has direct agonist action on excitatory thalamocortical projection neurons and local circuit neurons, although nicotine also stimulates GABAergic inhibitory interneurons, so that the relationship between nicotine stimulation and thalamocortical stimulation may be complex (Clarke 2004).

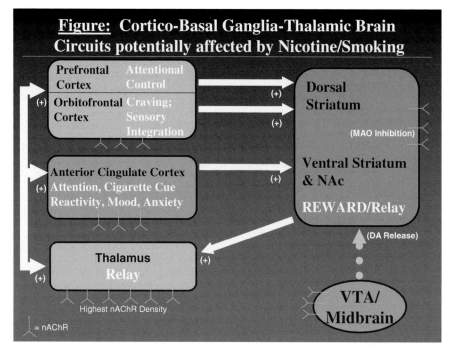

FIG. 1.   Simplified representation of cortico-basal ganglia-thalamic brain circuitry that mediates effects of nicotine/smoking on attentional control, craving, sensory integration, mood and anxiety. Potential targets for nicotine/smoking to enhance attention (and improve craving, mood, and anxiety) include: (1) direct stimulation of nicotinic acetylcholine receptors (nAChRs) in the prefrontal, orbitofrontal or anterior cingulate cortex, (2) stimulation of nAChRs in the nAChR-rich thalamus and basal ganglia (which function as relay stations for this circuitry), (3) activation of dopaminergic mesolimbic reward pathways originating in the ventral tegmental area and projecting to the striatum, and (4) monoamine oxidase (MAO) inhibition in the basal ganglia. NAc, nucleus accumbens; VTA, ventral tegmental area.

Enhancement of neurotransmission through prefrontal and paralimbic cortico-basal ganglia-thalamic circuits may account for the most commonly reported cognitive effect of cigarette smoking, namely improved attentional performance (Newhouse et al 2004), and also related effects, such as improvements in reaction times, arousal, motivation and sustained attention. The prefrontal (including both dorsolateral and ventrolateral) and anterior cingulate cortices are reported to activate during attentional control tasks (especially visuospatial tasks) (Pessoa et al 2003). Cigarette smoking may enhance attentional control through direct stimulation of nAChRs within these structures or perhaps through subcortical stimulation of nAChRs in the thalamus and via DA release and/or MAO inhibition in the basal ganglia.

In addition to these primary effects of nicotine and smoking, other functional imaging studies reviewed here focus on smoking-related states, such as cue-induced cigarette craving. Such studies are part of a large body of literature examining cue-induced craving for addictive drugs. Studies specific for cigarette cues/craving reveal that exposure to visual cigarette cues immediately activates mesolimbic (ventral tegmental area, amygdala and hippocampus) and visuospatial cortical attention areas of the brain, and acutely (over a 30 min period) activate paralimbic regions (ACC and OFC), and that this cue-induced activation may be diminished by a course of bupropion treatment. In addition, it has been posited that at least some of the activations seen with cigarette-related cues (cortical attention areas and OFC) are associated with an expectation of smoking in the non-treatment-seeking subjects who participated in these studies (Wilson et al 2004).

In summary, functional brain imaging studies of nicotine/cigarette smoking have demonstrated a link between nicotine/cigarette administration and brain circuitry that mediates visuospatial attentional processing and withdrawal symptoms. The brain mediation of tobacco dependence will undoubtedly be characterized more fully as functional brain imaging methodology improves.

Acknowledgement

The author would like to thank Sanjaya Saxena MD for his helpful comments on the manuscript. This work was supported by a Department of Veterans Affairs Type I Merit Review Award, the Tobacco-Related Disease Research Program (11RT-0024), the National Institute on Drug Abuse (R01 DA15059), and a National Alliance for Research on Schizophrenia and Depression Independent Investigator Award.

References

Alexander GE, Crutcher MD, DeLong MR 1990 Basal ganglia-thalamocortical circuits: parallel substrates for motor, oculomotor, 'prefrontal' and 'limbic' functions. Prog Brain Res 85:119–146

Baker RR, Massey ED, Smith G 2004 An overview of the effects of tobacco ingredients on smoke chemistry and toxicity. Food Chem Toxicol 42 Suppl:S53–83

Barrett SP, Boileau I, Okker J, Pihl RO, Dagher A 2004 The hedonic response to cigarette smoking is proportional to dopamine release in the human striatum as measured by positron emission tomography and [(11)C]raclopride. Synapse 54:65–71

Brody AL, Mandelkern MA, London ED et al 2002 Brain metabolic changes during cigarette craving. Arch Gen Psychiatry 59:1162–1172

Brody AL, Mandelkern MA, Lee G et al 2004a Attenuation of cue-induced cigarette craving and anterior cingulate cortex activation in bupropion-treated smokers: a preliminary study. Psych Res Neuroimaging 130:269–281

Brody AL, Olmstead RE, London ED et al 2004b Smoking-induced ventral striatum dopamine release. Am J Psychiatry 161:1211–1218

Carter BL, Tiffany ST 1999 Meta-analysis of cue-reactivity in addiction research. Addiction 94:327–340

Clarke PBS 2004 Nicotinic modulation of thalamocortical neurotransmission. Acetylcholine in the cerebral cortex. Prog Brain Res 145:253–260

Corrigall WA, Franklin KB, Coen KM, Clarke PB 1992 The mesolimbic dopaminergic system is implicated in the reinforcing effects of nicotine. Psychopharmacology (Berl) 107:285–289

Corrigall WA, Coen KM, Adamson KL 1994 Self-administered nicotine activates the mesolimbic dopamine system through the ventral tegmental area. Brain Res 653:278–284

Davila-Garcia MI, Houghtling RA, Qasba SS, Kellar KJ 1999 Nicotinic receptor binding sites in rat primary neuronal cells in culture: characterization and their regulation by chronic nicotine. Mol Brain Res 66:14–23

Dewey SL, Brodie JD, Gerasimov M, Horan B, Gardner EL, Ashby CRJ 1999 A pharmacologic strategy for the treatment of nicotine addiction. Synapse 31:76–86

Di Chiara G, Imperato A 1988 Drugs abused by humans preferentially increase synaptic dopamine concentrations in the mesolimbic system of freely moving rats. Proc Natl Acad Sci USA 85:5274–5278

Ding YS, Volkow ND, Logan J et al 2000 Occupancy of brain nicotinic acetylcholine receptors by nicotine doses equivalent to those obtained when smoking a cigarette. Synapse 35:234–237

Domino EF, Minoshima S, Guthrie S et al 2000a Nicotine effects on regional cerebral blood flow in awake, resting tobacco smokers. Synapse 38:313–321

Domino EF, Minoshima S, Guthrie SK et al 2000b Effects of nicotine on regional cerebral glucose metabolism in awake resting tobacco smokers. Neuroscience 101:277–282

Due DL, Huettel SA, Hall WG, Rubin DC 2002 Activation in mesolimbic and visuospatial neural circuits elicited by smoking cues: Evidence from functional magnetic resonance imaging. Am J Psychiatry 159:954–960

Ernst M, Matochik JA, Heishman SJ et al 2001 Effect of nicotine on brain activation during performance of a working memory task. Proc Natl Acad Sci USA 98:4728–4733

Fallon JH, Keator DB, Mbogori J, Turner J, Potkin SG 2004 Hostility differentiates the brain metabolic effects of nicotine. Brain Res Cogn Brain Res 18:142–148

Fowler JS, Logan J, Wang GJ, Volkow ND 2003 Monoamine oxidase and cigarette smoking. Neurotoxicology 24:75–82

Fujita M, Ichise M, van Dyck CH et al 2003 Quantification of nicotinic acetylcholine receptors in human brain using [I-123]5-I-A-85380 SPET. Eur J Nucl Med Mol Imaging 30:1620–1629

Ghatan PH, Ingvar M, Eriksson L et al 1998 Cerebral effects of nicotine during cognition in smokers and non-smokers. Psychopharmacology 136:179–189

Gioanni Y, Rougeot C, Clarke PB, Lepouse C, Thierry AM, Vidal C 1999 Nicotinic receptors in the rat prefrontal cortex: increase in glutamate release and facilitation of mediodorsal thalamo-cortical transmission. Eur J Neurosci 11:18–30

Jacobsen LK, D'Souza DC, Mencl WE, Pugh KR, Skudlarski P, Krystal JH 2004 Nicotine effects on brain function and functional connectivity in schizophrenia. Biol Psychiatry 55:850–858

Kimbrell TA, George MS, Parekh PI et al 1999 Regional brain activity during transient self-induced anxiety and anger in healthy adults. Biol Psychiatry 46:454–465

Kimes AS, Horti AG, London ED et al 2003 2-[18F]F-A-85380: PET imaging of brain nicotinic acetylcholine receptors and whole body distribution in humans. FASEB J 17:1331–1333

Klimek V, Zhu MY, Dilley G et al 2001 Effects of long-term cigarette smoking on the human locus coeruleus. Arch Gen Psychiatry 58:821–827

Koob GF 1992 Drugs of abuse: anatomy, pharmacology and function of reward pathways. Trends Pharm Sci 13:177–184

Koren AO, Horti AG, Mukhin AG et al 1998 2-, 5- and 6-halo-3-(2(S)-azetidinylmethoxy) pyridines: Synthesis, affinity for nicotinic acetylcholine receptors, and molecular modeling. Eur J Med Chem 41:3690–3698

Kumari V, Gray JA, Ffytche DH et al 2003 Cognitive effects of nicotine in humans: an fMRI study. Neuroimage 19:1002–1013

Lawrence NS, Ross TJ, Stein EA 2002 Cognitive mechanisms of nicotine on visual attention. Neuron 36:539–548

London ED, Connolly RJ, Szikszay M, Wamsley JK, Dam M 1988 Effects of nicotine on local cerebral glucose-utilization in the rat. J Neurosci 8:3920–3928

London ED, Waller SB, Wamsley JK 1985 Autoradiographic localization of [^{3}H]nicotine binding sites in the rat brain. Neurosci Lett 53:179–184

Lukas RJ 1998 Neuronal nicotinic acetylcholine receptors. In: Barrantes FJ (ed) The nicotinic acetylcholine receptor: current views and future trends. R.G. Landes Company, Georgetown, p 145–173

Marenco S, Carson RE, Berman KF, Herscovitch P, Weinberger DR 2004 Nicotine-induced dopamine release in primates measured with [C-11]raclopride PET. Neuropsychopharmacology 29:259–268

Naito E, Kinomura S, Geyer S, Kawashima R, Roland PE, Zilles K 2000 Fast reaction to different sensory modalities activates common fields in the motor areas, but the anterior cingulate cortex is involved in the speed of reaction. J Neurophysiol 83:1701–1709

Nakamura H, Tanaka A, Nomoto Y, Ueno Y, Nakayama Y 2000 Activation of fronto-limbic system in the human brain by cigarette smoking: evaluated by a CBF measurement. Keio J Med 49 Suppl 1:A122–124

Newhouse PA, Potter A, Singh A 2004 Effects of nicotinic stimulation on cognitive performance. Curr Opin Pharmacol 4:36–46

Nisell M, Nomikos GG, Svensson TH 1994 Systemic nicotine-induced dopamine release in the rat nucleus accumbens is regulated by nicotinic receptors in the ventral tegmental area. Synapse 16:36–44

Paterson D, Nordberg A 2000 Neuronal nicotinic receptors in the human brain. Prog Neurobiology 61:75–111

Pessoa L, Kastner S, Ungerleider LG 2003 Neuroimaging studies of attention: From modulation of sensory processing to top-down control. J Neurosci 23:3990–3998

Picciotto MR, Corrigall WA 2002 Neuronal systems underlying behaviors related to nicotine addiction: neural circuits and molecular genetics. J Neurosci 22:3338–3341

Pontieri FE, Tanda G, Orzi F, Di Chiara G 1996 Effects of nicotine on the nucleus accumbens and similarity to those of addictive drugs. Nature 382:255–257

Rolls ET, Critchley HD, Browning A, Hernadi I 1998 The neurophysiology of taste and olfaction in primates, and umami flavor. Ann N Y Acad Sci 855:426–437

Rose JE, Behm FM, Westman EC et al 2003 PET Studies of the influences of nicotine on neural systems in cigarette smokers. Am J Psychiatry 160:323–333

Rourke SB, Dupont RM, Grant I et al 1997 Reduction in cortical IMP-SPET tracer uptake with recent cigarette consumption in a young group of healthy males. San Diego HIV Neurobehavioral Research Center. Eur J Nucl Med 24:422–427

Rowell PP, Carr LA, Garner AC 1987 Stimulation of [^{3}H]dopamine release by nicotine in rat nucleus accumbens. J Neurochem 49:1449–1454

Salokangas RKR, Vilkman H, Ilonen T et al 2000 High levels of dopamine activity in the basal ganglia of cigarette smokers. Am J Psychiatry 157:632–634

Schilstrom B, Fagerquist MV, Zhang X et al 2000 Putative role of presynaptic alpha7* nicotinic receptors in nicotine stimulated increases of extracellular levels of glutamate and aspartate in the ventral tegmental area. Synapse 38:375–383

Schuh KJ, Stitzer ML 1995 Desire to smoke during spaced smoking intervals. Psychopharmacology (Berl) 120:289–295

Stapleton JM, Gilson SF, Wong DF et al 2003 Intravenous nicotine reduces cerebral glucose metabolism: A preliminary study. Neuropsychopharmacology 28:765–772

Stein E, Pankiewicz J, Harsch HH et al 1998 Nicotine-induced limbic cortical activation in the human brain: A functional MRI study. Am J Psychiatry 155:1009–1015

Thompson JC, Wilby G, Stough C 2002 The effects of transdermal nicotine on inspection time. Hum Psychopharmacol 17:157–161.

Tsukada H, Miyasato K, Kakiuchi T, Nishiyama S, Harada N, Domino EF 2002 Comparative effects of methamphetamine and nicotine on the striatal [C-11]raclopride binding in unanesthetized monkeys. Synapse 45:207–212

Valette H, Bottlaender M, Dolle F, Coulon C, Ottaviani M, Syrota A 2003 Long-lasting occupancy of central nicotinic acetylcholine receptors after smoking: a PET study in monkeys. J Neurochem 84:105–111

Wilson SJ, Sayette MA, Fiez JA 2004 Prefrontal responses to drug cues: a neurocognitive analysis. Nat Neurosci 7:211–214

Yamamoto Y, Nishiyama Y, Monden T, Satoh K, Ohkawa M 2003 A study of the acute effect of smoking on cerebral blood flow using 99mTc-ECD SPET. Eur J Nucl Med Mol Imaging 30:612–614

Zubieta J, Lombardi U, Minoshima S et al 2001 Regional cerebral blood flow effects of nicotine in overnight abstinent smokers. Biol Psychiatry 49:906–913

Zubieta JK, Heitzeg MM, Xu Y, Koeppe RA, Ni L, Guthrie S, Domino EF 2005 Regional cerebral blood flow responses to smoking in tobacco smokers after overnight abstinence. Am J Psychiatry 162:567–577

DISCUSSION

Shiffman: In your studies you are looking at people who are abstinent or smoking. Can you comment on the degree to which the findings should be interpreted as direct effects of nicotine or relief of withdrawal effects?

Brody: We are now doing treatment studies, where we scan people before and after treatment. So we are getting at least some people who are abstinent for a few weeks. There aren't quite as many studies on human functional brain imaging in former smokers; I can think of just two (Rourke et al 1997, Ernst et al 2001).

Shiffman: You discussed whether some of these effects seen in imaging mediate effects on cognitive performance or mood. There is a common point of view that those effects in humans are withdrawal relief effects rather than direct nicotine effects.

Brody: It is difficult to get approval to get non-smokers to smoke during scanning, or give them nicotine.

West: Occasional smokers are a great group to study for this sort of work, but rarely get looked at. They can take in nicotine but don't experience withdrawal symptoms. You would get ethics approval to give nicotine to occasional smokers.

Brody: Yes. I agree occasional smokers would be an important control group, but such studies have not yet been done.

Clarke: In scanning studies I notice that great emphasis is placed on 't' statistic maps and hence statistical significance. In a between-subject design you could have high statistical significance even with small drug effects. The areas that light up as red on your maps might not be the areas that show the biggest percentage difference from controls, but those which show the least between subject variability. In your studies do you find the biggest effects are also the most significant?

Brody: My guess is yes.

Markou: That also means that they are more reliable. They may be small but functionally they may be very important. That is, even a small change in one brain region may have a significant effect in mood or behaviour, for example.

Clarke: But you may be missing areas that could be important through a lack of statistical power.

Brody: That is the problem in this sort of research. When you study an fMRI scan you are looking at a million voxels (units of space). How do you draw a statistical threshold?

Clarke: I asked the question partly because of the correlation with craving. In some studies craving correlates with activity in the dorsal striatum or even the ventral putamen. This is not an area that I would think of naturally in terms of craving.

Brody: That is true. In our study we did find the correlation between dopamine release (measured indirectly) in the ventral striatum and craving.

Bizarro: I like the way you use a film as a cue. Why don't you use an appetitive control instead of a film of someone gardening? You could use the same person eating or drinking instead of smoking.

Brody: We could. There are groups that use emotionally positive and emotionally negative cues combined with cigarettes or not.

Stolerman: On that theme, I wonder whether seeing a cigarette cue but not being able to smoke is positive or negative. What stimuli would you use as controls for this?

Brody: I think my research subjects experience this as negative. I felt a little threatened by some of them when I was repeatedly asking them about their craving and presenting them with cigarette cues at the same time!

Shiffman: Michael Sayette at the University of Pittsburgh does experiments in which he manipulates whether people expect to actually get to smoke or not (Sayette et al 2003). Among other things, he codes facial expressions, which are readouts of emotional tone, and does imaging work. He finds that if you expect to smoke, exposure is experienced positively; if you don't expect to smoke, then it is a negative stimulus. This makes sense, but it complicates the work.

Brody: In our study we did the cues for 30 min and then we were going to scan them for 30 min. They knew there was going to be this 30 min where they weren't going to be allowed to smoke.

Changeux: You say that there is a smaller grey matter density in the people that smoked a lot. How do you explain this? Is it due to cell loss to shrinkage of neurons?

Brody: We did two analyses of pack year smoking history versus grey matter: one was positive, the other negative. Our group and others have proposed following these people over time to see whether this is the effect of chronic cigarette smoking. These were middle-aged people who had been smoking for a while. One of our analyses indicated that higher pack year smoking history was associated with lower grey matter density in the prefrontal cortex.

Changeux: What do you mean by lower grey matter density? Is this relative to white matter? Is there any expansion of the cortex? Is this fluid content or vascularization? I can't imagine it's similar to what happens in Alzheimer's disease: are you implying that there is loss of neurons?

Brody: That is the implication I have read about by people who invented this method of analysis. We use two methods of analysis, one of which is a computer method which shows the density.

Changeux: So this means that there is an absolute loss of matter. This could be looked at on histological slices at autopsy. It should be easy to check.

Chiamulera: It would be interesting to see the situation in long-term abstinent ex-smokers.

Bertrand: There was a report in *Nature* not so long ago showing juggle learning increased the grey matter density in some local area and that this change is reversible. (Dragansky et al 2004). I see many similarities with your study. As we are not expecting the number of neurons to grow and then decrease, something else must be happening!

Jarvis: It was striking that you saw a lot of nicotine receptors occupied at low blood nicotine levels. This was 1 ng/ml, which is well within the non-smoking range. Although it looked like a very nice dose–response curve, can it be imagined that some of this might be due to learned associations between cigarette stimuli and nicotine delivery? In other words, could it be secondary conditioning that is leading to some of the nicotine receptors being occupied, rather than a direct effect of the nicotine delivered by the cigarette?

Brody: It could be. One way to test this would be via using denicotinized cigarettes.

West: One of the issues with this kind of research is the specificity of associations, and whether the things that you are measuring that are associated with the other things you are measuring are really the things that are associated with each other. You measure craving, but they are experiencing other withdrawal symptoms at the same time which are correlated with this. Did you measure other withdrawal symptoms?

Brody: We did, but our subjects were really focused on the craving. They didn't report a lot of depression and anxiety.

West: They shouldn't report anxiety, because I don't think this is a withdrawal symptom from smoking. There is a general issue of the state they are in: even if they don't report irritability, for example, that is a clear-cut withdrawal symptom. I also have a very small complaint: you cite the relationship between craving and abstinence. Peter Hajek and I published the first study on this in 1989 (West et al 1989) on that and it never gets cited!

Peto: I have a couple of trivial statistical points. It is a bad idea to adjust to pack years, because this is correlated with age, and so many things change with age. If you are going to adjust, use age or the daily number of cigarettes usually smoked, but don't make a composite index such as pack years. Second, I find it very odd that these serious questions are being addressed by studies with such large random errors because of small numbers. By the standards of epidemiology these numbers just aren't adequate. The play of chance is producing fluctuations which are the same order of magnitude as the things being studied. Lastly, as a point of clarification, we heard a paper earlier emphasizing the fundamental importance of one receptor, the dopamine D_3 receptor. It suggested that this is the key to all sorts of things. Now you are emphasizing all these other receptors with nothing relating specifically to the D_3 receptor. Is the D_3 receptor in some way fundamental?

Corrigall: This question points out one of the reasons why we are here. The identity and nature of the neurochemical systems involved in nicotine addition started some decades ago with a focus on the dopamine system. We remain at the discovery stage, with research both broadening the focus to other neurochemical systems, as well as aiming to uncover which elements of the dopamine system—receptor subtypes, function, and cellular locales—are critical.

Peto: Do other people feel that the emphasis on D_3 was inappropriately narrow?

Stolerman: No, until someone looks at the role of D_3 receptors in depth we won't know their role. People haven't examined it before. Naturally, other targets need to be investigated as well.

Shiffman: There is nothing in Art Brody's work that rules out a D_3 effect. Art Brody is showing occupancy of these cholinergic receptors, which in turn could lead to the release of dopamine acting on the D_3 receptor. They are interconnected systems.

Brody: Our tracer does label D_2 and D_3 receptors. The raclopride studies label both because they are similar. Your point about these small studies is true, but this is a chronic problem in the brain imaging field. In one of the studies I talked about we did 80 PET scans. This is a large PET scan study and cost several hundred thousand dollars. If you really want to do these studies in the kinds of samples you are talking about the cost would be millions and millions of dollars or so for a single study. It's a tricky business.

Peto: The competition are spending six billion dollars a year advertising the stuff.

Balfour: I am concerned about the correlation between venous nicotine and displacement of ligands. The peak that would have gone through the artery to the brain would have been even higher.

Brody: The figures I presented were estimated on the low side. They were levels drawn some time after the person smoked.

Balfour: Is the ligand an agonist or an antagonist?

Brody: It is neither: we give it in trace amounts. Pharmacologically it is an agonist.

Balfour: So what you are showing is that an agonist stays there for three hours.

Brody: We have an infusion of the tracer taking place during the imaging.

Balfour: Nevertheless, the pulse of nicotine that has been inhaled has an effect that lasts three hours. This implies occupation by nicotine or acetylcholine for three hours.

Clarke: Or there is internalization of the nicotinic receptor as is thought to occur with radiolabelled raclopride and dopaminergic receptors (Ginovart et al 2004).

Balfour: What I am trying to get at is that you have not lost function for 3 h.

Brody: We don't know. This could be how nicotine exerts its effects.

Balfour: For the venous levels, I can tell you should not have lost function for 3 h. With regard to the effects of nicotine on dopamine release in conscious animals, we know what blood levels of nicotine you need to block the effects. You are occupying the receptor in doses which in animals would not completely block responses; this is an interesting finding.

Brody: All our study can tell you is whether the receptor is occupied or not.

References

Draganski B, Gaser C, Busch V, Schuierer G, Bogdahn U, May A 2004 Neuroplasticity: changes in grey matter induced by training. Nature 427:311–312

Ernst M, Matochik JA, Heishman S et al 2001 Effect of nicotine on brain activation during performance of a working memory task. Proc Natl Acad Sci USA 98:4728–4733

Ginovart N, Wilson AA, Houle S, Kapur S 2004 Amphetamine pretreatment induces a change in both D2-receptor density and apparent affinity: a [11C]raclopride positron emission tomography study in cats. Biol Psychiatry 55:1188–1194

Rourke SB, Dupont RM, Grant I et al 1997 Reduction in cortical IMP-SPET tracer uptake with recent cigarette consumption in a young group of healthy males. San Diego HIV Neurobehavioral Research Center. Eur J Nucl Med 24:422–427

Sayette MA, Wertz JM, Martin CS, Cohn JF, Perrott MA, Hobel J 2003 Effects of smoking opportunity on cue-elicited urge: a facial coding analysis. Exp Clin Psychopharmacol 11:218–227

West RJ, Hajek P, Belcher M 1989 Severity of withdrawal symptoms as a predictor of outcome of an attempt to quit smoking. Psychol Med 19:981–985

Pharmacogenetic approaches to nicotine dependence treatment

Caryn Lerman

University of Pennsylvania Transdisciplinary Tobacco Use Research Center (TTURC), 3535 Market Street, Suite 4100, Philadelphia, PA 19104, USA

Abstract. The emerging field of pharmacogenetics has the potential to advance the science of nicotine dependence treatment by generating new knowledge about genetic factors that influence therapeutic responses. The basic premise of this approach is that inherited differences in drug metabolism and drug targets have important effects on treatment toxicity and efficacy. This paper reviews evidence supporting the potential utility of a pharmacogenetic approach to smoking cessation treatment utilizing data from two completed pharmacogenetic trials: a placebo-controlled trial of bupropion and an open-label trial of alternate forms of nicotine replacement therapy (NRT). These data suggest that therapeutic response to bupropion and NRT is influenced by functional variants in *DRD2* and *COMT*. Further, response to nicotine patch is associated with functional genetic variation at *OPRM1* and individual variation in nicotine metabolic rate. Emerging health policy and bioethical issues related to the clinical integration of genetic testing to tailor nicotine dependence treatment are also addressed.

2005 Understanding nicotine and tobacco addiction. Wiley, Chichester (Novartis Foundation Symposium 275) p 171–183

Despite progress made in the treatment of tobacco dependence, currently available treatments are effective for only a fraction of smokers. Although current guidelines recommend the use of nicotine patch as a first-line treatment for tobacco dependence (Fiore et al 2000), about 70–80% of smokers treated with the patch relapse to their former smoking practices in the long-term (Fiore et al 1994, Transdermal Nicotine Study Group 1991). Bupropion has been shown to produce higher quit rates than nicotine replacement therapy (NRT) (Gold et al 2002), yet the majority of smokers do not quit and remain abstinent. Thus, research is needed to identify those smokers for whom smoking cessation pharmacotherapies will have the strongest beneficial effects on smoking behaviour, as well as to identify novel therapeutics.

The emerging field of pharmacogenetics has the potential to advance the science of nicotine dependence treatment by generating new knowledge about genetic factors that influence clinical treatment outcome. The basic premise of this approach is that inherited differences in drug metabolism and drug targets have important effects on treatment toxicity and efficacy (Evans & Relling 1999, Poolsup et al 2000). Efforts to increase our understanding of the role that inherited variation plays in response to pharmacotherapy for nicotine dependence may someday help practitioners to individualize treatment based on genotype, thereby maximizing its efficacy (Lerman & Niaura 2002, Lerman et al 2005). This paper reviews evidence supporting the potential utility of a pharmacogenetic approach to smoking cessation treatment utilizing data from two completed pharmacogenetic trials: a placebo-controlled trial of bupropion (Lerman et al 2002a) and an open-label trial of nicotine nasal spray versus nicotine patch (Lerman et al 2004a).

Pharmacogenetic investigation of NRT

We have completed an open-label pharmacogenetic trial of transdermal nicotine versus nicotine nasal spray. Nicotine is metabolized to cotinine, and then to 3'-hydroxcotinine (3-HC), predominantly by the liver enzyme CYP2A6. Genetic variation in CYP2A6 predicts cigarette consumption and smoking persistence (Schoedel et al 2004, Fujieda et al 2004), consistent with the premise that faster inactivation and elimination of nicotine requires higher levels of smoking to maintain the desired levels of nicotine in the body. In an analysis of 481 smokers in our NRT trial, the 3-HC:cotinine ratio derived from cigarette smoking (a phenotypic measure of CYP2A6 activity), predicted the effectiveness of transdermal nicotine at the end of treatment and at 6 month follow-up. The likelihood of abstinence was reduced by almost 30% with each increasing quartile of metabolic ratio. Higher metabolite ratios also predicted lower nicotine concentrations and more severe cravings for cigarettes after one week of treatment. The metabolite ratio did not predict cessation with use of nicotine nasal spray, suggesting that smokers titrated their intake of nicotine with this product (Lerman et al 2006a). Analyses underway are examining associations of genetic variation in CYP2A6 with response to NRT.

With regard to genetic variation in drug targets, nicotine stimulates release of dopamine from neurons in the ventral tegmental area, an action thought to underlie its rewarding effects (Pontieri et al 1996). Therefore, we have examined response to these alternate forms of NRT in relation to genetic variation in the dopamine pathway. We have focused our pharmacogenetic analysis on functional genetic variants in *DRD2*, specifically, two single nucleotide polymorphisms (SNPs) that may influence *DRD2* receptor expression by altering transcription or translation. An insertion/deletion variant in the *DRD2* promoter region (*DRD2* −141C *Ins/Del*) has been identified, with increased transcriptional efficiency observed with the more common −141C *Ins* C allele as compared to the −141C *Del* C allele (Arinami et al 1997). In addition, Duan et al (2003) recently identified a functional synonymous SNP in *DRD2* (C957T) that decreases mRNA stability and protein synthesis. As

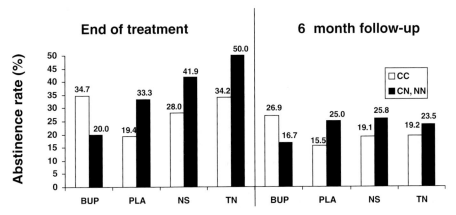

FIG. 1.   Abstinence rates by *DRD2* −141C *Ins/Del* genotype and treatment.

shown in Fig. 1, we found that smokers carrying the *Del* C allele or the −141C had statistically significantly higher quit rates on NRT compared to those homozygous for the *Ins* C allele, independent of NRT type (Lerman et al 2006b). The C957T variant was also associated with abstinence following NRT. Smokers carrying variants associated with reduced transcriptional efficiency or translation responded better to NRT, perhaps because of nicotine's effects on dopamine release.

We also examined the role of the catechol-*O*-methyltransferase (COMT) Val/Met functional polymorphism in response to NRT (Colilla et al 2005). COMT is the primary enzyme involved in the degradation and inactivation of the neurotransmitter dopamine (Cooper & Roth 1996). There is a polymorphism in the *COMT* gene that results in conversion of a Val high-activity allele to a Met low-activity allele, resulting in a three- to fourfold reduction in COMT activity. In the NRT trial, the Met/Met genotype was associated with a higher probability of abstinence with either nicotine nasal spray or nicotine patch, among women, but not in men (Colilla et al 2005). Consistent with the findings described above, this suggests that smokers carrying variants associated with lower levels of dopaminergic activity may respond better to NRT.

Another analysis from this investigation focused on the role of the *μ*-opioid receptor (OPRM1) gene (Lerman et al 2004b). The *μ*-opioid receptor is the primary site of action for the rewarding effects of the endogenous opioid peptide, *β*-endorphin (Zadina et al 1997) which is released following acute and short-term nicotine administration (Davenport et al 1990). Exon 1 of the human *OPRM1* gene includes a common Asn40Asp (A118G) mis-sense SNP. The Asp40 variant increases the binding affinity of *β*-endorphin for this receptor by threefold, relative to the wild-type Asn40 OPRM1 (Bond et al 1998). The Asp40 variant in OPRM1 is found in about 25–30% of individuals of European ancestry.

Among 320 smokers of European ancestry, smokers carrying the OPRM1 Asp40 variant were significantly more likely than those homozygous for the Asn40 variant to be abstinent at the end of the treatment phase. The differential treatment response was most pronounced among smokers receiving transdermal nicotine (quit rates of 52% vs. 33% for Asp40 and Asn40 groups, respectively, OR = 2.4), was modest and non-significant among smokers receiving nicotine nasal spray (OR = 1.28), and was non-significant in a group of 190 smokers treated with placebo in the bupropion clinical trial described above. Thus, smokers with the OPRM1 Asp40 variant appear to benefit most from the higher and consistent levels of nicotine delivered by transdermal nicotine.

Consistent with this pharmacogenetic hypothesis, a longitudinal analysis in the TN group revealed dose-response effects of transdermal nicotine, such that the genotype effect in the Asp40 group was greatest during 21 mg patch treatment, reduced as treatment was tapered, and disappeared after treatment was discontinued. Dose tapering did not appear to alter abstinence rates in the Asn40 group, which declined steadily from quit date. Further, event history analysis of lapse and recovery events showed that smokers with the Asp40 variant treated with transdermal nicotine were significantly more likely to *recover* from lapses than those with Asn40 variant during the 21 mg dose phase. There was no genotype effect on recovery from lapses during the 14 mg or 7 mg phase or after treatment was discontinued.

Consistent with the treatment outcome data from this trial, smokers with the Asp40 variant reported significantly less severe withdrawal symptoms and mood disturbance during the first two weeks of abstinence. Further, increases in negative affect during this period strongly predicted relapse. Smokers with the Asp40 variant also had significantly less weight gain at the end of treatment than those with the Asn40 genotype. OPRM1 genotype effects on these intermediate outcomes may be mediated by enhanced occupancy by β-endorphin at the μ receptor. While these results must be validated in future research, the findings suggest a hypothesis that smokers with the OPRM1 Asp40 variant may be candidates for extended high dose patch treatment, or even maintenance therapy, as an alternative to smoking.

Pharmacogenetic investigation of bupropion

We have conducted pharmacogenetic analyses as part of a bupropion placebo-controlled smoking cessation clinical trial (Lerman et al 2002a). The initial report from this trial focused on the *CYP2B6* gene, which has been implicated in bupropion kinetics (Kirchheiner et al 2003) as well as in brain metabolism of nicotine (Miksys et al 2003). In this trial, 426 smokers of European Caucasian ancestry provided blood samples and received bupropion (300 mg/day for 10 weeks) or placebo, plus counselling. Smokers with a decreased activity variant of *CYP2B6* (slower metabolizers) reported greater increases in cravings for cigarettes following the target quit date and had significantly higher relapse rates (Lerman et al 2002b). These effects were modified by a significant gender × genotype × treatment interaction, suggesting that bupropion attenuated the effects of genotype among female smokers. The finding of a significant association of *CYP2B6* genotype with smoking cessation in the placebo group and the absence of a genotype association with bupropion side-effects suggests that the genotype effect on treatment outcome is not attributable to bupropion pharmacokinetics. Rather, the greater relapse liability in the genetically slower metabolizers may be attributable to slower rates of inactivation of nicotine (by conversion to cotinine) in the CNS, and neuroadaptive changes that promote dependence and abstinence-induced craving.

Genetic variation in the dopamine pathway is a plausible target for pharmacogenetic studies of response to bupropion treatment. As mentioned above, there is abundant empirical support for the role of dopamine in the rewarding effects of nicotine (Pontieri et al 1996, Schultz 1998). Further, inhibition of dopamine reuptake is one putative mechanism for the beneficial effects of bupropion (Ascher et al 1995, Sanchez & Hyttel 1999). Therefore, we conducted an analysis of response to bupropion in relation to the functional genetic variants in *DRD2* described above. As shown in Fig. 1, we found a statistically significant interaction between the *DRD2* −141C *Ins/Del* genotype and treatment, at the end of the treatment phase, indicating a more favourable response to bupropion among smokers homozygous for the *Ins* C allele compared to those carrying a *Del* C allele (Lerman et al 2006b). The C957T variant was not associated with bupropion response. Given that the −141 *Ins* C allele results in higher transcriptional efficiency compared to the *Del* (N) allele (Arinami et al 1997), individuals with the −141C *Ins/Del* CC genotype may have more D2 receptors available to bind dopamine, yielding a more rewarding experience of the nicotine-induced dopamine release. Blockade of dopamine reuptake by bupropion may be more effective in promoting abstinence in the CC genotype group due to greater ability to bind dopamine.

Another analysis from this study tested whether genetic variation in the dopamine pathway moderated the effect of bupropion on abstinence-induced changes in the rewarding value of food (Lerman et al 2004c). Seventy-one smokers of European ancestry participated in this experiment, all of whom were genotyped for the *DRD2* Taq1 polymorphism and randomized to treatment with bupropion (300 mg) or placebo. They participated in two behavioural laboratory sessions during which the rewarding value of food was assessed using a behavioural economics measure: session 1 occurred prior to medication and before cessation of smoking; session 2 occurred following 3 weeks of bupropion and 1 week of sustained abstinence. Carriers of the *DRD2* A1 allele exhibited significant increases in the rewarding value of food following abstinence from smoking, and these effects were attenuated by bupropion treatment (a significant medication by genotype interaction). Further, higher levels of food reward at session 2 (post-quit) predicted a significant increase in weight by 6 month follow-up in the placebo group, but not the bupropion-treated group. These results provide new evidence that the increase in body weight that occurs following smoking cessation is related to increases in food reward, and that food reward is partly determined by genetic factors. Bupropion's efficacy in attenuating abstinence-induced weight gain may be attributable, in part, to decreasing food reward.

Implications of pharmacogenetics research for nicotine dependence

Pharmacogenetics research on nicotine dependence treatment is in the very early stages. Although the results of these initial studies are promising, there are several stages of research needed prior to translation to clinical practice. First, initial results from pharmacogenetic trials of nicotine dependence treatment must be validated in independent trials. Pooling of data across trials and centres would also be a critical step toward increasing the power to conduct analysis of multiple genetic effects on treatment response simultaneously. This is critical, as therapeutic response is a complex phenotype, resulting from the interplay of multiple genetic factors, and analyses of individual gene effects may not capture this complexity. In addition to these important steps, additional research should be conducted to examine the benefits, risks, and challenges of conveying genetic information about smoking predisposition to the patient, clinicians and the public. For example, recent research has highlighted barriers to the clinical integration of genetic information to tailor smoking treatment and suggests that health care providers may need additional training to be equipped to educate and counsel patients (Shields et al 2004, 2005). Economic analyses of the cost-effectiveness of using genotype to tailor smoking treatment would also be necessary. Although clinical and ethical issues arising from the clinical use of genotype data in the smoking context must still be addressed, pharmacogenetic research may provide an important step toward improving the delivery and outcomes of nicotine dependence treatment.

Acknowledgement

The following individuals collaborated on the projects mentioned in this paper: W.H. Berrettini, N. Benowitz, R. Tyndale, P. Shields, K. Perkins, M. Rukstalis, F. Patterson, E.P. Wileyto, J. Audrain and C. Jepson.

References

Arinami T, Gao M, Hamaguchi H, Toru M 1997 A functional polymorphism in the promoter region of the dopamine D2 receptor gene is associated with schizophrenia. Hum Mol Genet 6:577–582

Ascher JA, Cole JO, Colin JN et al 1995 Bupropion: a review of its mechanism of antidepressant activity. J Clin Psychiatry 56:395–401

Bond C, LaForge KS, Tian M et al 1998 Single-nucleotide polymorphism in the human mu opioid receptor gene alters beta-endorphin binding and activity: possible implications for opiate addiction. Proc Natl Acad Sci USA 95:9608–9613

Colilla S, Lerman C, Shields PG et al 2005 Association of catechol-O-methyltransferase with smoking cessation in two independent studies of women. Pharmacogenet Genomics 15:393–398

Cooper JB, Bloom FE, Roth R 1996 The biochemical basis of neuropharmacology. Oxford University Press, New York

Davenport KE, Houdi AA, Van Loon GR 1990 Nicotine protects against mu-opioid receptor antagonism by beta-funaltrexamine: evidence for nicotine-induced release of endogenous opioids in brain. Neurosci Lett 113:40–46

Duan J, Wainwright MS, Comeron JM et al 2003 Synonymous mutations in the human dopamine receptor D2 (DRD2) affect mRNA stability and synthesis of the receptor. Hum Mol Genet 12:205–216

Evans WE, Relling MV 1999 Pharmacogenomics: translating functional genomics into rational therapeutics. Science 286:487–491

Fiore MC, Smith SS, Jorenby DE, Baker TB 1994 The effectiveness of the nicotine patch for smoking cessation. A meta-analysis. JAMA 271:1940–1947

Fiore MC Bailey W, Cohen S 2000 Treating tobacco use and dependence. Clinical Practice Guideline. Rockville, MD, US Department of Health and Human Services. Public Health Service

Fujieda M, Yamazaki H, Saito T et al 2004 Evaluation of CYP2A6 genetic polymorphisms as determinants of smoking behavior and tobacco-related lung cancer risk in male Japanese smokers. Carcinogenesis 25:2451–2458

Gold PB, Rubey RN, Harvey RT 2002 Naturalistic, self-assignment comparative trial of bupropion SR, a nicotine patch, or both for smoking cessation treatment in primary care. Am J Addict 11:315–331

Kirchheiner J, Klein C, Meineke I et al 2003 Bupropion and 4-OH-bupropion pharmacokinetics in relation to genetic polymorphisms in CYP2B6. Pharmacogenetics 13:619–626

Lerman C, Niaura R 2002 Applying genetic approaches to the treatment of nicotine dependence. Oncogene 21:7412–7420

Lerman C, Roth D, Kaufmann V et al 2002a Mediating mechanisms for the impact of bupropion in smoking cessation treatment. Drug Alcohol Depend 67:219–223

Lerman C, Shields PG, Wileyto EP et al 2002b Pharmacogenetic investigation of smoking cessation treatment. Pharmacogenetics 12:627–634

Lerman C, Kaufmann V, Rukstalis M et al 2004a Individualizing nicotine replacement therapy for the treatment of tobacco dependence: a randomized trial. Ann Intern Med 140:426–433

Lerman C, Wileyto EP, Patterson F et al 2004b The functional mu opioid receptor (OPRM1) Asn40Asp variant predicts short-term response to nicotine replacement therapy in a clinical trial. Pharmacogenomics J 4:184–192

Lerman C, Berrettini W, Pinto A et al 2004c Changes in food reward following smoking cessation: a pharmacogenetic investigation. Psychopharmacology (Berl) 174:571–577

Lerman C, Patterson F, Berrettini W 2005 Treating tobacco dependence: state of the science and new directions. J Clin Oncol l 23:311–323

Lerman C, Tyndale RF, Patterson F et al 2006a Nicotine metabolite ratio predicts the efficacy of transdermal nicotine for smoking cessation, under review

Lerman C, Jepson C, Wiley E et al 2006b Role of functional genetic variation in the dopamine D2 receptor (DRD2) in response to bupropion and nicotine replacement therapy for tobacco dependence: Results of two randomized clinical trials. Neuropsychopharmacology 31:231–242

Miksys S, Lerman C, Shields PG, Mash DC, Tyndale RF 2003 Smoking, alcoholism and genetic polymorphisms alter CYP2B6 levels in human brain. Neuropharmacology 45:122–132

Pontieri F, Tanda G, Orzi F, Di Chiara G 1996 Effects of nicotine on the nucleus accumbens and similarity to those of addictive drugs. Nature 382:255–257

Poolsup N, Li Wan Po A, Knight TL 2000 Pharmacogenetics and psychopharmacotherapy. J Clin Pharm Ther 25:197–220

Sanchez C, Hyttel J 1999 Comparison of the effects of antidepressants and their metabolites on reuptake of biogenic amines and on receptor binding. Cell Mol Neurobiol 19:467–489

Schoedel KA, Hoffmann EB, Rao Y, Sellers EM, Tyndale RF 2004 Ethnic variation in CYP2A6 and association of genetically slow nicotine metabolism and smoking in adult Caucasians. Pharmacogenetics 14:615–626

Schultz W 1998 Predictive reward signal of dopamine neurons. J Neurophysiol 80:1–27

Shields A, Lerman C, Sullivan P 2004 Translating emerging research on the genetics of smoking into clinical practice: Ethical and social considerations. Nicotine Tob Res 6:675–688

Shields A, Blumenthal D, Weiss K et al 2005 Barriers to translating emerging genetic research on smoking into clinical practice: perspectives of primary care physicians. J Gen Intern Med 20:131–138

Transdermal Nicotine Study Group 1991 Transdermal nicotine for smoking cessation: Six-month results from two multicenter controlled trials. JAMA 266:3133–3138

Zadina JE, Hackler L, Ge LJ, Kastin AJ 1997 A potent and selective endogenous agonist for the mu-opiate receptor. Nature 386:499–502

DISCUSSION

[Note: Dr Caryn Lerman was not able to attend the meeting and the data were kindly presented by Dr Tyndale. After the meeting, Dr Lerman added her comments to this discussion.]

Peto: From a clinical trial technique point of view I am concerned as to which, if any, of these differences are real. Some of them are based on very small numbers. The way they are analysed and described makes it impossible to assess whether the apparent heterogeneity of effect is real. You can always produce a story that will account for any heterogeneity of effects that you find. But in most cases, the differences were absolutely non-significant. If you are going to look at heterogeneity of response in clinical trials then you need to use the techniques for assessing those subgroup results that are in the 30 page meta analysis of breast cancer trials in the May 14th *Lancet* (Early Breast Cancer Trialists' Collaborative Group 2005). Is there any serious evidence of heterogeneity of response? You aren't displaying the results in ways that lets even you assess it, let alone anyone who is reading this paper.

Lerman: First, to respond to the point about statistical significance, the *DRD2* − 141 by treatment interaction in the bupropion trial was statistically significant (odds ratio [OR] = 4.99, 1.42 − 17.62, $P = 0.01$) and the main effect of genotype in the NRT study was also significant (OR = 0.44, 0.25 − 0.79, $P = 0.006$). These data were included in the slide, but perhaps the text was too small to see. With regard to the data on the role of the 3-HC/cotinine ratio in response to patch vs. spray, there was also a statistically significant interaction effect (the ORs for each treatment were compared with a Wald Test [$P = 0.04$]). Having said that, we all agree that the numbers are small for a pharmacogenetics trial. As such, the results from these initial trials should be considered hypothesis generating. We are in the process of genotyping samples from comparable trials conducted by our colleagues for the purposes of replication, and to determine if the observed effects are 'real'. Another way to address small sample sizes is to combine study sets. However, the optimal approach would be to conduct a larger scale pharmacogenetic trial with 3000–5000 participants to test for interactions between treatment effects and candidate polymorphisms identified in these initial trials. One could genotype smokers prospectively in such a study and randomize by genotype.

Peto: You can do genetic analyses restrospectively or prospectively; it doesn't matter. What matters is that you display the results in a way that lets the variation be assessed both by you and those who read what you are presenting.

Tyndale: Odds ratios are a relatively common way to do this.

Peto: Odds ratios are fine, but they have to be displayed in ways that show the uncertainty. There are ways of looking at odds ratios that allow this (Early Breast Cancer Trialists' Collaborative Group 2005).

Shiffman: What you are asking for? In this case what I would want to see is the OR for the interaction, and ideally the confidence intervals.

Lerman: I agree, and as mentioned above, the ORs for the interactions presented are statistically significant.

Peto: I'd like to see the OR in each subgroup as well as the test of whether those ORs differ. The ORs in each subgroup should be done with squares and lines giving 99% confidence intervals, not 95%. You have also got to allow for the multiplicity of hypothesis, and even that if you have a single CT polymorphism you can analyse that three ways round. There is too much data-dependent selection possible and this has gone badly wrong with genetic epidemiology.

Lerman: These data are included in the original publications. In these initial pharmacogenetic trials of medications for nicotine dependence, there are indeed issues of multiple testing, as well as sample size limitations. This is why replication and larger scale trials are essential.

Bertrand: You presented some polymorphism in the *DRD2*. My understanding is that this is the D_2 dopamine receptor. On which chromosome is the D_2 receptor located?

Walton: I think it is 11q23. Why do you ask?

Bertrand: In some cases there are genetic polymorphisms that are positively associated with smoking behaviour. How distant is this polymorphism for all the other genes that could be implicated in the interaction?

Walton: It is quite some distance from any that could be a plausible biological candidate. There is very strong linkage disequilibrium in this region.

Lerman: The LD between the *DRD2* −141 and the *DRD2* Taq1A variant (in the nearby ANKK1 gene) is about 0.48 in our sample.

Tyndale: In vitro, the *DRD2* −141 and C957T variants have been shown to have an effect on the levels of transcription and translation. The use of functional variants in pharmacogenetic trials may reveal more information than use of markers of unknown function, as the latter will produce greater error depending on the distance from the marker to the functional variant.

Bertrand: We are touching on something that is even more difficult. You mentioned that perhaps there is a different stability of the environment, or maybe you have more D_2 receptors. This touches the problem of G protein-coupled receptors (GPCRs) where response and desensitization depend on the amount of receptor in the membrane and the receptor gets internalized.

Lerman: This is an excellent point. We are currently in the process of analysing data on genetic variation in dopamine receptor interacting proteins that regulate D_2 receptor desensitization and internalization. Ultimately, in a larger trial, it would be useful to examine genetic variation within and across relevant neurotransmitter signalling pathways.

Clarke: Given that some dopaminergic markers have been related to sensation seeking or risk taking, do people give sufficient thought to differential compliance in pharmacogenetic trials of medications for nicotine dependence? In other words, what may be associated with the genetic markers is compliance rather than the pharmacological effects of the medication.

Tyndale: Good point. However, there is limited evidence from these trials for effects of genotype on compliance or side effects. As such, the effects are likely to be mediated by other mechanisms.

Shiffman: You interpreted some of the patch/spray differences in part as a function of dose. There are other possibilities. Spray requires self-administration.

Tyndale: There are several possible explanations for the role of the 3-HC/cotinine ratio in response to spray versus patch. It may be the delivery or the dose.

Shiffman: This leads to other issues. In this design, which follows the normal course of clinical treatment, time in abstinence is confounded with dose. If you want to say that you drop down from 21 to 14 mg nicotine, it is also the passage of four weeks. Are you having an effect on primary acute withdrawal that might disappear in a time-bound way rather than in a dose-dependent way?

Tyndale: Robert Walton's study isn't tapered so there may be ways to answer this. Perhaps this question can be better addressed in the context of human laboratory studies.

Shiffman: That's what we need: studies that unconfound dose and time.

Jarvis: In the current state of the art, have any of the pharmacogenomic findings been replicated? Are there any which have stood up?

Tyndale: These are the initial pharmacogenetic studies of medications for nicotine dependence. As mentioned, attempts to replicate the findings across other trials are underway. It should be mentioned, however, that in case control studies of smoking behaviour, the effects of some of these variants have not been reproduced.

Walton: Caryn Lerman's work replicates to an extent what we have done. The effects are in the same direction. But there are only two rather small studies and much larger studies are needed.

Shiffman: As we are getting into the human clinical work, I have a comment I think needs making. We have seen data on animal studies with say nine animals per group that show statistically significant effects. It's wonderful to see programs of research with multiple related studies on a particular topic. However, we need to appreciate how difficult this is to do in human clinical research. One of the things we need to appreciate as we go into the human work is the cost and time of this sort of work. I envy animal researchers who can complete a study in a couple of weeks. The study I will be presenting in my paper took two or three years and in the region of two million dollars. One solution to the problem of low statistical power is to run bigger studies, but I don't think anyone is providing the sort of time and money needed for this. We need to be clever therefore: can some of these questions be answered in a simpler way?

Corrigall: We should be proceeding by choosing our targets for large studies based on data from smaller and earlier ones that provide a compelling rationale to commit the resources, in other words, the discovery-to-development pathway. While we might argue that this approach needs some rethinking with respect to some of the tactics by which we operate within it, as I will do in my presentation, such an approach nonetheless provides a logical way to chose a target for a major study. However, we do not always appear to proceed in this way. For example, regarding the opioid system, some years ago we published a body of data on naloxone and naltrexone in animals. Neither of these opiate antagonists had any effect on nicotine self-administration across a wide range of doses. Of course one could note, as again I will do in my presentation, that the predictive validity of the self-administration model for medication development has not been demonstrated. However, there is in addition limited evidence for the effectiveness of opiate antagonists in human subjects. Before I could argue for the allocation of extensive resources to investigate the opioid system in tobacco addiction, I would want to see more convincing data from small scale studies, and a coalescing of those data to a consistent conclusion. This in turn points the need for us to define go/no-go algorithms so that we can make decisions about when it might be valuable to continue to pursue a given line of investigation, and when it should be ended.

Shiffman: Part of what is so elegant about the preclinical research is that if you run something and get a result you can then say that you need a certain control, and proceed to run that control. While human clinical researchers think that way, they don't necessarily have the freedom and resources to operate that way.

Stolerman: The comparisons being made between clinical, preclinical and epidemiological studies aren't quite getting at one of the critical aspects: it isn't because work is in animal subjects that it is group sizes are smaller; the level of control is much higher because it is laboratory-based. One also sees good data with adequate statistical power in human laboratory studies with fairly small numbers of subjects where conditions are relatively well controlled; the numbers are not as small as needed for animal studies because the previous history of the people is not as well controlled.

Peto: I think the clinical trials do need to be 10 times larger. If we are trying to work out how to treat millions of people, we should be randomizing many thousands and not many hundreds. There isn't 10 times the money to do the trials so the only way to do this is by making the trials 10 times simpler. This has been a successful strategy in some areas. The idea is to get the numbers so big that the play of chance does average out. All the pressures in the regulation of trials go towards making them more complicated, which makes them yield less reliable results: extensive auditing reduces reliability.

Tyndale: The problem with this is that we would then lose some of the additional information you get from intensive study of smaller numbers of people, which gives us some idea of where to head.

Peto: Yes, but it won't be useful if it is wrong. We do need some large simple trials as well as some smaller, more intensive ones. The trouble is that the current trial strategies are driven by regulatory departments of companies who want FDA registration. The design is affected too much by the influence of manufacturers.

Clarke: How much bigger would such trials have to be? If you were polling voting intentions, surely you would not need to poll 10 times more people to represent a country 10 times as large?

Peto: Not at all. Quite small differences in long-term quit rates would be worth knowing about, and you can't pick up these differences in trials with only a few hundred people in them. You certainly need trials with at least a few thousand if you are going to do successful genetic subgroup analyses in trials. The problem is the fact that moderate differences are worth knowing about.

West: This is pie in the sky for those of us who have to get research grants from public sources and charities. We do our power calculations on the kind of effect size that we think we are going to get and then they give us half the money we ask for. The point you make is valid but it is violated by the real world economics of doing research. I think the whole history of nicotine in clinical research could have been completely different purely by chance. Over half the placebo-controlled randomized controlled trials on NRT didn't produce a statistically significant effect. If Mike Russell's first trial with 108 subjects had come out completely negative, we might not be sitting here. His 1979 brief advice trial was misanalysed, the true effect size isn't the claimed 5% but about 1–2%. We are dealing with a noisy world when it comes to looking at clinical trial data. There is a lot of noise and not very much signal, but we do what we can with it.

Shiffman: There is also an issue about the developmental stage of the research. The question we have to face each time is do we feel we have something new enough to be worth testing definitively in a large trial? Or, how much resource do you put into these sorts of exploratory studies that help nominate and develop treatments? At this stage of the research we very much need both.

Reference

Early Breast Cancer Trialists' Collaborative Group (EBCTCG) 2005 Effects of chemotherapy and hormonal therapy for early breast cancer on recurrence and 15-year survival: an overview of the randomised trials. Lancet 365:1687–1717

Pharmacogenomics and smoking cessation

Robert Walton

Department of Clinical Pharmacology, University of Oxford, Radcliffe Infirmary, Woodstock Road, Oxford OX2 6HE, UK and MRC Laboratories, The Gambia, West Africa

Abstract. Evidence is accumulating that genes affecting dopamine function may predict response to treatment for tobacco dependence. One important genetic variant in *ANKK1* near the *DRD2* gene, which encodes the dopamine D2 receptor, has been linked to tobacco dependence and smoking cessation. The effects of this variant seem to be greater in women. However these results need to be confirmed and other neurotransmitter systems are likely to be important. Recent evidence suggests that a genetic variation in the serotonin transporter affects serotonin binding in the human brain. Social drinkers with variant alleles at this locus have lower alcohol consumption and smokers with the same variant may be more dependent on tobacco. Further work is necessary to apply these scientific findings to develop more effective interventions for smoking cessation. This will require much more powerful studies than have currently been performed. Epidemiological case control and cohort studies need to be an order of magnitude greater than those conducted to date. Finer definition of smoking phenotype will be important thus new brain imaging techniques offer the prospect of investigating mechanisms underlying tobacco dependence with increased power and precision

2006 Understanding nicotine and tobacco addiction. Wiley, Chichester (Novartis Foundation Symposium 275) p 184 –196

Evidence is accumulating that genes affecting central neurotransmitter function may to a certain extent predict the development of dependence on tobacco and response to treatment. These same genes may also be linked to dependence on other substances. Studies in the past have focused on dopaminergic pathways. Here we present evidence from studies in humans that serotonin may also be important in governing to some extent the use of tobacco and alcohol. We have recently shown that serotonin transporter (5HTT) genotype may affect serotonin neurotransmission and that 5HTT genotype may be related to level of alcohol consumption and to nicotine dependence. Much of the work to date has focused on relatively crude measures of the smoking phenotype. New techniques in brain imaging could be an important advance in the investigation of genetic effects on tobacco dependence. This chapter examines only genetic effects on nicotine pharmacodynamics—the effects of genes on nicotine pharmacokinetics are discussed elsewhere (Lerman 2006, this volume).

The genetic basis for nicotine addiction

The pleasure derived from tobacco is linked to stimulation of neurotransmitter pathways in the brain, in particular in the mesolimbic system. The precise nature of this link remains controversial but interestingly many of the neurophysiological processes underlying nicotine addiction are common to other addictive drugs with diverse pharmacological actions such as opiates, cannabis, alcohol and cocaine. Some of these pathways are dependent on dopamine neurotransmission however it seems likely that other neurotransmitters such as serotonin are also involved.

Drugs stimulate receptors on the cell bodies of dopaminergic neurones causing dopamine release thus stimulating postsynaptic dopamine receptors in the nucleus accumbens, which is thought by some to result in perception of pleasure (Koob & Le Moal 1997). Other hypotheses suggest that these mesolimbic dopaminergic pathways are necessary for the associative learning necessary to link perception of pleasure with particular external stimuli (Spanagel & Weiss 1999, Robinson & Berridge 1993). The distinction between drug 'liking' (i.e. the pleasurable effects derived from its use) and drug 'wanting' (i.e. the cravings experienced in addiction) is conceptually important, and Robinson & Berridge (2000, 1993) suggest that it is the latter subcomponent of reward, rather than hedonic pleasure, which results from critical neuroadaptations in dopaminergic systems.

These underlying theories of dependence may in fact be complementary but clearly hypotheses resting on dopamine alone cannot give the whole picture when heavily abused drugs such as benzodiazepines, which have rewarding properties, cause no dopaminergic activation. Other neurotransmitters implicated in the development of addiction include serotonin, GABA, glutamate (Wickelgreen 1998) and noradrenaline (Delfs et al 2000).

Many people experience the pleasurable effects of addictive drugs but only a few persistently abuse them. This supports the distinction between drug liking and drug craving, and suggests that positive reinforcement associated with drug use is not sufficient for addiction to develop. The molecular mechanisms underlying the enhanced drug craving seen in addicts in withdrawal may be key to explaining why only some people become dependent (Robinson & Berridge 1993) and informing strategies to combat addiction. It is also worth noting that the negative reinforcement aspects of addiction (i.e. the suggestion that drug use persists to counter the effects of drug withdrawal) do not offer a sufficient explanation either, as some drugs which result in tolerance and withdrawal do not result in dependence, such as tricyclic anti-depressants.

In addition to changes in cellular biochemistry, neuroadaptations at the synaptic level may also play an important part in establishing the cycle of addiction (Koob & Le Moal 1997). Long-term drug use results in impairment of dopaminergic function that may be related to dopamine receptor down regulation. Adaptations to the glutaminergic system also seem to be important in the development of the negative affective state and noradrenaline in the ventral forebrain has a key role in the changes associated with drug withdrawal (Delfs et al 2000). Linking the unpleasant effects of drug withdrawal with environmental stimuli may occur in the basolateral amygdala, which has been shown in animal experiments to be responsible for conditioned responses to stimuli linked with acute withdrawal (Schulteis et al 2000). These neuroadaptive changes may be responsible for associative learning processes (i.e. the classical or Pavlovian conditioned responses) that occur in addicts in relation to environmental stimuli that are temporally related to drug use. Such learning processes could play a major part in the development of cravings (i.e. excessive 'wanting') initiated by environmental stimuli that have become associated with the addictive substance, which results in the drug user seeking out new drug supplies and either persisting in drug use (i.e. dependence) or beginning again the cycle of addiction (i.e. relapse).

Genetic variation and predisposition to tobacco use

In a the first large study of genetic effects on tobacco dependence Caporaso et al (1997) found that a polymorphism in the 3′ untranslated region of the dopamine D$_2$ receptor (*DRD2*) gene was about twice as common in smokers compared to non-smokers. Originally defined as a restriction fragment length polymorphism (Taq 1A RFLP) the polymorphism results from a C to T change at position 32806 in *DRD2*. These findings linking the polymorphism to smoking confirmed earlier work (Noble et al 1994) and recent studies suggest the same link although the sizes of the effects are smaller (Bierut et al 2000, Comings et al 1996, 1997, Lerman et al 1999, Noble et al 1994).

The Taq1A RFLP lies 10 kB downstream of *DRD2* and may therefore fall within a different coding region than the *DRD2* gene or within a regulatory region. Within this downstream region, we have identified a novel kinase gene, named ankyrin repeat and kinase domain containing 1 (*ANKK1*), which contains a single serine/threonine kinase domain and is expressed at low levels in placenta and whole spinal cord RNA. This gene is a member of an extensive family of proteins involved in signal transduction pathways. The *DRD2* Taq1A RFLP is a single nucleotide polymorphism (SNP) that causes an amino acid substitution within the 11th ankyrin repeat of ANKK1 (p.Glu713Lys), which, while unlikely to affect structural integrity, may affect substrate-binding specificity. If this is the case, then changes in ANKK1 activity may provide an alternative explanation for previously described associations

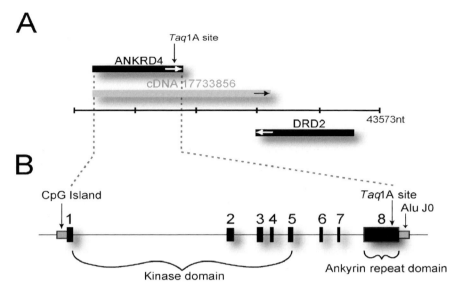

FIG. 1. The genomic organization and structure of the putative kinase gene. (A) Relative positions of transcripts around the *DRD2* locus. (B) Genomic structure of the putative kinase gene confirmed by RT-PCR. The kinase domain is highlighted in bold text and underlined, the ankyrin repeat domain is boxed, and alternate repeat units are highlighted in light and dark grey. The non-synonymous Taq1 ARFLP (dbSNP_rs1800497) causes a Glu713Lys amino acid substitution in the kinase gene.

between the *DRD2* Taq1A RFLP and neuropsychiatric disorders such as addiction.

The exact mechanism by which the allele exerts its effects on predisposition to tobacco addiction is not known. However, people with one or more of the variant alleles are believed to have reduced numbers of dopamine receptors in the corpus striatum (Thompson et al 1997). If these changes are also present in central dopaminergic reward pathways it may be that the allele is linked to impaired perception of reward. It has been suggested that an inherited dopamine deficit could be overcome by nicotine, which stimulates dopamine release thereby restoring dopamine function to normal levels (Blum et al 1996). In this way the polymorphism could confer susceptibility to tobacco use.

Several studies suggest a similar link between the nine-repeat allele of the dopamine transporter VNTR and smoking behaviour (Caporaso et al 1997, Lerman et al 1999, Sabol et al 1999). In this case the variant allele, which is related to low scores for novelty seeking and extraversion in personality questionnaires, seems to protect people from persistent smoking. The mechanism of action on a molecular level for this polymorphism has not yet been determined but it is thought to enhance dopaminergic transmission and therefore reduce the need to use nicotine to augment dopaminergic function.

A polymorphism in the dopamine D_4 receptor which results in reduced cAMP formation when the receptor is stimulated may also be linked with smoking but the strongest evidence comes from a small study in only one ethnic group and needs to be confirmed in larger studies (Shields et al 1998). Other studies on enzymes important in dopamine metabolism, such as monoamine oxidase, give further weight to the argument that dopaminergic pathways are important in tobacco dependence (McKinney et al 2000).

Genes linked with smoking predict cessation with nicotine replacement therapy

Polymorphisms in *DRD2* and in dopamine-β-hydroxylase (*DBH*) have been implicated in smoking and other reward-seeking behaviours. We therefore investigated whether these same genetic variants would predict outcome of nicotine patch therapy for smoking cessation.

In 1991–93, we performed a randomized controlled trial of the nicotine patch on 1686 heavy smokers (>15 cigarettes/day). In 1999–2000, we contacted 1532 of the 1612 subjects still available; 767 (50%) completed a questionnaire and gave a blood sample. In the 755 cases in which DNA was successfully genotyped, we examined associations between the polymorphisms in *DRD2* and *DBH*, and smoking cessation. At 1 week, the patch was more effective for smokers with *DRD2* 32806 CT/TT genotype [patch/placebo odds ratio (OR) 2.8, 95% confidence interval (CI) 1.7–4.6] than with CC (OR 1.4, 0.9–2.1; *P* for difference in ORs 0.04). Smokers with both *DRD2* CT/TT and *DBH* 1368 GA/AA genotypes had an OR of 3.6 (2.0–6.5) compared to 1.4 (1.0–2.1) for others (*P* = 0.01). At 12 weeks, the ORs for these genotypic groups were 3.6 (1.7–7.8) and 1.4 (0.9–2.3), respectively (*P* = 0.04). There was no association between patch effectiveness and the *DRD2* exon 8, 22316 polymorphism. We concluded that short-term effectiveness of the nicotine patch may be related to *DBH* and *DRD2* genotype.

In an investigation to determine whether the effects of the polymorphism were different in men and women, we measured effectiveness of the patches by the relative odds of abstinence for active and placebo patches over five cumulative time periods: one week, 12 weeks, 24 weeks, 52 weeks and to follow up. Treatment by genotype and sex, and their interaction, was examined in a full logistic regression model. The three way interaction by genotype by sex was significant for all time periods (*P* = 0.009, *P* = 0.03, *P* = 0.006, *P* = 0.006, *P* = 0.004, respectively). In women, the effectiveness of the patches differed with genotype at all time points. In men, the genotype groups did not differ significantly at any time. In both sexes, when active and placebo groups were combined, the quit rate was not related to genotype.

An association between the *DRD2* Taq1A (C32806T) polymorphism and social alcohol consumption in the opposite direction to that reported for alcoholism has recently been reported in a male Finnish sample. We attempted to replicate these findings in two independent samples, and extend on previous work by including female participants. The *DRD2 A1* allele was significantly associated with reduced alcohol consumption in sample one ($P < 0.004$) and sample two ($P < 0.015$). In sample two there was a significant genotype by sex interaction ($P < 0.016$), with the association of the *A1* allele and reduced alcohol consumption significant in men only. This interaction was marginally significant ($P < 0.042$) in a meta-analysis of combined data from both samples, and the main effect of genotype highly significant ($P = 0.001$). Age at time of data collection and cigarette consumption were entered as covariates in all analyses. These results replicate recent previous findings and suggest a possibility that this association may exist in men only, or be stronger in men.

Serotonin transporter genotype affects serotonin binding in human brain

In humans, 5-HT$_{1A}$ serotonin receptors have been implicated in affective disorders and their treatment. However, the physiological and genetic factors controlling 5-HT$_{1A}$ receptor expression have not yet been determined in health and disease. We assessed the influence of two genetic factors on 5-HT$_{1A}$ receptor expression in the living human brain using the 5-HT$_{1A}$-selective positron emission tomography (PET) ligand [^{11}C]WAY 100635. 140 healthy volunteers were genotyped to find frequencies of known SNPs in the *5HT1A* gene.

The influence of the common SNP (−1018) C > G on *5HT1A* expression was then examined in a group of 35 healthy volunteers scanned with [^{11}C]WAY 100635. We also studied the influence of a common variable number tandem repeat (VNTR) polymorphism [short (S) and long (L) alleles] of the serotonin transporter (*5HTT*) gene on 5-HT$_{1A}$ receptor density. Whereas, the *5HT1A* genotype did not show any significant effects on [^{11}C]WAY 100635 binding, 5-HT$_{1A}$ receptor binding potential values were lower in all brain regions in subjects with *5HTT-LPR* short (SS or SL) genotypes than those with long (LL) genotypes (Fig. 2). This is the first demonstration that a functional polymorphism in the *5HTT* gene, but not the *5HT1A* receptor gene, affects 5-HT$_{1A}$ receptor availability in human. The results may offer a plausible physiological mechanism underlying the association between *5HTT-LPR* genotype, behavioural traits and mood states.

In view of this demonstration of the effects of the polymorphism in the serotonin transporter on serotonin binding, we sought to replicate previous studies reporting a moderating effect of the *5HTT* gene on the association between trait

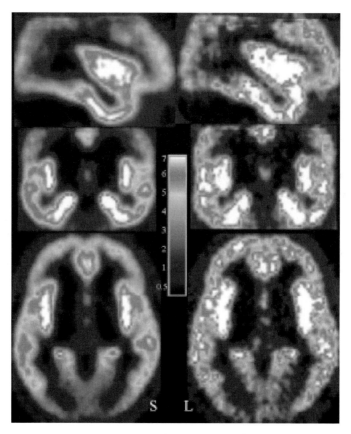

FIG. 2.   Mean positron emission tomography (PET) images of the brain showing the differential genetic effects of a functional VNTR polymorphism of the *5HTT-LPR* gene on [^{11}C]WAY 100635 binding in healthy human volunteers. Mean images of S (SS+SL) allele group (*n* = 24) is shown on the left and that of L (LL) allele group (*n* = 5) on the right. Images shown are (from the top) in the sagittal, coronal and transverse planes. The top portion of the brain is missing in these images because they were obtained using ECAT953 scanner, which has a smaller field of view (10 cm). The mean image of S allele group appears smoother than that of L allele because of larger sample size. Reproduced with permission from David et al (2005a).

neuroticism and smoking behaviour, and extend on this work by including a formal test of this interaction, in a sample of 141 heavy smokers. Nicotine dependence was measured using the Fagerstrom Test for Nicotine Dependence; trait neuroticism was assessed using the Eysenck Personality Questionnaire. All participants were genotyped for the *5HTT-LPR* polymorphism. Analysis of variance of nicotine dependence score, with genotype (L/L, L/S, S/S) and neuroticism (high, low) as between-subjects factors, indicated a significant main effect of genotype

(F[2, 135] = 3.13, $P < 0.05$) in the predicted direction, with the short allele of the *5HTT* gene being associated with higher nicotine dependence score. There was a marginal effect of neuroticism (F[1, 135] = 3.01, $P = 0.08$) in the predicted direction, with high trait neuroticism being associated with higher nicotine dependence score. The interaction effect was non-significant (F < 1). These data suggest that *5HTT* genotype is associated with nicotine dependence independently of any association between this gene and trait neuroticism that may modulate smoking behaviour.

New techniques in brain imaging offer the fine definition of phenotype necessary for genetic investigation of smoking behaviour

Converging evidence from several theories of the development of incentive sensitization to smoking-related environmental stimuli suggests that the ventral striatum plays an important role in the processing of visual and other cues related to the development of tobacco dependence. We examined 26 healthy, right-handed volunteers (16 smokers and 12 non-smoking controls) with functional magnetic resonance imaging (fMRI) during which neutral and smoking-related images were presented. We then examined changes in fMRI signal related to brain activation within the ventral striatum/nucleus accumbens to compare the effects of smoking-related and neutral cues (Fig. 3). Preferential brain activation for smoking-related cues was observed in smokers but not in non-smokers in medial orbitofrontal cortex, superior frontal gyrus, anterior cingulate cortex and posterior fusiform gyrus, and in the ventral striatum and nucleus accumbens. This is the first demonstration of greater brain activation in this important part of the central reward pathway in addicted smokers compared to non-smokers presented with smoking-related cues. These finding are consistent with cue reactivity studies of other drugs of abuse and constitute an fMRI-determined phenotype that could usefully be examined in relation to genetic variations in future studies on tobacco dependence.

Summary

Some evidence exists that inherited differences affect the propensity to develop substance use although the effects of single genes appears to be relatively small (Munafo et al 2004). These or other genetic differences may also affect response to therapy for tobacco dependence and thus could lead to the development of personalized therapy for tobacco dependence. ANKK1 and the 5HTT are currently lead candidates to explain the genetic component of the pharmacodynamic effects of nicotine. More powerful studies are needed to dissect the underlying mechanisms more fully and particularly to explore the interaction between different genes. Larger case control studies may be an option but these are expensive and resources for

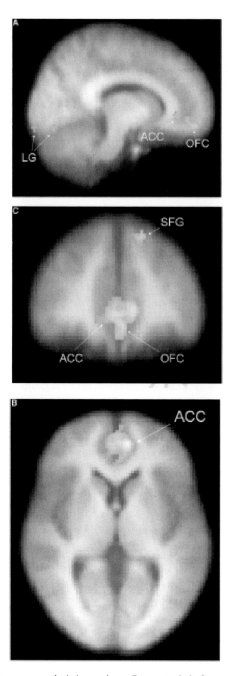

FIG. 3.   Mixed-effects group analysis in smokers. Group statistical map of three activation clusters within the mixed-effects group analysis of smokers only. Colour of clusters corresponds to increasing *Z*-statistic from dark to light yellow, but here this is shown in grey scale only. Structural image is a group-averaged T1 structural scan from all subjects in the study registered to standard space. (A) Clusters for lingual gyrus (LG), anterior cingulate gyrus (AC), and orbitofrontal gyrus (OFC) are indicated with white arrows in sagittal slice (x_ _ 2). (B) Bilateral ACC activation in axial slice (z _ _2). (C) Bilateral ACC, OFC, and left superior frontal gyrus (SFG) activation in coronal slice (y_ _42). (Reproduced from David et al 2005b, with permission from Elsevier.)

research are scarce. New techniques in brain imaging may have potential for answering more complex questions on the mechanisms of tobacco dependence. Finer definition of phenotype using these methods will enable small but important effects of individual genes to be more precisely defined, thus leading to a better understanding of these complex pathways which may in turn lead to new treatments for dependence and more accurately targeted use of existing therapies.

References

Bierut LJ, Rice JP, Edenberg HJ et al 2000 Family-based study of the association of the dopamine D2 receptor gene (DRD2) with habitual smoking. Am J Med Genet 90:299–302

Blum K, Sheridan PJ, Wood RC et al 1996 The D2 dopamine receptor gene as a determinant of reward deficiency syndrome. J R Soc Med 89:396–400

Caporaso N, Lerman C, Main D et al 1997 The genetics of smoking: The Dopamine receptor (DRD2) and transporter polymorphisms in a smoking cessation study. Proc Am Assoc Cancer Res 38:168

Comings DE, Gade R, Muhleman D et al 1996 Exon and intron variants in the human tryptophan 2,3-dioxygenase gene: potential association with Tourette syndrome, substance abuse and other disorders. Pharmacogenetics 6:307–318

Comings DE, Gade R, Wu S et al 1997 Studies of the potential role of the dopamine D1 receptor gene in addictive behaviors. Mol Psychiatry 2:44–56

David SP, Murthy NV, Rabiner EA et al 2005a Functional genetic variation of the serotonin (5-HT) transporter affects 5-HT1A receptor binding in humans. J Neurosci 25:2586–2590

David SP, Munafò MR, Johansen-Berg H et al 2005b Ventral striatum/nucleus accumbens activation to smoking-related pictorial cues in smokers and nonsmokers: A functional magnetic resonance imaging study. Biol Psychiatry 58:488–494

Delfs JM, Zhu Y, Druhan JP, Aston-Jones G 2000 Noradrenaline in the ventral forebrain is critical for opiate withdrawal-induced aversion. Nature 403:430–434

Koob GF, Le Moal M 1997 Drug abuse: hedonic homeostatic dysregulation. Science 278:52–58

Lerman C 2006 Pharmacogenetic approaches to nicotine dependence treatment. In: Understanding nicotine and tobacco addiction. Wiley, Chichester (Novartis Found Symp 275) p 171–183

Lerman C, Caporaso NE, Audrain J et al 1999 Evidence suggesting the role of specific genetic factors in cigarette smoking. Health Psychol 18:14–20

McKinney E, Walton RT, Yudkin P et al 2000 Association between polymorphisms in dopamine metabolic enzymes and tobacco consumption in smokers. Pharmacogenetics 10:1–9

Munafo M, Clark T, Johnstone E, Murphy M, Walton R 2004 The genetic basis for smoking behavior: a systematic review and meta-analysis. Nicotine Tob Res 6:583–597

Noble EP, St Jeor ST, Ritchie T et al 1994 D2 dopamine receptor gene and cigarette smoking: a reward gene? Med Hypotheses 42:257–260

Robinson TE, Berridge KC 1993 The neural basis of drug craving: an incentive-sensitization theory of addiction. Brain Res Brain Res Rev 18:247–291

Robinson TE, Berridge KC 2000 The psychology and neurobiology of addiction: an incentive-sensitization view. Addiction 95 Suppl 2:S91–117

Sabol SZ, Nelson ML, Fisher C et al 1999 A genetic association for cigarette smoking behavior. Health Psychol 18:7–13

Schulteis G, Ahmed SH, Morse AC, Koob GF, Everitt BJ 2000 Conditioning and opiate withdrawal. Nature 405:1013–1014

Shields PG, Lerman C, Audrain J et al 1998 Dopamine D4 receptors and the risk of cigarette smoking in African- Americans and Caucasians. Cancer Epidemiol Biomarkers Prev 7:453–458

Spanagel R, Weiss F 1999 The dopamine hypothesis of reward: past and current status. Trends Neurosci 22:521–527

Thompson J, Thomas N, Singleton A et al 1997 D2 dopamine receptor gene (DRD2) Taq1 A polymorphism: reduced dopamine D2 receptor binding in the human striatum associated with the A1 allele. Pharmacogenetics 7:479–484

Wickelgreen I 1998 Teaching the brain to take drugs. Science 280:2045–2047

DISCUSSION

Stolerman: I have a naïve pharmacological point. With regard to both nicotine and alcohol you found a genomic variation correlates with or predicts a certain type of outcome in terms of use of a substance or success in treatment. How do you interpret this? Is it due to differences in response to the drugs under study, or is there something else like a personality variation such as impulsivity (which is linked with serotonin) that might account through that variable for a change in tendency to use any substance?

Walton: That's a good question. It's easy to be wise at the end of the study: I wish we had collected personality data in this study. We did discuss it, but we chose not to collect it because there would be too much in the questionnaire. We have, however, conducted a meta analysis of genetic effects on personality (Munafo et al 2004) which implicated to an extent both *DRD2* and *5HTT* although the effects are relatively small.

Stolerman: What always puzzles me is that I see these sophisticated genetic studies, and then I think that in a year or two I am going to find out something about the relative sensitivity of these genetically distinct populations to the target drug, which may or may not be relevant to differences in use. I never seem to get this information. People don't seem to go from doing this kind of study to laboratory psychopharmacology, which only requires a comparatively small number of subjects.

Walton: Our next move with the fMRI is to take people who are homozygous for some of these variants and give them a scan.

Stolerman: I hope you will be looking at them with and without the drug (i.e. doing some pharmacology).

Bertrand: Nicotine receptors have been shown to be very sensitive to steroids (Paradiso et al 2001, Curtis et al 2002, Valera et al 1992). Your studies show male–female differences: does this have anything to do with the oestrous cycle? Is there a change with hormone replacement therapy?

Walton: I started out fairly sceptical about these male–female differences in smoking. I am coming round to believe them, and there are plausible biological mechanisms. One thing we are looking at is the promoter of the *DRD2* gene to see whether there are steroid hormone response elements, or polymorphisms that might predict responses to steroid hormones at transcription factor binding sites.

Changeux: I was not clear about the strategy that led you to look at these particular genes. Is there a general approach for selecting genes, or do you just choose some that might be related to dopamine? You know dopamine is a strategic molecule. If you look at other, irrelevant areas of the brain would you see similar effects?

Walton: It's the latter approach. The Taq1a variant which was previously used in connection with the dopamine D_2 receptor (now shown to be in ANKK1) is associated with reduced numbers of receptors.

Changeux: Is there any general genetic approach which led you to select the dopamine receptor gene, or did you look at dopamine receptor related genes?

Walton: The latter. We went for the dopamine D_2 receptor because it seemed like the most plausible candidate mechanistically.

Changeux: You could take the opposite approach which is to start from an epidemiological study and restrict the number of subjects to the heaviest smokers to see whether there is a genetic predisposition for smoking. Is this approach feasible?

Walton: Yes, certainly. That would essentially be a whole-genome study. I haven't planned such a study because the analysis would be complex and the methodologies not yet completely worked out. It would be an interesting experiment to do.

Changeux: There is a heavy bias here towards the dopamine system.

Walton: We are starting to get the tools now: we can get large numbers of single nucleotide polymorphism (SNPs) done simultaneously using chips.

Changeux: You could have a large set of samples and within this sample test for occurrence of particular genes that you suspect already may be involved.

Walton: The chances of throwing up something by chance in that kind of exercise would be high.

Hajek: Have you looked at any other genes?

Walton: We have looked at catechol-*O*-methyltranferase, and a variety of other dopamine related genes. There seems to be no relationship between catechol-*O*-methyl transferase and smoking behaviour (David et al 2002). We found some evidence that monoamine oxidase and DBH are linked to high level of tobacco consumption (McKinney et al 2000) and unpublished data suggesting no link with the dopamine transporter.

Hajek: When you were looking at male–female differences did you look at other differences, such as high and low dependence?

Walton: Yes we analysed the data, using a regression model including these factors.

Clarke: In a study like this where you are screening for a lot of measures taken from the same individuals, is there a way of protecting against false positives?

Walton: We address this by setting α at a particular level, say 0.01. If we are doing odds ratios we use 99% confidence intervals rather than 95%. We can use a Bonferroni correction, which involves dividing the P value by the total number of comparisons: this gives a more conservative α—thought by some to be overly conservative

Clarke: The problem with the Bonferroni correction is that it assumes that the measures are independent of each other. This may not be the case.

Walton: Arbitrary selection of a relatively low α value seems like a relatively straightforward way of taking multiple comparisons in to account.

Stolerman: If you have a large number of variables, 0.01 is not a very small value for α.

Peto: You need a difference of about five standard errors rather than two. To go from 2.5 standard errors ($P = 0.01$) to five standard errors only involves a fourfold increase in sample size, but it will filter out all sorts of things that aren't true.

Walton: From the pharmacogenetics perspective it would be nice if we could construct one large study of a few thousand people.

Tyndale: I was interested in your association of the serotonin polymorphism with the Fagerstrom score. Was there any particular question in the Fagerstrom that was driving the association?

Walton: It's an interesting observation but I wouldn't push it too far—there were only 120 people in this group for whom we had questionnaire data. But the story hangs together in that people with the short form of the transporter polymorphism (associated in some studies with neuroticism) have lower 5-HT$_{1A}$ binding potential, a higher Fagerstrom score and tend to drink a little more alcohol.

References

Curtis L, Buisson B, Bertrand S, Bertrand D 2002 Potentiation of human alpha4beta2 neuronal nicotinic acetylcholine receptor by estradiol. Mol Pharmacol 61:127–135

David SP, Johnstone E, Griffiths SE et al 2002 No association between functional catechol O-methyl transferase 1947A > G polymorphism and smoking initiation, persistent smoking or smoking cessation. Pharmacogenetics 12:265–268

McKinney EF, Walton RT, Yudkin P et al 2000 Association between polymorphisms in dopamine metabolic enzymes and tobacco consumption in smokers. Pharmacogenetics 10:483–491

Munafo M, Clark T, Johnstone E, Murphy M, Walton R 2004 The genetic basis for smoking behavior: a systematic review and meta-analysis. Nicotine Tob Res 6:583–597

Paradiso K, Zhang J, Steinbach JH 2001 The C-terminus of the human nicotinic alpha4beta2 receptor forms a binding site required for potentiation by an estrogenic steroid. J Neurosci 21:6561–6568

Valera S, Ballivet M, Bertrand D 1992 Progesterone modulates a neuronal nicotinic acetylcholine receptor. Proc Natl Acad Sci USA 89:9949–9953

General discussion II

Power in studies

West: Power in studies is a really tricky problem. I don't think we are necessarily going to solve it by larger studies. It is a classic signal:noise issue. Perhaps the way to address it is by more traditional signal detection type approaches across studies, or some sort of Bayesian statistical approach. This would involve coordinated efforts across studies and research groups, in which you can take a more strategic approach to the detection of the signal from the noise in this situation where you are starting out with a wide range of hypotheses. Is a Bayesian approach feasible here?

Markou: Could you elaborate what you mean by 'Bayesian'?

West: Rather than going down the standard route of significance testing, you start with an a priori probability and you adjust the odds of the hypothesis being true incrementally on the basis of each new result that comes in. It is a probability adjustment process. It has been advocated for many years by statisticians.

Peto: Almost all conclusions are in one sense 'Bayesian'. We start off with some idea of how plausible they are, then we get evidence and in the light of this evidence we modify our prior judgement as to how plausible it is to get our conclusions. Almost all sensible thought is Bayesian, if that is what Bayesian means. In the past the term 'Bayesian' got itself into disrepute, however, because peoples' prior hypotheses were often so silly that they were producing silly conclusions. You need sensible priors. I don't think this is going to help much in the particular case of dealing with multiple results from genetic analyses. Probably, most genes aren't importantly relevant, but there may be some that are. There are so many single nucleotide polymorphisms (SNPs) conveniently available that just by the play of chance we are going to get some of them seeming at first sight to be strikingly associated with any characteristic you like. There are so many different diseases and so many different genotypes, we are going to get hundreds of thousands of potential associations flowing through the computers of the world and generating publishable papers with false-positive results. I think the rough general rule is that if something is real in a not-very-preselected gene then you need something of the order of four or five standard errors before you should start believing it. Using two standard errors ($P = 0.05$) has been a disaster: it generates so many false positives.

Perkins: The biggest problem is that we have a dichotomous outcome: quit or not quit. When an interaction is added to the analysis, this results in the explosion of the necessary sample size. One way around this is to go to a continuous variable, if you can, such as survival analysis of days to relapse. Otherwise I don't see any way around this.

Peto: It doesn't make much difference to the problem. There are so many different medical questions that could have genetic correlates; and there are so many false-positive genetic correlates that will come flooding out of these multiple SNP machines.

Perkins: I am talking about a trial with a treatment by genetic comparison. This involves a two by two interaction (at least), which requires a much greater sample.

Peto: I think it would be better to ask for at least three standard errors on a trial result, because even if you have three standard errors the 95% confidence interval still goes down to only one third of your apparent results, indicating fivefold uncertainty as to how real the effect is.

Perkins: That is fine, but if you have a dichotomous outcome you reduce the power of most samples. I am saying that to try to solve the conundrum caused by the dichotomous dependent variable you could try to go to a continuous variable.

Peto: It could be slightly more sensitive but it makes little difference to power. It doesn't deal with the subgroup problem.

Shiffman: It is interesting that we are mixing up what are almost opposites. That is, power deals with false negatives, which we want to avoid, but the problem you are pointing to is one of false positives.

Peto: Large numbers help in both respects.

Markou: Five standard deviations would be a really nice effect. However, would you advocate this high standard also for new compounds that could make it in the market with lower standards and still be very helpful to clinical populations? In psychiatry there is a desperate need for new treatments. We'd be happy with even one standard deviation there, if indeed it was reliable.

Peto: I think the desperate need is for new treatments that *work*. If you look at Chinese traditional medicine there are loads of new treatments, but do they work? For antidepressants, for example, can you prevent major relapse with antidepressants? We know that the answer is yes, because so many patients have been randomized in so many trials. If we put all these randomized trial results together we now have a 10 standard error difference between treatment and control: such antidepressants do, on average, work. Patients need clear evidence like this, but still, many doctors who should know better aren't offering them to patients who need to be offered them. It takes serious evidence, seriously disseminated, to change practice on a large scale.

Markou: Maybe lowering the standard would lead to advancement in the field.

Peto: No, it would be a massive step backwards. You'd have a deluge of financially motivated adverts for all sorts of things, and no one would have a clue what was real and what wasn't. Things that did work would be underutilized and lots of money would be spent on things that don't work. Lewis Thomas, who was head of the Sloan Kettering Institute in New York for a time and who observed medicine for more than half a century, from the 1930s to 1980s, said that he felt the greatest breakthrough of 20th century medicine wasn't the structure of DNA or the discovery of penicillin, but the realization that most of the things that were being done probably didn't do any good at all, and there was no way of knowing which of the things did do good. With serious evidence you can transform worldwide medical practice.

Clarke: I think Athina Markou's point is that where a false negative is very expensive, then maybe the trade-off between false positives and false negatives has to be readjusted, at least in preliminary trials.

Peto: In preliminary trials you don't know whether things are going to work so you have to take a guess as to what is plausible. But if we want to change medical practice we need strong results from large-scale randomized evidence.

Walton: I wonder if a two-step procedure is helpful: we could do an explanatory study, say with imaging, as a surrogate. Then, if a particular genetic marker is positive in that study we can carry it through into a clinical study.

Receptor desensitization

Bertrand: I'd like to raise the issue of receptor desensitization. There are two types, fast and slow. When you apply nicotine for a long time (minutes), the receptors will desensitize and progressively do not respond, even to 10 nM nicotine. The question is whether in animal models or humans receptor activation or desensitization is occurring. Which one is mediating the effect of nicotine?

Clarke: Animal studies as they are conducted tend to favour behavioural effects that are the result of nicotinic receptor stimulation rather than desensitization. It is hard to find any effect of nicotine in the animal literature that is not blocked by mecamylamine. But this may not reflect the human condition. Let's consider the nicotinic receptors that control dopamine release. David Balfour has shown nicely that if you give a rat 24 h exposure to nicotine via osmotic minipump, at the level found in the daytime in a moderate/heavy smoker, then acute nicotine challenge no longer induces dopamine release in the nucleus accumbens. I don't believe there are any human studies in non-abstinent smokers that would tell us whether nicotine or smoking during the daytime in a free-smoking individual would increase dopamine release. I believe all the studies done to date were done in abstinent smokers.

Brody: In our study, smokers were abstinent for 2 h prior to smoking, so that the abstinence period may explain why we were able to indirectly demonstrate dopamine release with smoking.

Clarke: There are also some interesting animal studies, again with minipumps, which ask what are the remaining functional nicotinic receptors in rats that are chronically infused with nicotine (Salminen et al 1999, 2000). The answer is that not all nicotinic receptors shut off under these conditions. It depends which brain area is being examined. The rate of recovery after continuous nicotine infusion also depends on brain area.

Picciotto: It is not clear at all that this is an either/or question. Both desensitization and activation can be going on simultaneously, and both can contribute to behavioural effects of nicotine in animal studies as well as in smokers. Perhaps a more nuanced question is which aspects of behaviour that we are looking at are most influenced by desensitization and which are most influenced by activation.

Changeux: I think the question of the action of nicotine on activation versus desensitization is a crucial one, if one wants to relate molecular properties of receptors to behaviour. Nicotine as an agonist may act on both depending on the mode of application and with different time-scales. Brief application (milliseconds) yields activation; prolonged exposure results in desensitization. One should also be aware of a few characteristic aspects of desensitization. First, the kinetic parameters of desensitization may vary with the subunit combination of the receptor oligomers. Some types of receptor oligomers desensitize very quickly, others very slowly. Second, the timescales of desensitization range between 100 ms to a few minutes. Under the conditions of standard pharmacological experiments *in vivo*, these are very short times. Moreover when a drug like nicotine is injected in the organism, its dynamics of access to the target receptors is much slower and prolonged compared with the dynamics of the release of the neurotransmitter. As Marina says, and in agreement with Langley (1905)'s and Katz & Thesleff (1957)'s early experiments, one can have activation together with desensitization in a sequential fashion. For instance, a puff of nicotine causes first activation and then desensitization. A brief activation may then trigger a cascade of effects at the level of second messenger systems which may last a longer time. It might then be difficult to sort out what is due to activation, to the secondary consequences of activation and to desensitization. I think one should at least make a clear distinction between the acute effects of nicotine and the long-term exposure effects.

Moreover, with the long-term effects another problem is raised. We know that on top of desensitization, chronic exposure to nicotine leads to an up-regulation of receptor sites (see Sallette et al 2005). Does it result in a loss or in an increase in receptor function after long-term exposure? We have compared knockout mice without exposure to nicotine and wild-type mice that have been chronically exposed to nicotine. We have done this twice. The first time was by following the respiratory reflex after a stress response by anoxia in the adult. In this kind of stress response, the knockout animals respond less efficiently. If the same experiment is done with animals chronically exposed to nicotine the result is quite similar (Cohen et al 2002). This experiment has been repeated with newborn mice, looking at their respiration after the mothers have been chronically exposed to nicotine. The wild-type pups that have been chronically exposed to nicotine have the same phenotype as the knockout pups (Cohen et al 2005). It looks as if the chronic exposure to nicotine gives a negative phenotype as far as the nicotine receptors are concerned. This is supporting the idea that chronic exposure to nicotine results in some kind of functional inactivation. But then this raises the issue of the contribution of up-regulation to these processes. Is there a functionally positive effect of up-regulation? The timescale of the experiments we have been using is a rather long one: several weeks. Is up-regulation playing a positive role in an intermediate scale or does it have a negative role? This has to be further understood.

Balfour: What Marina Picciotto was saying is correct: as an injection of nicotine is given there is stimulation and then desensitization. The plasma level of nicotine matters, with respect to what desensitizes. We have argued that different subtypes of receptor desensitize at different concentrations. What I didn't show yesterday is that if you use the lowest dose of nicotine that we used in the minipumps, which gives a venous blood nicotine concentration of about 10 ng/ml, it sensitizes the dopamine system to an acute challenge in an otherwise drug naïve animal. It not only doesn't block the sensitized response, it evokes it. We have speculated as to how this happens, but what it demonstrates is that different receptors desensitize at different concentrations. As you inject, you go through all of these concentrations and come back down again.

As I was listening to Christian Heidbreder's paper I began to see commonalities between what I was trying to suggest earlier and hypotheses for the D_3 receptor. I was trying to argue that what was important was a paracrine release of dopamine that was acting as a hormone within the nucleus accumbens, and having to travel to the receptors. What we are hearing this morning is that blockade of D_3 receptors seems to influence responding for drugs of abuse, where there is a large, sustained increase in dopamine overflow, but not that important for natural reinforcers. My speculation is that we might have been talking about the same thing: these D_3 receptors are located on cells, and what the drugs are doing is allowing the dopamine to get to these receptors. This doesn't happen under normal physiological circumstances because the burst firing is too short, or it doesn't happen at all. When you get pathological over-eating, what you might be seeing is a pathological burst firing which mimics what is happening with the drug of dependence. My prediction is that the D_3 receptors are almost hormonal receptors as opposed to strictly transmitter receptors. They only come into play when the dopamine is allowed to diffuse to those receptors.

Heidbreder: This is an interesting point. At a resting dopamine concentration of 5 nM, relative affinities predict that the D_3 receptor is 14% occupied, while occupancies of D_1 and D_2 receptors are approximately 0.2%. At a dopamine concentration of 250 nM, low affinity state D_3 receptor occupancy is 90%, while D_1 and

D_2 receptor low affinity state occupancy is approximately 10%. Intracerebral microdialysis studies and fast-scan cyclic voltammetry generally report basal extracellular dopamine levels between 3 and 5 nM. Measurements of transient stimulated extracellular dopamine concentrations range from 120 nM during high frequency stimulation trains to approximately 250 nM following a single-stimulus pulse, suggesting transient synaptic dopamine concentrations as high as 1.6 mM, taking into account the geometry of the synaptic cleft. When the dopamine transporter is blocked by stimulant drugs such as cocaine or amphetamine, clearance is slowed, and the decline in dopamine concentration is slowed. This leads to prolonged periods of elevated dopamine concentrations, with average concentrations in the range of 750 nM as determined by microdialysis. Thus, the 70-fold greater affinity for dopamine dictates low-affinity state D_3 occupancy of 96% at this dopamine concentration, compared to occupancy of 25% for D_1 and 27% for D_2 receptors.

Clarke: I'd say it is very difficult to guess the extent of occupancy of the D_3 receptor. 5 nM has been reported to be a basal level of dopamine, but the latest data would perhaps put this figure an order of magnitude higher (Wightman & Robinson 2002). Do spare receptors occur with D_3 receptors? In some systems you only need to occupy a few percent of the receptors to get maximal response. Raising occupancy from x to y may not have any functional consequence.

Bertrand: Autocrine versus paracrine is an important issue that touches on our work. If you take the example of the GABA receptor, it has been shown that they are expressed as an extrasynaptic receptor which is supposed to respond to responses. The difference that you need for an autocrine-type receptor is that the desensitization should not be too high. This means that the release of neurotransmitter in the extrasynaptic cleft is going to be sustained over a long period. One of the questions we have to ask ourselves is how much it desensitizes and how much internalized. For some of the G protein receptors, if you internalize the receptors they disappear for a long time. The question is how much receptor is available and how the transmission is mediated.

Peto: Even if you have the mechanism dead right, and these D_3 receptors are fundamental, and you can get something very specific binding, then if what you said is true that the difference between 20% occupancy and 96% occupancy might mean only a moderate difference in cellular function, this emphasizes that it would be a dreadful thing to lose something of moderate value because it wasn't of colossal value. It would be such a pity to lose something to a false negative in the trials because the design was too complicated and the trial wasn't big enough. There are circumstances when things are picked up in large, simple trials that are missed in smaller, more complicated trials, and vice versa. We need both strategies when we have a compound that seems promising enough to take into trials.

References

Cohen G, Han ZY, Grailhe R et al 2002 β2 nicotinic acetylcholine receptor subunit modulates protective responses to stress: A receptor basis for sleep-disordered breathing after nicotine exposure. Proc Natl Acad Sci USA 99:13272–13277

Cohen G, Roux JC, Grailhe R, Malcolm G, Changeux JP, Lagercrantz H 2005 Perinatal exposure to nicotine causes deficits associated with a loss of nicotinic receptor function. Proc Natl Acad Sci USA 102:3817–3821

Katz B, Thesleff S 1957 A study of the 'desensitization' produced by acetylcholine at the motor endplate. J Physiol (Lond) 138:63–80

Langley JN 1905 On the reaction of cells and of nerve-endings to certain poisons, chiefly as regards the reaction of striated muscleto nicotine and curari. J Physiol (Lond) 33:374–413

Sallette J, Pons S, Devillers-Thiery A et al 2005 Nicotine upregulates its own receptors through enhanced intracellular maturation. Neuron 46:595–607

Salminen O, Seppä T, Gäddnäs H, Ahtee L 1999 The effects of acute nicotine on the metabolism of dopamine and the expression of Fos protein in striatal and limbic brain areas of rats during chronic nicotine infusion and its withdrawal. J Neurosci 19:8145–8151

Salminen O, Seppa T, Gaddnas H, Ahtee L 2000 Effect of acute nicotine on Fos protein expression in rat brain during chronic nicotine and its withdrawal. Pharmacol Biochem Behav 66:87–93

Wightman RM, Robinson DL 2002 Transient changes in mesolimbic dopamine and their association with 'reward'. J Neurochem 82:721–735

What limits the efficacy of current nicotine replacement therapies?

Peter Hajek

Barts and The London, Queen Mary's School of Medicine and Dentistry, University of London, Turner Street, London E1 2AD, UK

Abstract. Nicotine replacement therapy (NRT) represents the first real breakthrough in treatment of tobacco dependence. The current nicotine replacement products double the efficacy of behaviour treatments alone and are widely used. However, even with the best current treatments, NRT or others, most smokers fail in their quit attempt. The presentation discusses the following riddle: if smokers smoke for nicotine, why are nicotine replacement treatments not 100% effective? A range of possible explanations is considered, including the effect of other chemicals in tobacco smoke, insufficient dosing, insufficient speed of delivery, insufficient duration of use, lack of targeting types of smokers likely to benefit from NRT, and limitations of focusing on withdrawal relief alone. There exists limited experimental evidence for at least some of these pointers. There may well be scope for improving efficacy of the existing NRT products e.g. via improving the targeting of treatment, NRT pre-loading prior to smoking cessation, and prolonged NRT use. Developing faster and higher delivery products for long-term use which would replace some of the subjectively positive effects of smoking (enhanced nicotine replacement, ENRT) is likely to further improve the reach and impact of treatment.

2005 Understanding nicotine and tobacco addiction. Wiley, Chichester (Novartis Foundation Symposium 275) p 204–218

This presentation concerns a simple question which I have heard asked by students and patients long before being invited to contemplate it at this Symposium. It is a good question, and it goes: 'If people smoke for nicotine, why are nicotine replacement treatments not more effective?'

Before we start to consider some of the possible answers, one clarification is needed. It is not the intention of this article to imply that nicotine replacement treatment (NRT) is ineffective. NRT has been the first important breakthrough in treating tobacco dependence. There is no doubt about its efficacy, and it remains the reference treatment to be improved upon. Sustained abstinence rates of treatments combining NRT and behavioural support are around 50% short-term (one month) and 15% long-term (one year) even when practiced in routine care on a large scale with highly dependent and predominantly disadvantaged smokers (Judge et al 2005, Ferguson et al 2005). Quit rates in untreated smokers are a small fraction of this (RCP 2000). Nevertheless, as positive as these results may be in this notoriously difficult field, there is of course a substantial scope for improvement.

Throughout the rest of the article, we will be encountering gaps in our knowledge of optimal use of NRT. We have only limited data available on essential and easily researched issues such as whether NRT efficacy can be improved by faster nicotine delivery, higher doses, prolonged use prior to quitting smoking, or prolonged use of oral products after quitting smoking. In fact, since nicotine chewing gum was developed in the 1970s (Ferno et al 1973) and nicotine spray and patch in the early 1980s (Russell et al 1983, Rose et al 1984), there have only been small marketing-oriented additions such as new oral products mimicking the gum effects (inhalator, microtab and lozenges), changes in flavouring and tinkering with the patch. Some critics say there has been no new development in NRT for over 20 years (Fagerstrom 2005).

One obstacle to the full development of the nicotine replacement idea seems to be the long-standing attitudes to recreational use of nicotine, mixed with, by now largely irrational, safety concerns. The prevailing view considers the evils of smoking virtually identical with nicotine use and insists that patients must stop using nicotine, rather than just stop using it in a way which is dangerous to health. Although this outlook is weakening, by and large it still dominates the field and it may explain the reluctance to look into improving NRT products. Smoking behaviour is driven by positive reinforcement generated by immediate effects of smoking which are perceived as pleasant, and negative reinforcement generated by discomfort which dependent smokers experience during periods of abstinence. An ideal NRT product would provide both of these effects. The existing products mostly focus on withdrawal relief. In a somewhat puritanical way, NRT seems acceptable only as long as quitting smoking remains painfully difficult. Designing NRTs aiming at an effortless switch from cigarettes to a safe long-term alternative is still considered a highly controversial (though no longer a totally irresponsible) idea.

The history of NRT research may perhaps suggest another possible reason for the slowing down of development in this area after the early discoveries. The first nicotine replacement product, nicotine chewing gum, was launched by a small Swedish company, AB Leo. As its products for smokers grew in stature and presumably in profits, the company has been taken over by ever larger partners, becoming Kabi (1984), Pharmacia (1990), Pharmacia Upjohn (1995) and Pfizer (2003). During the Leo and early Kabi years, the company collaborated with leading Swedish, UK and US researchers who were designing, running and analysing their own trials with the company's eager collaboration but without any interference. Despite several factors acting against more adventurous projects, including limited resources and worry that NRT may produce adverse health effects, the progress was swift, driven largely by independent scientists. With passing years, the resources of NRT manufacturers grew and the fear of nicotine subsided as it was becoming increasingly obvious that the product is one of the safest treatments in the whole of the pharmacopoeia. Research, however, seems to have become increasingly conservative, designed exclusively in-house, with marketing considerations the dominant research priority.

We shall visit the following hypothetical answers to the question of what limits the efficacy of existing NRT treatments.

1. There may be other substances in tobacco smoke apart from nicotine which contribute to compulsive self-dosing.
2. Current NRT products provide nicotine in too small doses and/or too slowly to mimic effects of smoking.
3. Current NRT labelling reduces NRT efficacy by not allowing sufficient duration of use, preventing use prior to quitting, and reducing product use by unnecessary precautionary warnings.
4. Current NRTs target primarily withdrawal relief and thus only work for some smokers.

We shall also consider some of the general problems likely to accompany any attempt to disable an acquired motivational drive.

There may be other substances in tobacco smoke apart from nicotine which contribute to compulsive self-dosing

There is little doubt that for most smokers, smoking behaviour aims at self-admin-istering nicotine. Pure nicotine is a reinforcing agent for animals and humans (smokers can transfer their dependence to NRT), changes in nicotine content of cigarettes lead to changes in smoking behaviour, and nicotine replacement helps with tobacco withdrawal and with stopping smoking (RCP 2000). This however does not exclude a possibility that other chemicals in tobacco smoke may contribute to its reinforcing properties either by enhancing nicotine effects, or independently. The tobacco industry is known to spike cigarettes with chemicals facilitating nico-tine uptake. Ammonia has received the most publicity, but several other additives have been suspected to enhance nicotine bioavailability and/or to potentiate effects of nicotine (Bates et al 1999). One substance which may act as an independently reinforcing agent as well as an enhancer of nicotine effects is acetaldehyde. It acts as a primary reinforcer in animal studies and has been recently shown to enhance nicotine self-administration in rats (Belluzzi et al 2005). Monoamine oxidase inhibitors in tobacco smoke may be another contributing chemical (Villegier et al 2003). Other less hopeful candidate chemicals include carbon monoxide (an unpub-lished study did not find any effect of carbon monoxide inhalations on abstaining smokers; N. Benowitz 2005, verbal communication) and nor-harman (Van Den Eijnden et al 2003). There are little data available on whether any of these candidate substances improve NRT effects. This may yet prove to be a relevant area of enquiry.

Current NRTs provide insufficient dose of nicotine and/or administer it too slowly

This is the most obvious common-sense hypothesis. NRT was initially formulated to deliver less nicotine than smoking, and warnings on its packaging still emphasize the maximum recommended dose which must not be exceeded. As the fear of nicotine subsided, the allowance for the 'maximum dose' doubled (e.g. from 15 pieces of 2 mg gum to 30 pieces of 2 mg Microtab per day), but the products still typically deliver only about half of the average daily nicotine dose from cigarette smoking.

With nicotine patches, achieving higher nicotine levels is easy. Putting on additional patches can match any nicotine delivery from cigarettes. One large trial found higher patch dose leading to slightly higher quit rates (Tonnessen et al 1999), but several other smaller studies found little or no effect (Paoletti et al 1996, Jorenby et al 1995, Hughes et al 1990, Killen et al 1999, Dale et al 1995). The available evidence suggests that it is unlikely that increased patch delivery would generate dramatically increased success rates.

Looking at the oral products, there is some evidence to suggest that higher dose delivers better outcomes, although this too may just reflect under-dosing with low use or weaker products. Firstly, higher NRT use is typically associated with better outcomes (e.g. Shiffman et al 2002). Self-selection may play a role here. Better evidence can be found in studies comparing 2 mg and 4 mg gum, where 4 mg gum showed superior efficacy (Silagy et al 2004). The fly in the ointment is patient behaviour. In theory, users of oral NRT can titrate their nicotine intake to match their need, but in practice it is a hard task to encourage them to use even the modest recommended dose. In patients allowed to experiment with different strengths of NRT, individual levels of dependence or habitual nicotine intake do not predict the choice of NRT strength (Hajek et al 1988). It seems that for most NRT users any positive NRT effects are too weak or too slow to reinforce product use. Other contributing factors may involve the unattractiveness of the products, the still widespread fear of nicotine, and the tenor of the medical presentation of the products with strict warnings against excessive use (see below).

The speed of nicotine delivery is another factor of prominent interest. Nicotine from cigarettes reaches the brain in a high concentration in a discreet 'bolus' within seconds of inhalation. This is considered the key to its perceived positive effects, including hypothetical associated processes mediating reinforcing properties of smoking such as release of cortisol (Kirschbaum et al 1992). For most smokers reinforcing effects of smoking are likely to be related to the post-inhalation nicotine bolus more closely than to the systemic nicotine levels. Current NRT products cannot match the speed of nicotine delivery or the bolus provided by smoking. However, they differ in the rate in which they deliver nicotine and this may provide some pointers as to whether this is important, and to possible product improvements.

Unfortunately, in the existing NRT products, there is a close relationship between speed of nicotine delivery and the initial unpleasantness of product use. The fact that there are no substantial differences between products in efficacy (Hajek et al 2002) could be due to the trade off between product's efficacy and patients' adherence. For example nicotine nasal spray is the fastest nicotine delivery device available so far, but it is also the least user friendly of the available products. It is worth noticing that it is achieving parity with the other products despite the much lower product compliance, and in fact the absolute quit rates and the odds ratio for spray-placebo difference are larger (although not significantly so) than for the other NRT products (Silagy et al 2004).

Another indirect indicator of the importance of speed of nicotine delivery can be found in between-product differences in the likelihood that patients would want to use them long-term. The faster the nicotine absorption, the higher the 'dependence potential' of the product (West et al 2000). It is likely that in a hypothetical trial only including subjects who can tolerate and fully use any of the products, the spray would prove to be the most effective, followed by the oral products, followed by patches.

Apart from developing new products, there is a scope for improving the existing ones with regards to both speed and volume of nicotine delivery, but the product manufacturers seem reluctant to take this route. For instance the existing nicotine inhalator only allows modest nicotine delivery at a cost of vigorous and frequent puffing. The volume of nicotine vapour can be easily increased by using more or larger cartridges and a wider inhalation aperture. Such a device has been developed and its enhanced delivery well documented (R. West 2003, verbal communication), but it has generated no obvious interest from NRT manufacturers so far. A device allowing genuine inhalation of nicotine could be expected to significantly surpass the efficacy of the existing products.

In summary, there is some evidence that NRT efficacy may be limited by current restrictions on nicotine dose and especially on the speed of its delivery. It is likely that more efficient nicotine delivery systems would be more effective.

Current NRT labelling restricts NRT efficacy

Current NRT labelling restricts its use in several ways which may be detrimental to NRT efficacy. We already discussed the various restrictions on NRT dose. This may prevent patients who may require a higher dose from benefiting fully. Another labelling quirk concerns the prohibition to use product combinations. Like several other labelling restrictions (e.g. use in pregnancy, use in smokers under 18, use in a whole range of medical conditions) this is seen increasingly as unnecessary and it is being overridden by other recommendations (McNeill et al 2001, McRobbie & Hajek 2002, Benowitz et al 2004, NICE 2002). However, even where local regulation manages to override such restrictions, the heavily over-cautious presentation of the products is conveying a message that these are dangerous medications which should be used sparingly and only when necessary. This may have a general effect on limiting patient adherence to treatment and may be one of the reasons why oral products are notoriously underused.

There are two other labelling restrictions which have already been shown to limit NRT efficacy. One concerns duration of use. NRT products include recommended maximum treatment duration (usually three months). This is despite the fact that long-term NRT use has no known negative effects (e.g. Murray et al 1996). Duration of withdrawal discomfort varies highly (Piasecki et al 1998) and dependent smokers may benefit from much longer product use. Long-term users of oral NRT products are predominantly long-term treatment successes, characterized by high levels of dependence, and continuous use may assist in preventing relapse (Hajek et al 1998, 2005).

The final labelling issue concerns the start of product use in relation to quit date. The product labelling includes strict warnings regarding concurrent NRT use and smoking, and NRT is only allowed to be used after smoking cessation. Yet there are good theoretical reasons to expect that NRT use prior to quitting smoking could be helpful, e.g. it may assist in de-conditioning some of the effects of smoking, make smoking less attractive, reduce smoking frequency, help users to habituate to NRT use, and with oral products allow time for conditioned reinforcers of NRT use to develop. There is some evidence that even a short term NRT pre-loading may increase NRT efficacy (Schuurmans et al 2004), and a longer pre-quit use could be even more helpful.

Relaxing the various unnecessary restrictions on NRT use could improve its efficacy.

NRT works primarily for some types of smokers and its efficacy would improve with better targeting

Current NRTs only work for some smokers. Among those with identical baseline smoke intake using the same product in the same dose, some report no effect at all, while others describe substantial benefits. In theory, the efficacy of NRT would improve if only those who react to it were targeted.

We have already discussed the focus of current NRT products on withdrawal relief rather than on positive reinforcement factors. Withdrawal relief and replacement of pleasurable effects of smoking can be expected to be of different importance to different smokers. Severity of withdrawal is usually considered a function of dependence, but our measures of tobacco dependence are rather crude and only manage weak predictions of the outcome of a quit attempt and of the actual post-cessation withdrawal discomfort (Hajek 1992, Piasecki et al 2003). It could be hypothesized that NRT products, especially patches, would be more effective for smokers driven primarily by negative reinforcement ('trough maintainers' in Mike Russell's memorable terminology; Russell & Feyerabend 1978), while faster-acting products providing some positive feedback may be more useful for those who are more dependent on positive reinforcement ('peak seekers'). A related typology could divide smokers into those for whom the primary trigger to smoking relates to blood nicotine levels, and those who react more strongly to conditioned environmental stimuli. Again, the former may react better to nicotine replacement than the latter. A number of other genetically determined factors such as individual dopamine response to smoking (Johnstone et al 2004) or speed of nicotine metabolism (Malaiyandi et al 2005) may prove to be relevant. It is feasible that better targeting of NRT treatment would improve its efficacy.

Future of NRT

It is likely that even with all the improvements to existing products discussed so far, we would still remain a considerable way off from a 100% effective treatment. Addiction has been characterized as an acquired drive, with drug-specific salient stimuli triggering the largely automated drug taking behaviour. Where the conditioned reinforcers are of critical importance, NRT would need to provide sufficiently strong and fast reinforcement signalled by a new set of sensory cues to replace the older set of signals. Most of the existing NRT products provide some sensory cues, but NRT effects seem too weak and their onset too slow to lend the cues the necessary salience. There may also be insufficient time allowed for the associative processes to take place. Smoking becomes reinforced over many years and an enormous number of repetitions. For NRT to replace smoking cues with its own set of secondary reinforcers, both fast nicotine delivery and prolonged use may be needed.

Throughout this article, the issue of NRT therapeutic target has emerged repeatedly. We currently do not have a full understanding of what exactly mediates NRT effects. Another presentation (Shiffman et al 2006, this volume) covers this topic. NRT has been formulated primarily to suppress withdrawal discomfort and it indeed reduces the severity of practically all withdrawal symptoms (West & Shiffman, 2001). The relief is only partial and it is possible that more effective NRT products can be formulated with better withdrawal relief efficacy. However, negative reinforcement is only one of the forces driving smoking behaviour and a withdrawal relief medication, however good at its task, is unlikely to provide the final answer in treatment of tobacco dependence. Other nicotine effects perceived as rewarding by smokers may need to be replaced.

A product to fulfil such needs, including fast nicotine delivery and strong sensory cues which would generate positive subjective effects possibly comparable to smoking, could be labelled an enhanced nicotine replacement treatment (ENRT). It would probably significantly improve existing long-term success rates, at a cost of long-term use. As nicotine alone does not seem to pose more health risks than e.g. caffeine, this may not present any more challenges in future than drinking tea and coffee does today, but the level of safety and the likely prevalence of use would require careful consideration.

In view of the current negative attitudes to recreational nicotine use, and pharmaceutical industry's cautious stance, it seems likely that the next breakthrough in nicotine replacement will come from tobacco industry. Smokeless tobacco (Tilashalski et al 1998) and especially Swedish snus (Foulds et al 2003) are the possible contenders at the moment. It is probably only a matter of time for a safe inhalable nicotine delivery system attractive to smokers to emerge. Such future ENRT products may not be marketed as treatments, but their effects in enabling smokers to quit and thus dramatically reducing tobacco related morbidity and mortality could be much larger than any achieved by existing NRTs so far.

Acknowledgment

I am grateful to John Hughes for helpful comments.

References

Bates C, Jarvis M, Connoly, G 1999 Tobacco additives: cigarette engineering and nicotine addiction. Ash Publications, London

Belluzzi JD, Wang R, Leslie FM 2005 Acetaldehyde enhances acquisition of nicotine self-administration in adolescent rats. Neuropsychopharmacology 30:705–712

Benowitz N, Dempsey D 2004 Pharmacotherapy for smoking cessation during pregnancy. Nicotine Tob Res 6(Suppl 2):S189–202

Dale L, Hurt R, Offord K, Lawson G, Croghan I, Schroeder D 1995 High dose nicotine patch therapy. JAMA 274:1353–1358

Fagerstrom K 2005 The past, present and future of tobacco dependence. 11th SRNT Annual Meeting, Prague

Ferguson J, Bauld L, Chesterman J, Judge K 2005 The English smoking treatment services: one year outcomes. Addiction 100:59–69

Ferno O, Lichtneekert S, Lundgren C 1973 A substitute for tobacco smoking. Psychopharmacologia 31: 201–204

Foulds J, Ramstrom L, Burke M, Fagerstrom K 2003 Effect of smokeless tobacco (snus) on smoking and public health in Sweden. Tob Control 12:349–359

Hajek P, Belcher M, Feyerabend C 1988 Preference for 2mg versus 4mg nicotine chewing gum. Br J Addict 83:1089–1093

Hajek P, Jackson P, Belcher M 1988 Long-term use of nicotine chewing gum. Occurrence, determinants, and effect on weight gain. JAMA 260:1593–1596

Hajek P 1992 Why can some smokers quit while others cannot? Journal of Smoking Related Disorders 3:61–68

Hajek P, West R, Foulds J, Nilsson F, Burrows S, Meadow A 1999 Randomised comparative trial of nicotine chewing gum, transdermal patch, nasal spray, and inhaler. Arch Intern Med 159:2033–2038

Hajek P, Stead LF, West R, Jarvis M 2005 Relapse prevention interventions for smoking cessation. The Cochrane Database of Systematic Reviews, Issue 1

Hughes J, Lesmes G, Hatsukami D et al 1990 Are higher does of nicotine replacement more effective for smoking cessation? Nic Tob Res 1:169–174

Johnstone EC, Yudkin PL, Hey K et al 2004 Genetic variation in dopaminergic pathways and short-term effectiveness of the nicotine patch. Pharmacogenetics 14:83–90

Jorenby D, Smith S, Fiore M et al 1995 Varying nicotine patch dose and type of smoking cessation counseling. JAMA 274:1347–1352

Judge K, Bauld L, Chesterman J, Ferguson J 2005 The English smoking cessation services: short term outcomes. Addiction 100:46–58

Killen J, Fortmann S, Strausberg L, Varady A 1999 Do heavy smokers benefit from higher dose nicotine patch therapy? Exp Clin Psychopharmacol 7:226–233

Malaiyandi V, Sellers EM, Tyndale RF 2005 Implications of CYP2A6 genetic variation for smoking behaviors and nicotine dependence. Clin Pharmacol Ther 77:145–58

McNeill A, Foulds J, Bates C 2001 Regulation of nicotine replacement therapies (NRT): a critique of current practice. Addiction 96:1757–1768

McRobbie H, Hajek P 2001 Nicotine replacement therapy in patients with cardiovascular disease: guidelines for health professionals. Addiction 96:1547–1551

Murray RP, Bailey WC, Daniels K et al 1996 Safety of nicotine polacrilex gum used by 3,094 participants in the lung health study. Lung Health Study Research Group. Chest 109:438–445

NICE (National Institute of Clinical Excellence) 2002 Guidance on the use of nicotine replacement therapy (NRT) and bupropion for smoking cessation. NICE, London (*http://www.nice.org.uk/page.aspx?o=30631*)

Paoletti P, Fornai E, Maggiorelli F et al 1996 Importance of baseline cotinine plasma values in smoking cessation: results from a double-blind study with nicotine patch. Eur Respir J 9:643–651

Piasecki TM, Fiore MC, Baker TB 1998 Profiles in discouragement: two studies of variability in the time course of smoking withdrawal symptoms. J Abnorm Psychol 107:238–251

Piasecki TM, Jorenby DE, Smith SS, Fiore MC, Baker TB 2003 Smoking withdrawal dynamics: III. Correlates of withdrawal heterogeneity. Exp Clin Psychopharmacol 11:276–285

Pomerleau OF, Pomerleau CS, Marks JL et al Prolonged nicotine patch use in quitters with past abstinence-induced depressed mood. J Subst Abuse Treat. 2003 24:13–18

Rose J, Jarvik M, Rose K 1984 Transdermal administration of nicotine. Drug Alcohol Depen 13:209–213

Royal College of Physicians 2000 Nicotine addiction in Britain. RCP, London

Russell MA, Feyerabend C 1978 Cigarette smoking: a dependence on high-nicotine boli. Drug Metab Rev 8:29–57

Russell M, Jarvis M, Feyerabend C, Ferno O 1983 Nasal nicotine solution: a potential aid to giving up smoking? BMJ 286:683–684

Schuurmans MM, Diacon AH, van Biljon X, Bolliger CT 2004 Effect of pre-treatment with nicotine patch on withdrawal symptoms and abstinence rates in smokers subsequently quitting with the nicotine patch: a randomized controlled trial. Addiction 99:634–640

Shiffman S, Khayrallah M, Nowak R 2000 Efficacy of the nicotine patch for relief of craving and withdrawal 7–10 weeks after cessation. Nicotine Tob Res 2:371–378

Shiffman S, Dresler CM, Hajek P, Gilburt SJ, Targett DA, Strahs KR 2002 Efficacy of a nicotine lozenge for smoking cessation. Arch Intern Med 162:1267–1276

Shiffman S, Ferguson S, Scharf D 2006 Exploring behavioural mechanisms of nicotine replacement therapy for smoking cessation. In: Understanding nicotine and tobacco addiction. Wiley, Chichester (Novartis Found Symp 275) p 219–234

Silagy C, Lancaster T, Stead L, Mant D, Fowler G 2004 Nicotine replacement therapy for smoking cessation. Cochrane Database Syst Rev CD000146

Tonnesen P, Paoletti P, Gustavsson G et al 1999 Higher dosage nicotine patches increase one-year smoking cessation rates: results from the European CEASE trial. Collaborative European anti-smoking evaluation. European Respiratory Society. Eur Respir J 13:238–246

Van Den Eijnden R, Spijkerman R, Fekkes D 2003 Craving for cigarettes among low and high dependent smokers: impact of norharman. Addict Biol 8:463–472

Villegier S, Blanc G, Glowinski J, Tassin P 2003 Transient behavioral sensitization to nicotine becomes long-lasting with monoamine oxidases inhibitors. Pharmacol Biochem Behav 76:267–274

West R, Hajek P, Foulds J, Nilsson F, May S, Meadows A 2000 A comparison of abuse liability and dependence potential of nicotine patch, gum, spray and inhaler. Psychopharmacology 149:198–202

West R, Shiffman S 2001 Effect of oral nicotine dosing forms on cigarette withdrawal symptoms and craving. Psychopharmacology 155:115–122

DISCUSSION

Bertrand: There are at least two studies with partial agonist-like compounds (Cohen et al 2003, Coe et al 2005). Do we have any evidence showing that they would be better or worse than nicotine patches and NRT substitutes currently on the market?

Hajek: There were some preliminary results showing that varenicline, which is a selective partial nicotinic receptor agonist, is more effective than bupropion, but there are no comparisons of varenicline or rimonabant with NRT in the public domain yet.

Stolerman: It would be helpful if we could understand better where the failure occurs. Is it that people restart smoking while they are using NRT, having quit? Or is it that after they have stopped NRT, they resume some time later? Our approach needs to be different if we know where the problem lies.

Shiffman: It is both. There is some evidence that prolonging treatment improves outcome, but a good deal of failure occurs on treatment.

Stolerman: With regard to the longer term aspects of coming off, the way I would look at this is a parallel with the use of methadone. Methadone maintenance is quite effective, yet methadone as a detoxifying agent is ineffective—it's very hard to come off it. It may have no benefit at all over the longer term.

Corrigall: What is the strength of the evidence with regard to the safety and toxicity of nicotine long-term? Is it strong enough to satisfy regulatory agencies?

Hajek: One source of information on this is the long-term NRT users. There are quite a few of them and the long term use of nicotine seems to be safe.

Incidentally, they also present another pointer to the importance of speed of nicotine delivery. Among a few thousand people on our database, about 13% of nasal spray users still use it one year later, whereas the figure is 8% for oral products and 2% for the patch. There are people who use nicotine for many years and we don't know of any harmful effects.

Jarvis: The epidemiology on this is difficult because usually nicotine delivery is confounded with other things. The best evidence comes from Swedish snus, where there is a substantial proportion of the adult population using it. The evidence is convincing that it is hard to detect a cancer risk associated with snus use. There is no chronic respiratory disease. The evidence on cardiovascular effects is a little bit less clear. The risks associated with long-term nicotine use are very much smaller than those associated with cigarette use.

Shiffman: I agree that oral tobacco users are the best natural control. They get high levels of nicotine—often higher than those achieved by smokers. Where there is pathology, it is very local. The nicotine circulates everywhere but we only see cancers locally. One other study which has some limits but is more of a traditional clinical study is the US government-sponsored Lung Health Study. This was intended not as a study of smoking cessation. Cessation was the independent variable, and they wanted to see what effect it had on progression of obstructive lung disease. Because they needed to produce cessation they pulled out all the stops and despite regulatory constraints encouraged the smokers to use nicotine gum as much and for as long as they wanted to. They had a cohort that used it for five years. Those people were followed, and not only was there no evidence of any harm, but also the trends were that the smokers who used gum had better health outcomes than those who hadn't (Murray et al 1996).

Corrigall: If we believe that we are 'there' with respect to nicotine replacement as an approach, but we want to move NRT further along by making a higher yield or faster delivery system for nicotine, we will need to convince regulatory bodies at some point. How do we do this?

Balfour: There are two issues. One is toxicity, which we can deal with to some extent. The second is whether regulatory authorities would accept a drug that causes dependence.

Corrigall: We have methadone. There will always be walls to scale.

Balfour: I accept this, but the real hurdle for us is to say that we intend to transfer addiction from one preparation to another.

West: This does differ from country to country. The climate in the UK has changed quite a bit in recent years and I don't perceive that it has changed sufficiently in the USA. The pharmaceutical companies are very concerned. Pharmaceutical companies see NRT primarily as an over-the-counter (OTC) product. It has to pass the regulations. In the USA the nasal spray isn't even OTC. If you come up with a product that is even as good as the nasal spray, it will have to go on prescription, so many companies won't consider this worthwhile. There needs to be quite a major shift. In terms of taking this forward, organizations such as the SRNT (Society for Research on Nicotine and Tobacco) must play a role.

Corrigall: There's a point in which we have to decide whether to proceed or not. I agree the driving is tough.

Perkins: Is the rate-limiting step the lack of new products? Or should we be thinking of more effective use of current products?

Shiffman: I think it is both. The current products are used so poorly that we are nowhere close to reaching their potential.

Perkins: What is the priority?

Shiffman: There is a lot of concern about long-term use, which limits appropriate use of current nicotine treatments. We studied duration of use and found that 6% of people who take gum use it for at least six months, which is considered a horror; in the USA it is approved for three months. The reality is that 78% use it for less than a month. We have much more of a problem with too-little use. Even if you look at groups who use it in ways that are regarded to be appropriate and likely to be effective, the efficacy is limited. I think there are significant technical problems with getting nicotine absorbed through the lungs. There are companies working on this. I think the FDA is way behind. Their worry is about smoking while using NRT. We have to take a long-term view: in some ways the FDA views a period of being Rx as a way to get some experience with a product destined to be OTC in large populations. This is not a cemetery, but a way station for such a product.

Jarvis: We also have to see this issue in the context of the current broader nicotine market. It is the efficacy of the product in the context of cigarettes being widely available and very little regulated. As we have already touched on, the biggest predictors of failure to quit are not dependence, but they are the social context in which use occurs. If you have a smoking partner, or come from a poorer socioeconomic background, then it's harder to quit. This speaks to the competing pressures from effective nicotine delivery devices, typically cigarettes. It is not just a question of getting the alternative treatments right—it is regulating the broader nicotine market.

Powell: I wanted to return to the subject of why nicotine replacement is of only limited effectiveness. There is an intrinsic limitation. Given that one of the obvious effects of nicotine is to promote activity within the reward pathways and enhance responsivity to reward cues, logically one might argue that NRT, as well as substituting for some of the indirect or direct reinforcing effects of nicotine, would also increase the person's reactivity to social and other environmental cues indicating cigarette availability. This might increase their tendency to engage in automatic smoking patterns, and so to relapse. Perhaps the way forward with NRT is to look at combining it with psychological therapies, focusing on how people respond to the cue-elicited craving which might be being promoted or prolonged by NRT. In experimental studies of cue reactivity, we have found that smokers' reactions to drug-related cues were not attenuated by NRT.

Shiffman: They are not accentuated, either.

Powell: In one of our studies they were. It varied.

Hajek: It is an interesting hypothesis. The fact that NRT does help some people quit contradicts this somewhat, but it may be a factor undermining the effectiveness of this therapy. When NRT first emerged, one of the first things we wanted to do was to study a combination of NRT and herbal cigarettes.

Brody: I wanted to ask about the combination of smoking and NRT. There is another side, which is nicotine toxicity. In your paper you say that smoking combined with patches is OK. I have five patients a week tell me that they do this, but once every year or two someone has a stroke or a myocardial infarction (MI) in my clinic when they do this.

Shiffman: But probably once or twice every year one of your patients has a stroke when they are not doing this.

Brody: Is it a coincidence?

Shiffman: Yes. You have just replicated one of the big stories in the history of really bad press coverage of science. The reason everyone thinks that smoking in combination with patches causes heart attacks is that in 1992 a hospital in Boston reported that they had seen six heart attacks in patients who were on patch and who had smoked. This made the front page of the *New York Times*. The FDA convened a hearing and someone did epidemiology 101: they looked at how many patients were under care, how many were smokers, and what the expected rates of MI should be. It turned out that the six observed were *lower* than expected in that population. This also got published, in page 32 next to the underwear adverts. To this day, when I give a talk to practising physicians they ask whether patients on the patch will get heart attacks if they smoke. In addition to this a thorough case control study was done and there is not a shred of evidence that there is any risk.

Walton: It is quite clear that strokes and heart attacks are caused by large vessel disease, which is caused by smoking.

Shiffman: Exactly. Mahmarian et al (1997) did a thalium scan study of coronary perfusion on patients with compromised cardiovascular systems on patch or off patch, smoking or not smoking. This study finds improved coronary perfusion in patients on patch and smoking. I have a completely different question. Oral tobacco is an interesting case because it is not much more rapid than patches, yet there are populations who find it reinforcing enough to use long term.

Jarvis: The evidence from Swedish snus is that the venous blood nicotine levels after use are almost identical to those achieved from cigarettes. With the products that succeed in the marketplace people can get the kind of blood nicotine levels that they want. It is not quite as fast with oral products.

Shiffman: Snus doesn't have the arterial bolus that we sometimes think is important.

West: The attachment of the nicotine effect to behavioural and sensory cues is quite significant. Also, we need to consider the dissociation you might get between the sensation of enjoyment and the level of dependence. My hypothesis would be that if you are comparing like with like, and the motivation not to use snus were the same as with smoking, people would find it easier not to use snus. For those reasons, snus is not as dependence forming but this may not purely be to do with the rate of nicotine delivery; it could be due to the way the behaviour and sensory stimuli interact with the nicotine.

Shiffman: This has important implications: if we could create an NRT product that has the PK (pharmacokinetics) profile of snus without the tobacco, but which also has a richness to accompanying stimuli, this could be successful.

Caggiula: I'd like to raise a couple of points, and relate them to the belief that speed of nicotine delivery is important. At the beginning of your paper you said that it is clear that people smoke to get nicotine. I am not sure this is the whole story. Equally true, I believe, is the idea that nicotine makes people smoke, which is a very different thing. The fast delivery of nicotine is probably important for the primary reinforcing effects of the drug. This is one component of nicotine's actions. The process by which neutral cues become conditional reinforcers because of their association with nicotine probably also depends on rapid delivery of nicotine, although none of this has been thoroughly tested in a rat model. But nicotine's effectiveness in enhancing the reinforcing effects of stimuli that are part of the self-administration or smoking context does not require rapid delivery of nicotine and we think that this reinforcement-enhancing effect of nicotine is an important part of the drug's role in self-administration and smoking. Thus, depending on which of nicotine's effects we are talking about, the kinetic profile can be very different.

Balfour: In animal work we give nicotine subcutaneously and compared with smoking this is absorbed slowly: the peak is 15 min after injection. Yet this raises brain extracellular dopamine. Why does rapidity matter? We have called a stimulus paired with nicotine a conditioned reinforcer. Years ago I was taught by a psychologist who called it a feedback signal. It may be that the rapid signals associated with the delivery of nicotine are a feedback signals saying yes you have done the right thing—15 minutes down the line life is going to be very pleasurable.

Caggiula: What you are calling a 'feedback' signal is relevant to the primary reinforcing effects of nicotine. When I talk about conditioned reinforcement I am referring to the ability of nicotine to endow neutral stimuli with reinforcing properties.

Picciotto: As far as I know, none of the animal models produce dependence. The idea that NRT in humans is relieving withdrawal is something that wouldn't be applicable to these points.

Caggiula: Athina Markou yesterday talked about moving the animal model into the area of dependence by looking at withdrawal after long-term exposure.

Hajek: In humans, smoking is typically triggered by low blood nicotine levels.

References

Coe JW, Brooks PR, Vetelino MG et al 2005 Varenicline: an alpha4beta2 nicotinic receptor partial agonist for smoking cessation. J Med Chem 48:3474–3477

Cohen C, Bergis OE, Galli F 2003 SSR591813, a novel selective and partial alpha4beta2 nicotinic receptor agonist with potential as an aid to smoking cessation. J Pharmacol Exp Ther 306:407–420

Mahmarian JJ, Moye LA, Nasser GA et al 1997 Nicotine patch therapy in smoking cessation reduces the extent of exercise-induced myocardial ischemia. J Am Coll Cardiol 30:125–130

Murray RP, Bailey WC, Daniels K et al 1996 Safety of nicotine polacrilex gum used by 3094 participants in the Lung Health Study. Lung Health Study Research Group. Chest 109:438–445

Exploring behavioural mechanisms of nicotine replacement therapy for smoking cessation

Saul Shiffman, Stuart Ferguson and Deborah Scharf

Department of Pyschology, University of Pittsburgh, Pittsburgh, PA 15260, USA

Abstract. Discussions of the 'mechanisms' by which medications help smokers quit usually focus on neuropharmacological mechanisms, with nicotine replacement therapy (NRT) considered simply as an agonist replacement. However, understanding the behavioural mechanisms by which proven therapies influence cessation can guide both basic research and treatment development. NRT is thought to promote abstinence by reducing craving and withdrawal. However, new analyses show that this does not fully mediate NRT's effects. It is also important to distinguish how treatment affects different milestones of cessation: i.e. promoting initial abstinence, preventing lapses from abstinence, or keeping lapses from progressing to relapse. New analyses show that NRT does all three. Surprisingly, its strongest effect is on preventing progression from lapse to relapse. This effect is apparently not mediated by reduction in hedonic response to the initial lapse. Different forms of nicotine delivery may also involve different behavioural mechanisms. For example, whereas nicotine patch (slow, steady administration) does not prevent the provocation of craving by smoking-related cueing stimuli that can trigger lapses, nicotine gum (acute administration) can rapidly relieve craving associated with these cue exposures, possibly preventing lapses. Behavioural mechanisms of other treatments are relatively unexplored.

2005 Understanding nicotine and tobacco addiction. Wiley, Chichester (Novartis Foundation Symposium 275) p 219–234

Discussions about the mechanisms by which medications assist in smoking cessation usually revolve around the neurochemical processes activated by the drug— what kind of action, at which receptors, in which neural system. While this level of analysis is important, it is also incomplete. Smoking cessation involves a complex chain of behavioural changes, and thus understanding how a drug affects cessation requires understanding what behaviours it affects, and how. Even when the neurochemical basis of a medication's actions is well understood, we need to understand its behavioural mechanisms of action.

Discussion of the mechanism of action for nicotine replacement therapy (NRT) provides a good foundation for exploring issues of behavioural mechanism, for several reasons. NRT is the oldest and most widely used medication for smoking cessation, being used in approximately 18% of quit efforts (Levinson et al 2004). The efficacy of NRT is very well established in over 100 randomized clinical trials (Silagy et al 2004). Most importantly, the neurochemical mechanism of NRT is considered simple and well-established: NRT is an agonist replacement therapy. The standard account of its mechanism is that smokers smoke in order to get nicotine and experience craving and withdrawal when they are deprived. Providing smokers with nicotine via NRT is intended to mitigate drug deprivation, subdue craving and withdrawal, and thus reduce the pressure to resume drug-taking, i.e. relapse. No novel pharmacological mechanism need be posited. Nicotine from NRT simply substitutes for what nicotine from cigarettes was doing (whatever that is!).

In this paper, we explore how NRT works to promote abstinence from smoking, and consider new evidence for various behavioural mechanisms. We suggest a framework for thinking about the different stages of the cessation process at which drugs might exert therapeutic effects. Our framework is based on different modes of failure in smoking cessation, which we divide into three successive milestones: failure to quit, lapsing and relapsing. First, the smoker has to quit smoking—making the initial behaviour change from regular smoking to initial abstinence. Some 5–20% of smokers fail to establish abstinence for even one day, thus failing immediately (Garvey et al 1992). For the majority who do achieve initial abstinence, the next challenge is avoiding lapsing to smoking. Most smokers who achieve initial abstinence 'lapse' by re-initiating smoking. Lapses—limited smoking episodes in which smoking is re-initiated—are key milestones on the road to treatment failure: smokers who don't have that first cigarette can't resume smoking. Most smokers who quit, resume regular smoking (i.e. relapse, Kenford et al 1994). However, the lapse in itself doesn't compel failure. If the smokers could recover abstinence following the lapse, success is still possible. Thus, understanding progression from a lapse to a relapse is critical. Thus, this analysis identifies three milestones on the road to cessation failure: failing to quit, lapsing and relapsing.

Using the milestones allows us to ask where NRT exerts its therapeutic influence. It is possible for pharmacological agents to impact specific milestones. For example, naltrexone is thought to have no effect preventing lapses to drinking, but to prevent lapses from progressing to relapse (Volpicelli et al 1995).

To study the mechanism by which NRT works, we conducted a randomized trial of high-dose (35 mg) nicotine patches (NPs), in which we analysed the effect of treatment at each milestone (Shiffman et al 2006a). Subjects in the study used palmtop computers to provide real-time accounts of their smoking and their experience during the quit process, thus avoiding the problems of retrospective data (Stone & Shiffman 1994). We used survival analysis to examine treatment efficacy, separately examining how NP influenced the risk of reaching each milestone—quitting, lapsing and relapsing—among the smokers who are 'at risk' for each milestone (e.g. only those who lapse are at risk to progress to relapse).

We found that treatment with active nicotine patch facilitated success at each milestone. Figure 1 shows the results, illustrated by survival curves.

Improving initial abstinence

A priori, we had not expected nicotine patch to offer smokers help in initial quitting. Since blood levels from the patch used in the study don't reach maximal levels until 4 hours after application (Fant et al 2000), active treatment was not expected to give smokers much help in the initial transition to abstinence. In fact, treatment did help smokers establish initial 24 h abstinence. One explanation is that motivated smokers can maintain abstinence for the first few hours on their own (S. Shiffman et al, unpublished work 2005) but encounter more serious difficulty maintaining it past this time, by which time the patch has developed therapeutic levels and provides assistance in abstaining. (We found that those who failed to quit on the quit day first smoked after a median of 7.8 waking hours of abstinence; S. Shiffman et al unpublished work.) Other patch formulations don't reach C_{max} until 10 hours (Fant et al 2000); it would be interesting to see whether they are less helpful in establishing initial abstinence. Of course, nicotine patches may provide therapeutic benefit before reaching maximum blood levels.

Preventing lapses

We expected NP to have its greatest effect in preventing lapses, since this is the effect that has been best documented (outcome measures based on continuous abstinence essentially assess avoidance of lapses). Indeed, we found that active patch reduced the daily risk of lapsing by 38%. But how does NP prevent lapses? It is widely accepted that NRT reduces lapsing by reducing craving and withdrawal, which have been linked to lapsing (Hughes 1993). Surprisingly, however, this mechanism has never been systematically tested. The hypothesis involves three postulates: (1) NRT reduces craving and withdrawal; (2) Craving and withdrawal promote lapsing; and (3) NRT's effects on lapse prevention are mediated by #2.

It is very well established that NP reduces craving and withdrawal (West & Shiffman 2001, Shiffman et al 2000). There is also evidence that craving and withdrawal are associated with lapse risk (West et al 1989), though this evidence is not as strong as it might be; many studies fail to show the effect (see Tiffany 1990). Thus, the building-blocks of the mediational hypothesis are established, but the actual mediational link (#3) has not, to our knowledge, even been tested.

To test the mediational hypothesis, we tested whether the effects of NP could be accounted for by relief of craving and withdrawal (Shiffman et al 2006b). Symp-

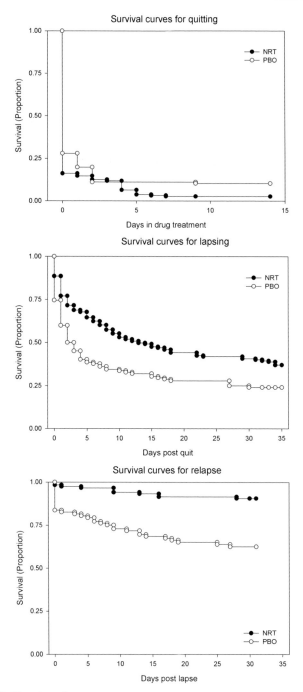

FIG. 1.   NRT effects by milestone.

toms were assessed intensively, five times per day at random times selected by the electronic diaries, which 'beeped' subjects for assessments (see Shiffman et al 1997). NP very significantly reduced craving and withdrawal, even totally eliminating some symptoms. Symptom-relief—particularly craving relief—did mediate some of the effects of NP, as illustrated by the fact that the NP effect was reduced when symptom-relief was accounted for. However, the mediation was far from complete. This is illustrated in Fig. 2, which shows survival curves for NP and placebo groups,

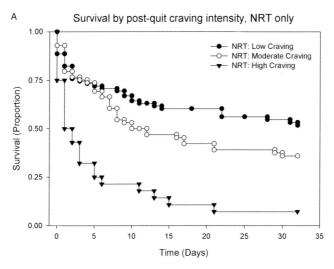

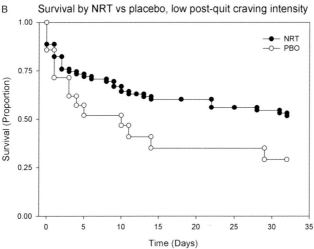

FIG. 2A,B.   Survival curves showing effect of NRT and craving reduction. (A) Survival by post-quit craving intensity, NRT only. (B) Survival by NRT vs. placebo, moderate post-quit craving intensity.

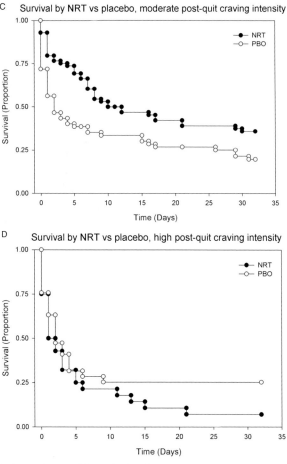

FIG. 2C,D.   (C) Survival by NRT vs placebo, low post-quit craving intensity. (D) Survival by
NRT vs placebo, high post-quit craving intensity.

stratified by craving intensity on the first day of quitting. Subjects on active NP had
lower lapse risk, even when the groups had similar craving. (The exception is the
high-craving group, where subjects who had high craving despite treatment with
high-dose patch fared particularly poorly.)

   These analyses might be criticized on the grounds that they only addressed the
effects of NP on symptoms at one early time-point, and would not account for
later symptom experience. Accordingly, we also tested the influence of daily
symptom intensity on subsequent lapse risk. The analysis again showed that
increases in symptom intensity were associated with greater lapse risk, and that NP

reduced symptoms, but again showed only partial mediation of NP effects through symptom relief. Thus, craving and withdrawal symptom relief does not completely mediate the effect of nicotine patches in reducing lapse risk.

Lapses as acute, precipitated episodes of smoking

If NRT does not work by relieving symptom intensity, how might it prevent lapses? One possibility we considered is that it might reduce smokers' reactions to situational stimuli that provoke craving and precipitate lapsing. Lapses are not random events. Rather, they are triggered by situational cues such as negative affect, alcohol consumption and exposure to others smoking (Shiffman et al 1996). (These same cues have also been shown to provoke immediate craving in laboratory research; Carter & Tiffany 1999) These phasic, proximal influences, appear to be the dominant factors in precipitating smoking (Shiffman 2005). Thus, nicotine patches might prevent lapses if they reduced smokers' reactions to such cues, even if they did not change smokers' average levels of craving outside these provocative situations.

We tested whether patches could buffer smokers' reactions by experimentally exposed smokers, who had been randomized to active or placebo patches, to a smoking cue (a cigarette; Waters et al 2004). As Fig. 3 shows, patch reduced the background levels of craving, but had no effect on the 'boost' due to cue exposure, nor did it affect recovery following the provocation (see also Tiffany et al 2000). It appears that nicotine patches do not protect smokers from the provocative effects of smoking cues. Notice, though, that the patch so reduced craving intensity that the craving of smokers on patch was actually lower *after* cue exposure than smokers on placebo experienced *before* cue exposure. Thus, if lapses are potentiated by the absolute intensity of craving, nicotine patch may help prevent lapses simply by lowering the baseline, even if it does not block the increase in craving following a provocative cue.

Whereas patch seemed to have no effect on recovery from cue-provoked craving, it appears that acute administration of nicotine, via forms such as nicotine gum, can 'treat' provoked craving rapidly. In a separate study (Shiffman et al 2003), we had subjects chew nicotine gum or inert gum after they had been exposed to a provocative cue (a lit cigarette). As shown in Fig. 4, craving in the active gum group began to separate from that in the placebo group after about 15 minutes—roughly the time frame in which nicotine gum begins to achieve significant blood nicotine levels (Benowitz et al 1987). A subsequent study showed that faster nicotine administration yielded faster craving relief (Niaura et al 2005). Clearly, acute administration of nicotine can reduce craving, even when the craving has been behaviourally instigated.

If patch does not protect smokers against cue-induced craving, and its effects are not mediated by its reduction of 'background' tonic craving, how does patch prevent lapses?

Cue Reactivity by Patch Condition

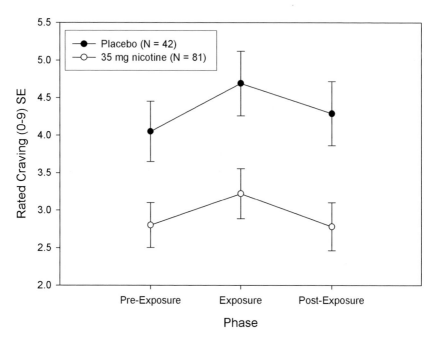

FIG. 3.   Null effect of patch on provoked craving (after Waters et al 2004).

Our data do not suggest alternative mechanisms for NRT's effects. One possibility is that subjectively-reported motivation (e.g. craving) does not fully capture the motivational influences of nicotine deprivation or replacement. There is considerable evidence that many important motivational processes operate outside of awareness, and thus may be incapable of capture by self-report (McCusker 2001). This mechanism is speculative, and it is not clear what data could be brought to bear to prove or disprove it. In any case, it is clear that the ability of nicotine patches to prevent lapses is not completely accounted for by reductions in craving and withdrawal symptoms, and not at all accounted for by blunting of cue-provoked craving.

The ability of nicotine patch to dramatically reduce background, tonic craving, and the complementary ability of acute NRT forms (such as gum or lozenge) to treat cue-provoked craving, suggests why combining patch with acute forms of NRT may provide incremental efficacy. While studies suggests that simply increasing the nicotine dose, by using higher-dose patches, does not substantially increase efficacy (Jorenby et al 1995), other studies suggest that supplementing patch with

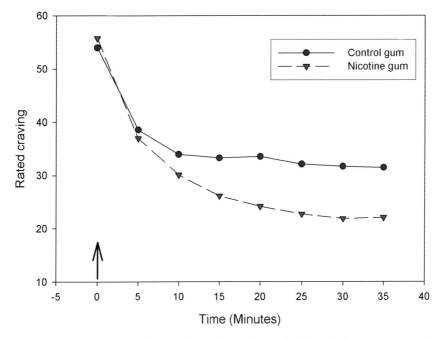

FIG. 4. Effect of gum on reduction of craving, rated on a 0–100 scale. Arrow represents time of exposure to lit cigarette. Data are adjusted for baseline craving (after Shiffman et al 2003).

an acute NRT form, does contribute to incremental efficacy (Sweeney et al 2001). The potential for synergistic actions from two forms of NRT needs to be further explored, and also suggests the possibility of other synergistic combinations of mechanisms as more diverse medications for smoking cessation become available.

Preventing progression from lapse to relapse

The literature on progression from lapse to relapse has emphasized the role of psychological, rather than pharmacological factors in this progression (Marlatt & Gordon 1985). Accordingly, we expected modest effects on relapse. Surprisingly, however, NP had very large effects in preventing progression from a lapse to relapse, reducing the daily risk of relapse by 86%—the largest patch effect we observed. This is particularly striking because the clinical literature on NRT and cessation does not emphasize the use of NP for preventing progression. (Indeed, instructions for NRT warn against using NRT while smoking, which might imply discontinuing treatment after a lapse.) Below, we consider whether one theoretically important mechanism that might underlie this effect.

The hedonic value hypothesis

One hypothesis is that having high circulating nicotine levels might reduce the hedonic or reinforcing value of smoking in the lapse, perhaps even making it aversive, thus disrupting an important mechanism by which lapses promote progression to relapse. This mediational hypothesis has three postulates: (1) that the hedonic value or pleasantness of smoking in a lapse promotes progression to further smoking and relapse; (2) treatment with NRT reduces the hedonic value of smoking in a lapse; and (3) #2 mediates the beneficial effect of NRT on progression to relapse.

We began by testing the first postulate (Shiffman et al 2006c). Smokers who had just experienced their first lapse rated the hedonic value or pleasantness of smoking in the lapse and any aversive symptoms experienced in the lapse. Aversive symptoms were unrelated to progression. However, subjects who rated smoking as more pleasant were at greater risk of progressing to a second episode of smoking and also at greater risk of progression to relapse. The latter is illustrated in Fig. 5. For each one-point increase in rated pleasantness (0–10 scale), the daily risk of progression to relapse was increased by 26%.

We next addressed the second postulate, and found that treatment with nicotine patch was unrelated to the hedonic value of smoking in the lapse. Smokers on active patch did not find smoking any less pleasant than smokers who were wearing placebo patches (both = 4.8 on a 0–10 scale). Since there was no treatment effect on hedonic value, this can't explain the effects of patch on progression.

Importantly, we have only examined how NP affects reactions to the very first lapse, on the reasoning that this is the pivotal event in relapse. However, it is possible that the effects of NP only become evident progressively over the course of multiple lapses. We also have not assessed the role of other variables, such as

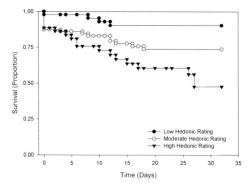

FIG. 5.   Effect of hedonic responses to a lapse on progression to relapse.

craving, in driving progression from an initial lapse to relapse. In other words, the results presented here are preliminary and the questions we addressed need to be explored in greater detail.

Summary

Our analysis of NP effects based on distinguishing among effects on quitting, lapsing and relapsing showed that NP affects all three milestones, though the effects differed in magnitude. Surprisingly, the analysis showed that NP had its greatest effect on preventing lapses from progressing to relapse. This effect has not been previously known. It suggests that treatment effects might be optimized by encouraging smokers to persist on treatment after a lapse, in contrast to the current policy that implicitly discourages persistence on NRT after a lapse. As further research and analysis suggests the mechanisms for this (and other) effects, this may suggest further ways to optimize NP effects.

Analysis of efficacy and mechanisms by milestones can also help guide the development and application of new drugs. As an example, consider the nicotine vaccines being developed for smoking cessation (Cerny 2005). The vaccines work by binding nicotine in the periphery and keeping it from reaching the brain, essentially creating a central blockade. How can this help a smoker to quit? It seems unlikely to have any effect on preventing lapses, since smokers have no circulating nicotine to be attacked by the immune system when they are at risk for lapsing (i.e. when they are abstinent). Conversely, the vaccination strategy might be best targeted to preventing a lapse from progressing to relapse, on the theory that nicotine re-exposure during lapses promotes progression to relapse through reinforcement mediated by nicotine receptors in the brain. Thus, a vaccinated smoker who lapses would fail to experience such reinforcement, and thus not progress to relapse. Our finding that hedonic responses to lapses do predict the risk of progression suggests the potential for this strategy to succeed. In any case, this illustrates the importance of thinking about the behavioural mechanisms by which drugs exert their effects and the cessation milestones where the effects are relevant.

Our study of high-dose nicotine patches has not suggested an account of the mechanisms by which NRT promotes successful cessation. The findings have been more useful in eliminating some putative mechanisms than in suggesting or validating the mechanisms by which NRT might operate. Accordingly, we offer this work, not as a definitive statement on the mechanisms of NRT, but as an illustration of the kind of process-mechanism research that needs to be done if we are to understand how NRT—or any other medication—works. If we are to understand drug effects on cessation, it is essential that pharmacological and neurobiological mechanisms be translated into specific behavioural mechanisms that operate at each stage of the quitting process. Such insights are essential for optimizing the effects of currently available medications, and for guiding the development of new medications to address the leading public health problem in the world.

References

Benowitz NL, Jacob P, Savanapridi C 1987 Determinants of nicotine intake while chewing nicotine polarex gum. Clin Pharmacol Ther 41:186–200

Carter BL, Tiffany ST 1999 Meta-analysis of cue-reactivity in addiction research. Addiction 94:349–351

Cerny T 2005 Anti-nicotine vaccination: where are we? Recent Results Cancer Res 166:167–175

Fant RV, Henningfield JE, Shiffman S, Strahs KR, Reitberg DP 2000 A pharmacokinetic crossover study to compare the absorption characteristics of three transdermal nicotine patches. Pharmacol Biochem Behav 67:479–482

Garvey A, Bliss R, Hitchcock J, Heinold J, Rosner B 1992 Predictors of smoking relapse among self-quitters: a report from the normative aging study. Addictive Behav 17:367–377

Hughes JR 1993 Pharmacotherapy for smoking cessation: unvalidated assumptions, anomalies, and suggestions for future research. J Consult Clin Psychol 61:751–760

Jorenby DE, Smith SS, Fiore MC et al 1995 Varying nicotine patch dose and type of smoking cessation counseling. JAMA 274: 1347–52

Kenford SL, Fiore MC, Jorenby DE, Smith SS, Wetter D, Baker TB 1994 Predicting smoking cessation. Who will quit with and without the nicotine patch. JAMA 271:589–594

Levinson AH, Perez-Stable EJ, Espinoza P, Flores ET, Byers TE 2004 Latinos report less use of pharmaceutical aids when trying to quit smoking. Am J Prevent Med 26:105–111

Marlatt GA, Gordon JR 1985 Relapse prevention. Guildford Press, New York

McCusker CG 2001 Cognitive biases and addiction: an evolution in theory and method. Addiction 96:47–56

Niaura R, Sayette M, Shiffman S et al 2005 Comparative efficacy of rapid-release nicotine gum versus nicotine polacrilex gum in relieving smoking cue-provoked craving. Addiction 100:1720–1730

Shiffman S 2005 Dynamic influences on smoking relapse process. J Pers 73:1715–1748

Shiffman S, Paty JA, Gnys M, Kassel JA, Hickox M 1996 First lapses to smoking: within-subjects analysis of real-time reports. J Consult Clin Psychol 64:366–379

Shiffman S, Engberg JB, Paty JA et al 1997 A day at a time: predicting smoking lapse from daily urge. J Abnorm Psychol 106:104–116

Shiffman S, Elash C, Paton SM et al 2000 Comparative efficacy of 24-hour and 16-hour transdermal nicotine patches for relief of morning craving. Addiction 95:1185–1195

Shiffman S, Shadel WG, Niaura R, Khayrallah MA, Jorenby DE, Ryan CF, Ferguson CL 2003 Efficacy of acute administration of nicotine gum in relief of cue-provoked cigarette craving. Psychopharmacology 166:343–350

Shiffman S, Scharf D, Shadel WG et al 2006a Analysing milestones in smoking cessation: illustration in a nicotine patch trial in adult smokers. Journal of Clinical and Consulting Psychology, in press

Shiffman S, Ferguson SG, Gwaltney CJ, Balabanis MH, Shadel WG 2006b Reduction of abstinence induced withdrawal and craving using nicotine replacement therapy. Psychopharmacology, in press

Shiffman S, Ferguson SG, Gwaltney CJ 2006c Immediate hedonic response to smoking lapses: Relationship to smoking relapse, and effects of nicotine replacement therapy. Psychopharmacology, in press

Silagy C, Lancaster T, Stead T, Mant D, Fowler G 2004 Nicotine replacement therapy for smoking cessation. Cochrane Database Syst Rev 3:CD000146

Stone AA, Shiffman S 1994 Ecological Momentary Assessment (EMA) in behavioral medicine 16:199–202

Sweeney CT, Fant RV, Fagerstrom KO, McGovern JF, Henningfield JE 2001 Combination nicotine replacement therapy for smoking cessation. CNS Drugs 15:453–467

Tiffany ST 1990 A cognitive model of drug urges and drug use behavior: Role of automatic and non-automatic processes. Psychol Rev 97:147–168

Tiffany ST, Cox LS, Elash CA 2000 Effects of transdermal nicotine patches on abstinence-induced and cue-elicited craving in cigarette smokers. J Consult Clin Psychol 68:233–240

Volpicelli JR, Watson NT, King AC, Sherman CE, O'Brien CP 1995 Effect of naltrexone on alcohol 'high' in alcoholics. Am J Psychiatry 152:613–615

Waters AJ, Shiffman S, Sayette MA, Paty JA, Gwaltney CJ, Balabanis MH 2004 Cue-provoked craving and nicotine replacement therapy in smoking cessation. J Consult Clin Psychol 72:1136–1143

West RJ, Shiffman S 2001 Effect of oral nicotine dosing forms on cigarette withdrawal symptoms and craving: a systematic review. Psychopharmacology 155:115–122

West RJ, Hajeck P, Belcher M 1989 Severity of withdrawal symptoms as a predictor of outcome of an attempt to quit smoking. Psychol Med 19:981–985

DISCUSSION

Tyndale: In our discussions yesterday, we focused on the vaccine concept in the relapse model. But in terms of lapsing moving to relapsing and this being the primary component that is causing the lack of abstinence, you still had a tremendous patch effect. Doesn't this suggest that they do need nicotine for the cessation.

Shiffman: I don't see it as either/or. That is, the vaccine would presumably help mitigate the response to a lapse. The processes that were present before lapse are still there. That is, to the extent that people experience craving and provocative stimuli, these happen after the lapse as well. One way to think of this is that the first lapse is not so special. It is stimulated by environmental stimuli and craving, and then along comes another one. In this sense, a nicotine medication that helps keep you from smoking in the first place is likely to keep you from progressing.

Brody: I know you are very sensitive to this issue of patient reporting. It seemed to me that having a palm pilot would affect the subjective experience: it is a bit like being on camera 24 h a day.

Shiffman: It is a tough issue. We have done some experimental studies, and it is surprisingly difficult to see any reactivity. In the pain area we did a study in which we randomized people to have different degrees of intensity of monitoring. We found no difference in the ratings. It is a bit like reality TV: when it is intense and ever-present, the monitoring fades into the background. There is probably an interaction here with individual differences. We noticed this in people who dropped out early: there are some people who deal with quitting smoking by a mental process of not thinking about it or denying that is there. We give them a computer which five times a day is effectively saying, 'So, do you like smoking?' These people throw the device back at us right away!

Clarke: The rapid effects of the nicotine patch on the first day prompts a question. Is it possible that the people in the nicotine patch group feel the nicotine right at the site of the patch, and therefore have a pretty good idea of which group they are in? If so, this would play on their expectation that the patch will be effective. I am aware of a study by John Hughes (Hughes et al 1985) in which the placebo group was deliberately told that they might be in a group that had a new improved gum with no side effects. In this study, the instructions had a clear effect on self-administration of the gum.

Shiffman: The issue of how unblinding affects treatment isn't worked out. A recent paper (Mooney et al 2004) shows that in some cessation studies where the effect was modest, it seemed to be due to people who were aware of their patch condition. A feature of this patch is that there is a little bit of nicotine in the adhesive. Even the placebo has the nicotine smell, so it is a little harder to unblind. I guess the more plausible explanation is that if we look at when the failures happened, they were late enough that it was well past the time when the patch would be kicking in substantially. This is why it is plausible that it is a pharmacological effect.

Clarke: I am not saying that it is not pharmacological; I am questioning where the nicotine is acting: skin or brain.

Shiffman: In studies of normal patches, patches are almost indiscriminable.

Walton: I think you have a really good way of examining the effects of nicotine in precise detail. However, within it you still have a confounder, which is nicotine metabolism.

Shiffman: The average nicotine blood levels while on patch was 125% of baseline, but 14% were below their baseline nicotine. There is certainly variability due to dosing, with metabolism not being the only source. Permeability of skin is another. The way I read this is that it suggests that we should have some modest expectations about how much we are going to account for by the crude random assignment of people to patch or not, because as you say there is variability. The patch is not a homogeneous treatment.

Walton: I suppose the answer is that as Rachel Tyndale gets her assays more and more defined, it is not going to be so expensive to type people for nicotine metabolism.

Tyndale: If you have pre-treatment smoking plasma data on these people, you could retrospectively look at the 3-hydroxycotinine to cotinine ratio as a relatively good surrogate for rates of nicotine metabolism (Dempsey et al 2004).

Shiffman: We tried correlating the degree of symptom relief with the degree of nicotine replacement. Our interpretation is that having achieved 100% or better for most people, the variations are not consequential in terms of symptoms, but this is not to say they aren't consequential in terms of outcomes.

Tyndale: We have found the same thing. The genetic slow metabolizers in the NRT study who had substantially higher nicotine replacement (>100%) didn't show a better outcome, although when you look at the general relationship between rates of metabolism, levels of nicotine and outcome you can see some improvement for those who are slower and have higher nicotine levels.

Jarvis: There is a literature about NRT: several studies say that any smoking after day 1 of a quit attempt is associated with long-term failure. This is at variance with your findings. Do you think that all that is coming out here is that if you study the processes in detail you find there are great deficiencies in the data on which those conclusions are based?

Shiffman: I am not sure they are contradictory. Those studies are based, for example, on six month outcome. It is quite possible that the people who showed low daily risk of relapsing will be back to smoking after six months.

Hajek: This approach may disentangle a very important issue. We talk about lapses triggering relapse, which is the received wisdom, but the logic of this is a bit like saying that the first sneeze gave you the cold.

West: There must be data on this. I seem to remember Stan Schachter doing naturalistic studies on the extent to which people stutter into abstinence (Schachter 1982). From an epidemiological point of view, the simple question is what proportion of long term ex-smokers stopped and have never had another cigarette since, and what proportion of quitters had lapses and so on? My recollection is that in the majority of cases they stuttered into abstinence.

Shiffman: We have great data. Ken Perkins, working with Cynthia Conklin, is doing some analysis of relapse patterns. What is important about this is not only does it help us to understand the process, but also it presents opportunities for interventions. Even if the failure is statistically inevitable, it is clear from our data that the process of getting there is prolonged and intermittent. People flop around like a fish pulled into a boat for a long time. We ought to think about how we can intervene during this period. The fact that the process is so chaotic suggests that some people could be rescued.

Perkins: Everyone used to think that lapse was similar to the effects of a priming dose in animal research. This is clearly incorrect. The median duration between the lapse and relapse is at least a month. We looked at the progression to regular smoking (Conklin et al 2005). We tracked these people and found a number of different subgroups, but they almost all end up either fully resuming smoking or returning to abstinence; we don't have many people in intermediate positions for very long.

Shiffman: The second lapse, which might be what is most relavant, often happens the same or next day.

West: This parallels the data with alcohol. A recent study (Mann et al 2005) involved long-term follow up of people who have had treatment for alcoholism, and found a bifurcation following a chaotic pattern.

Perkins: We have two subgroups in each direction. One group is quickly back to high-rate smoking, and the other is slowly back. There is the same thing in reverse (i.e. quickly abstinent versus slow return to abstinence).

Shiffman: Naltrexone for drinking is a good example. My understanding is that the mechanism is thought to be strictly to keep lapses from turning into relapse. Among people who maintain abstinence there is no effect, but for people who start drinking, those on naltrexone are less likely to progress. This is an example of a drug and a mechanism that works in a particular place behaviourally.

Balfour: We are returning to the issue of comparing using a high-dose nicotine patch with using a nicotine vaccine. One of the important issues is whether the patch provides a necessary pharmacological effect, or is it blocking by desensitization the effects of a subsequent nicotine dose? If it is doing the latter, we might expect the vaccine to do something similar. If it is the former there may be a problem with the vaccine, because people may smoke more with the vaccine as they seek to experience the effects of the nicotine they would anticipate from the smoke.

Shiffman: I don't see the two in opposition. It is ambiguous: it goes back to our discussion about receptor desensitization rather than activation. With this much nicotine floating around chronically I would think it is more desensitization than activation. It is a blockade. Both mechanisms are plausible. With the vaccine one has to struggle to think of a plausible mechanism. If it is to work at all it will be by knocking out the response to that re-exposure and reducing the progression from lapse to relapse.

Stolerman: If the vaccine is to be useful, it will have to be very highly effective in terms of blocking nicotine. Otherwise we will see the sorts of things that we saw with mecamylamine: compensatory smoking to get the nicotine in. The concept of the vaccine will then be prematurely killed because of an inadequate product reaching the market.

References

Conklin CA, Perkins KA, Sheidow AJ et al 2005 The return to smoking: 1-year relapse trajectories among female smokers. Nicotine Tobacco Res 7:533–540

Dempsey D, Tutka P, Jacob P 3rd et al 2004 Nicotine metabolite ratio as an index of cytochrome P450 2A6 metabolic activity. Clin Pharmacol Ther 76:64–72

Hughes JR, Pickens RW, Spring W, Keenan RM 1985 Instructions control whether nicotine will serve as a reinforcer. J Pharmacol Exp Ther 235:106–112

Mann K, Schäfer DR, Längle G 2005 The long-term course of alcoholism, 5, 10 and 16 years after treatment. Addiction 100:797–805

Mooney M, White T, Hatsukami D 2004 The blind spot in the nicotine replacement therapy literature: assessment of the double-blind in clinical trials. Addict Behav 29:673–684

Schachter S 1982 Recidivism and self-cure of smoking and obesity. Am Psychol 37:436–444

Modifying the metabolism of nicotine as a therapeutic strategy

Rachel F. Tyndale and Edward M. Sellers[1]

Centre for Addiction and Mental Health, Department of Pharmacology, 1 King's College Circle, Rm 4326, University of Toronto, Toronto, M5S 1A8, Canada

Abstract. CYP2A6 is the enzyme responsible for the metabolic inactivation of around 90% of nicotine to cotinine. Individuals with genetically decreased *CYP2A6* have slower rates of nicotine inactivation. We have found that slow nicotine inactivators are roughly twice less likely to be current adult smokers and those who are smoke 7–10 fewer cigarettes per day than people with normal metabolic rates. Slow nicotine inactivators also smoke for a shorter duration before quitting and may have increased success in quitting. Recently we have shown that imitating the protection offered by the slow metabolism, by inhibiting CYP2A6 activity *in vivo*, can decrease smoking. CYP2A6 is also involved in the activation of tobacco-smoke nitrosamines. Slow metabolizes are at lower risk for lung cancer and we have shown that CYP2A6 inhibitors can also decrease the nitrosamine activation (rerouting them to detoxified glucuronides). CYP2A6 inhibitors can be used alone, or with nicotine to make a nicotine oral pill, to inhibit the first-pass metabolism. CYP2A6 inhibitors can also increase nicotine plasma levels (and bioavailability) of nicotine when given with nicotine patch or gum. These approaches together may provide a better understanding of smoking behaviour and provide novel therapeutic approaches to smoking reduction and cessation.

2005 Understanding nicotine and tobacco addiction. Wiley, Chichester (Novartis Foundation Symposium 275) p 235–248

Nicotine is the major psychoactive compound in tobacco, and is the component in cigarettes which is primarily responsible for establishing and maintaining dependence on cigarette smoking (McMorrow & Foxx 1983, Henningfield et al 1985). Nicotine inhaled from cigarette smoke moves rapidly through the lungs to the brain. It has a distribution half-life of 15–20 min and an elimination half-life of 1–2 h (Hukkanen et al 2005). The short elimination half-life of nicotine results in

---

[1] Declaration of conflict of interest. Rachel F. Tyndale and Edward M. Sellers are shareholders in Nicogen Inc., a company focused on the development of smoking cessation and exposure reduction treatments. Nicogen has provided partial funding for some of the human experimental work included in this review.

nicotine-dependent smokers smoking regularly to replenish nicotine levels. Thus we hypothesized that slow rates of nicotine metabolism would result in lower levels of smoking. This review will describe the role of genetically variable CYP2A6-mediated nicotine metabolism in various smoking behaviours and our approaches to smoking reduction and cessation based on the rationale provided by the *CYP2A6* genetic studies.

Nicotine dependence, via smoking, is a complex behaviour produced by nicotine and influenced by both genetic and environmental factors. Estimates of the genetic contribution to the different aspects of smoking, derived from twin, family and adoption studies, are in general around 60–70% (Tyndale 2003). The primary addictive substance in tobacco smoke is nicotine and smokers have been shown to modulate their smoking to maintain nicotine levels (McMorrow & Foxx 1983). Factors that alter nicotine clearance can alter smoking behaviour, thus we have focused on genetic variation in nicotine metabolism (Hukkanen et al 2005, Malaiyandi et al 2005).

Genetic variation in the rates of nicotine metabolic inactivation

In humans approximately 80% of nicotine is metabolized to cotinine (Hukkanen et al 2005) and roughly 90% of this conversion is mediated by CYP2A6 (Nakajima et al 1996a, Messina et al 1997). Cotinine is further metabolized, specifically by CYP2A6, to 3-hydroxycotinine (Nakajima et al 1996b, Dempsey et al 2004). Substantial variation in CYP2A6 activity results in profound interindividual and interethnic variation in nicotine metabolism; this variability can be largely attributed to genetic polymorphisms in the *CYP2A6* gene.

Currently there are over 25 genetic variants of *CYP2A6* identified (*http://www.imm.ki.se/CYPalleles/cyp2a6.htm*); variants continue to be identified at a rapid rate. Of the variants that have been characterized, many alter enzyme activity or regulation. Genetic variation in *CYP2A6* has been shown to dramatically alter the rates of nicotine metabolic inactivation to cotinine. In *CYP2A6* genetically slow inactivators, defined as those with two decreased activity alleles or one or more inactive alleles, nicotine metabolism is reduced by 50% or more (Xu et al 2002, Schoedel et al 2004).

Factors that alter the removal of nicotine (e.g. acidification of urine to increase nicotine clearance) affect smoking behaviours (Hukkanen et al 2005). Since decreases in the rate of nicotine metabolism, due to *CYP2A6* genetic polymorphisms, increase the duration of nicotine in the body (Xu et al 2002) we hypothesized that this would reduce the urge to smoke among dependent smokers and lengthen the times between cigarettes. This impact on smoking has now been demonstrated in a number of studies, although in our work we have generally seen this effect only in those who are dependent smokers, where the smoking behaviour is more tightly regulated (Schoedel et al 2004). Caucasian slow inactivators (50% or more reduction in activity) smoke 5–10 cigarettes fewer per day relative to normal inactivators (100% activity). Plasma nicotine levels are similar between the slow and normal inactivators while carbon monoxide (CO) levels, a non-self-report of smoking, are significantly reduced in slow inactivators (Rao et al 2000). Individuals with fully inactive CYP2A6 (no CYP2A6 activity, poor inactivators) are rare in Caucasians but more common in Asian populations, especially Japanese (Schoedel et al 2004). While the levels of smoking vary by ethnicity, due to environmental, social or other genetic factors, within ethnic groups a *CYP2A6* gene-dose effect has been observed. For example, among Japanese men, who are heavy smokers, *CYP2A6* poor and slow inactivators smoked less per day and had a reduced risk for lung cancer (Fujieda et al 2004). These data are consistent with the relationship found between CYP2A6 activity, indicated by the metabolic ratio of 3-hydroxycotinine to cotinine, and the number of cigarettes smoked per day (Benowitz et al 2003).

CYP2A6 genetic variation and risk for being an adult smoker

A number of studies in adults have demonstrated that *CYP2A6* genetic variation, causing reduced or absent enzyme activity, is associated with a reduced risk for smoking, lower amount smoked, altered smoking intensity and increased quitting; however, not all studies are in agreement (recently reviewed by Malaiyandi et al 2005). We recently investigated several study variables that may alter the relationship between *CYP2A6* genetic variation and smoking behaviour (Schoedel et al 2004, Malaiyandi et al 2005). Briefly, we found that slow inactivators were more frequent among non-smokers than smokers regardless of whether the smokers were tobacco dependent (DSM IV) or not (OR = 0.52, 95% CI = 0.30–0.91, $P = 0.027$). Nicotine-dependent slow inactivators smoked fewer cigarettes per day compared to normal inactivators (21.3 versus 28.2 cigarettes per day, $P = 0.003$) but this effect was found only among those defined as current DSM IV *dependent* smokers. Reduced cigarette consumption is associated with better cessation outcomes, therefore slow inactivators might be able to quit sooner (Hymowitz et al 1997, Breslau & Johnson 2000). We found that the proportion of slow inactivators was the greatest among non-smokers, followed by short duration current smokers (<10 years) and was the lowest among long duration smokers (>30 years) (Schoedel et al 2004). This suggests that slow inactivator smokers (DSM IV dependent or not) may be quitting sooner. This is supported by some data from cessation trials as well as one study where smokers with a *CYP2A6*2* allele (slow inactivators) were more likely (OR = 1.75, 95% CI = 1.17–2.61) to quit compared to those without *CYP2A6*2* (Gu et al 2000). These studies provide support that smokers with a slow inactivator genotype may be quitting sooner and consequently are under-represented in smoker groups, particularly as the duration of smoking increases. However, a residual number of slow inactivators remain among long duration smokers, thus it will be important to determine whether these slow inactivators are resistant to quitting or have not yet made serious attempts to stop smoking. Several aspects of smoking related to cessation appear to be influenced by *CYP2A6* genetic variation; slow inactivators are less likely to be current smokers, if dependent they smoke less per day, and they appear more able to quit smoking.

CYP2A6 genetic variation and tobacco-related cancers

CYP2A6 can also metabolize tobacco-specific nitrosamines including 4-(methylnitrosamino)-1-(3-pyridyl)-1-butanone (NNK) and N'-nitrosonornicotine (NNN), to form active lung carcinogens (Yamazaki et al 1992, Patten et al 1997, Smith et al 2003). Some studies have found that those with reduced *CYP2A6* activity alleles (slow and poor metabolizers) have a lower risk of developing lung cancer (Miyamoto et al 1999, Ariyoshi et al 2002) although not all studies agree (Loriot et al 2001, Tan et al 2001). This reduced risk may be due to lower levels of smoking, as cancer risk is related to amount smoked (Law et al 1997), and/or to reduced procarcinogen activation. A very large study in Japanese men (Fujieda et al 2004) demonstrated a *CYP2A6* gene-dose reduction in amount smoked and risk for lung cancer (when controlling for smoking levels). We also observe a gene-dose effect on pack-years of cigarette procarcinogen exposure prior to lung cancer diagnosis. Slow CYP2A6 metabolism likely reduces lung cancer risk by reducing the amount and duration of smoking (Gu et al 2000, Schoedel et al 2004), thereby reducing the exposure to procarcinogens, in addition to reducing procarcinogen activation. Below we describe how we have inhibited CYP2A6 metabolism to reduce smoking behaviours and procarcinogen activation.

Mimicking *CYP2A6* genetic impairment: novel therapeutic strategies

Nicotine replacement therapy (NRT), including nicotine patch, nasal spray, gum, inhaler and lozenges, is the most commonly used treatment for smoking cessation (Sellers et al 2003a). However while effective, the vast majority of those treated relapse, suggesting the need for new treatments (Fiore et al 1994, Silagy et al 2000). Based on the premise that dependent smokers regulate their smoking to maintain target nicotine concentrations (McMorrow & Foxx 1983) and *CYP2A6* slow inactivators smoke less (Rao et al 2000), we postulated that inhibition of the CYP2A6 enzyme would slow nicotine inactivation, prolong brain nicotine levels, and reduce smoking.

In some populations, such as the Japanese, large numbers of individuals have no CYP2A6 at all, suggesting that it does not play an essential role in normal endogenous functions. In addition, CYP2A6 exhibits a narrow substrate and inhibitor spectrum, metabolizing only a very few pharmaceutical compounds (e.g. coumarin, halothane, valproic acid, disulfiram and the antineoplastic agent Tegafur®) and tobacco-specific nitrosamines (Hukkanen et al 2005). Thus, inhibiting CYP2A6 is unlikely to have substantive endogenous or clinical consequences, and the risk for clinically important drug interactions is also very low.

CYP2A6 inhibition of nicotine kinetics *in vitro* and *in vivo* (subcutaneous, oral, patch and gum delivery)

To mimic, or 'phenocopy', the genetically based reduction in smoking *in vivo* we searched for selective CYP2A6 inhibitors that could be given to humans. We established *in vitro* kinetic assays for each of the major drug metabolizing CYPs, CYP1A2, -2A6, 2B6, -2C9, -2C19, -2D6 and -3A4. Using cDNA-expressed CYPs, as well as human liver microsomes, we identified two CYP2A6 inhibitors that could be used in humans, methoxsalen and tranylcypromine (Zhang et al 2001). Both compounds have relatively high CYP2A6 specificity and selectivity (60–5000-fold for tranylcypromine, 3.5–200-fold for methoxsalen). In human liver microsomes, both had considerably higher affinity than nicotine ($K_m = 65\,\mu M$) with K_i values of 0.08–0.2 μM indicating they are potent inhibitors of nicotine metabolism (Sellers et al 2000, Zhang et al 2001). Due to the potential difficulty in interpreting pharmacodynamic data using tranylcypromine, a centrally active monoamine oxidase inhibitor antidepressant, much of our proof of concept work used methoxsalen. Methoxsalen, used to treat psoriasis, has no activity within the CNS.

We had a number of goals for these studies. We wanted to use CYP2A6 inhibitors to reproduce/corroborate the effects of genetically reduced metabolism. In addition, nicotine is not currently available as an oral pill medication due to the extensive hepatic first pass metabolism of nicotine following oral administration; only about 25–30% of nicotine is orally bioavailable (Hukkanen et al 2005). We were also interested in testing whether CYP2A6 inhibition could improve the nicotine plasma levels of existing NRTs such as the patch and the gum, and lastly we wanted to determine if CYP2A6 inhibition could reduce the activation of procarcinogens.

In overnight abstinent smokers methoxsalen (30–50 mg) was administered 30 minutes before three subcutaneous nicotine injections given at hourly intervals (Sellers et al 2003b). Each nicotine injection alone (31 µg/kg) resulted in an increase in plasma nicotine of 10–15 ng/ml, approximately the amount obtained from one cigarette. Nicotine was delivered subcutaneously to kinetically mimic the systemic delivery of nicotine from cigarettes. Methoxsalen increased the mean plasma nicotine levels by 47% ($P < 0.01$), the mean nicotine area under the curve (8 hour AUC) by 63% ($P < 0.0001$) while decreasing clearance by 39% ($P < 0.0001$).

Methoxsalen also inhibits metabolism of orally delivered nicotine. Nicotine (4 mg) was given to healthy abstinent tobacco-dependent smokers with placebo, or methoxsalen (3.5, 10 or 30 mg) followed by blood sampling for 3 hours (Sellers et al 2000). Placebo inhibitor plus oral nicotine increased the 3-hour plasma nicotine by 4 ng/ml, while methoxsalen (10 or 30 mg) increased nicotine by 9.7–10 ng/ml ($P < 0.01$). Methoxsalen also reduced the subjects' self-rated current desire to smoke relative to placebo inhibitor ($P < 0.01$).

CYP2A6 inhibition also increases nicotine plasma levels when nicotine is delivered via the transdermal patch or as nicotine gum. Nicotine patch (22 mg/day) and gum (4 mg) at therapeutic dosages result in nicotine plasma concentrations of about 50% of those achieved from smoking *ad libitum* (Benowitz et al 1987, Gorsline et al 1993), suggesting that reduced rates of removal of nicotine might improve these NRTs. Using a randomized double-blind crossover comparison, we compared methoxsalen (10 mg t.i.d.) versus placebo in dependent smokers using nicotine patch (21 mg/day) for four days or nicotine gum (one piece of 4 mg gum chewed for 30 min, hourly for 5 h) for three days. Methoxsalen, relative to placebo inhibitor, increased mean plasma nicotine levels by 24% (23 vs. 29 ng/ml, $P < 0.05$) with the nicotine patch and 52% ($P < 0.05$) with nicotine gum. The patch delivers nicotine directly into the systemic circulation, while with nicotine gum approximately 23% enters directly (via buccal absorption) while 25% is swallowed and the remaining nicotine is left in the gum or is expectorated (Benowitz et al 1987, Hukkanen et al 2005). The swallowed nicotine undergoes 60–80% first pass metabolism, thus CYP2A6 inhibition can dramatically increase the bioavailability of the swallowed nicotine from the gum, resulting in the relatively larger impacts of CYP2A6 inhibition on nicotine gum than patch.

Together these data indicate that *in vitro* inhibition of CYP2A6 can be used to predict the impact on nicotine metabolism *in vivo*, with inhibitors blocking nicotine metabolism from systemic (subcutaneous, patch and gum) as well as oral (oral and gum) deliveries, mimicking the increased/prolonged plasma nicotine levels seen in genetically slow inactivators.

CYP2A6 inhibition: effect on smoking and procarcinogen metabolism

The goals of the following study were (1) to determine if CYP2A6 inhibition increased the plasma nicotine to smoke exposure ratio and (2) to determine if inhibition of CYP2A6-mediated metabolic activation of NNK would reroute a larger portion of the inhaled NNK to the detoxified NNAL. Dependent smokers were instructed to maintain their same number of cigarettes smoked on the first day of study (day 1 placebo inhibitor) while receiving methoxsalen (10 mg t.i.d.) for three subsequent days during *ad libitum* smoking (Sellers et al 2003b). On day 3 of methoxsalen treatment there was a decrease in breath CO levels (indicating reduced smoking) and an increase in plasma nicotine levels (indicating accumulation of nicotine acquired from smoking during CYP2A6 inhibition). This resulted in a 32%

($P < 0.03$) increase in plasma nicotine to expired-air CO (an index of smoke exposure). Methoxsalen also decreased urinary 3-hydroxycotinine by 45% ($P < 0.0001$) and increased NNAL-glucuronide by 25% ($P = 0.01$) and free NNAL by 37% ($P = 0.07$) relative to placebo on day 1 (controlling for reduced smoking using breath CO). The inhibition of NNK hydroxylation, rerouting NNK to NNAL, may involve some inhibition of CYP1A2 as CYP1A2 can metabolize NNK and can be inhibited by methoxsalen, at least *in vitro*. Together this provides further evidence of CYP2A6 inhibition of nicotine (derived from cigarette smoke) to cotinine, and cotinine to 3-hydroxycotinine, metabolism as well as the inhibition of the metabolism of NNK and successful rerouting of this procarcinogen to a detoxification pathway (NNAL). Consistent with this, a study in mice used methoxsalen inhibition of CYP2A-mediated activation of NNK to demonstrate a substantial inhibition of lung tumorigenesis (Takeuchi et al 2003). These data suggest that CYP2A6 inhibition alone (in the absence of additional medicinal nicotine) may have potential as an exposure/harm reduction and/or cessation strategy in tobacco dependence.

CYP2A6 inhibition: a novel oral NRT and reduction in smoking

We tested whether the combination of oral nicotine and methoxsalen could reduce smoking. Based on a study with nicotine gum (Nemeth-Coslett et al 1987), overnight abstinent, nicotine-dependent smokers were assigned to individual hotel rooms, allowed to smoke one cigarette and then were given one of four oral drug combinations in a double-blind crossover design: methoxsalen (30 mg) or placebo, combined with nicotine (4 mg) or placebo. Drug administration was followed by 60 min of smoking abstinence, 90 min of *ad libitum* smoking (while being videotaped), and then 30 min of abstinence. Smoking during the methoxsalen/nicotine condition was lower than the placebo/placebo condition ($P < 0.01$) as indicated by breath CO, numbers of cigarettes smoked, latency to second cigarette and total puffs taken. In addition the ratio of plasma nicotine to breath CO during methoxsalen/nicotine was more than twice the placebo/placebo condition ($P < 0.01$) indicating a substantial improvement in the smoke exposure cost of nicotine acquisition. The decrease in CO was larger than the decrease in number of puffs (CO per puff, $P < 0.01$) suggesting that they were taking shallower or shorter puffs. The magnitude of reduction in smoking, measured by breath CO, was larger than seen previously with the nicotine gum (Nemeth-Coslett et al 1987). This is likely to be due to the inhibition of both the first pass nicotine metabolism and some contribution to systemic inhibition resulting in higher levels of nicotine for prolonged durations. This study has limitations, such as the smoking sessions being performed for short periods of time in an experimental setting, however the previous study using nicotine gum had very high predictive validity of clinical efficacy (Nemeth-Coslett et al 1987).

This study was not designed to detect the impact of CYP2A6 inhibition alone, however the rank order of effects (methoxsalen/nicotine > methoxsalen/placebo > placebo/nicotine > placebo/placebo) suggests that methoxsalen alone had effects on nicotine (derived from smoking) clearance and smoking behaviour. The rank order was apparent for the number of cigarettes smoked, latency to second cigarette ($P < 0.05$), number of puffs, and nicotine increase per CO increase. This suggests that CYP2A6 inhibition alone (in the absence of medicinal nicotine), if assessed over longer time periods, will have an impact on smoking behaviour due to the inhibition of nicotine metabolism from cigarette smoking. This exposure reduction might be particularly useful in smokers who cannot successfully quit smoking. CYP2A6 inhibition could be used to reduce the rates of smoking and exposure to harmful constituents of tobacco smoke (as well as potentially reducing the activation of tobacco-smoke procarcinogens) and/or as a part of a step-care reduction in smoking leading to cessation.

Together these genetic and biochemical studies indicate that having lower CYP2A6 activity reduces nicotine metabolism, the amount smoked, the activation of tobacco-specific procarcinogens, while increasing quitting. The identification and development of potent, selective and safe CYP2A6 inhibitors could be of great therapeutic utility. CYP2A6 inhibition, in the presence or absence of additional nicotine, could provide new and needed approaches to smoking reduction and cessation.

Acknowledgements

Supported by the Centre for Addiction and Mental Health, a grant from the Canadian Institutes of Health Research (MOP53248) and a Canada Research Chair (RFT). RFT thanks the members of her laboratory for careful review.

References

Ariyoshi N, Miyamoto M, Umetsu Y 2002 Genetic polymorphism of CYP2A6 gene and tobacco-induced lung cancer risk in male smokers. Cancer Epidemiol Biomarkers Prev 11:890–894

Benowitz NL, Jacob P 3rd, Savanapridi C 1987 Determinants of nicotine intake while chewing nicotine polacrilex gum. Clin Pharmacol Ther 41:467–473

Benowitz NL, Pomerleau OF, Pomerleau CS, Jacob P 3rd 2003 Nicotine metabolite ratio as a predictor of cigarette consumption. Nicotine Tob Res 5:621–624

Breslau N, Johnson EO 2000 Predicting smoking cessation and major depression in nicotine-dependent smokers. Am J Public Health 90:1122–1127

Dempsey D, Tutka P, Jacob P 3rd et al 2004 Nicotine metabolite ratio as an index of cytochrome P450 2A6 metabolic activity. Clin Pharmacol Ther 76:64–72

Fiore MC, Smith SS, Jorenby DE, Baker TB 1994 The effectiveness of the nicotine patch for smoking cessation. A meta-analysis. JAMA 271:1940–1947

Fujieda M, Yamazaki H, Saito T et al 2004 Evaluation of CYP2A6 genetic polymorphisms as determinants of smoking behavior and tobacco-related lung cancer risk in male Japanese smokers. Carcinogenesis 25:2451–2458

Gorsline J, Gupta SK, Dye D, Rolf CN 1993 Steady-state pharmacokinetics and dose relationship of nicotine delivered from Nicoderm (Nicotine Transdermal System). J Clin Pharmacol 33:161–168

Gu DF, Hinks LJ, Morton NE, Day IN 2000 The use of long PCR to confirm three common alleles at the CYP2A6 locus and the relationship between genotype and smoking habit. Ann Hum Genet 64:383–390

Henningfield JE, Miyasato K, Jasinski DR 1985 Abuse liability and pharmacodynamic characteristics of intravenous and inhaled nicotine. J Pharmacol Exp Ther 234:1–12

Hukkanen J, Jacob P 3rd, Benowitz NL 2005 Metabolism and disposition kinetics of nicotine. Pharmacol Rev 57:79–115

Hymowitz N, Cummings KM, Hyland A, Lynn WR, Pechacek TF, Hartwell TD 1997 Predictors of smoking cessation in a cohort of adult smokers followed for five years. Tob Control 6 (Suppl 2):S57–62

Law MR, Morris JK, Watt HC, Wald NJ 1997 The dose-response relationship between cigarette consumption, biochemical markers and risk of lung cancer. Br J Cancer 75:1690–1693

Loriot MA, Rebuissou S, Oscarson M et al 2001 Genetic polymorphisms of cytochrome P450 2A6 in a case-control study on lung cancer in a French population. Pharmacogenetics 11:39–44

Malaiyandi V, Sellers EM, Tyndale RF 2005 Implications of CYP2A6 genetic variation for smoking behaviors and nicotine dependence. Clin Pharmacol Ther 77:145–158

McMorrow MJ, Foxx RM 1983 Nicotine's role in smoking: an analysis of nicotine regulation. Psychol Bull 93:302–327

Messina ES, Tyndale RF, Sellers EM 1997 A major role for CYP2A6 in nicotine C-oxidation by human liver microsomes. J Pharmacol Exp Ther 282:1608–1614

Miyamoto M, Umetsu Y, Dosaka-Akita H et al 1999 CYP2A6 gene deletion reduces susceptibility to lung cancer. Biochem Biophys Res Commun 261:658–660

Nakajima M, Yamamoto T, Nunoya K et al 1996a Role of human cytochrome P4502A6 in C-oxidation of nicotine. Drug Metab Dispos 24:1212–1217

Nakajima M, Yamamoto T, Nunoya K et al 1996b Characterization of CYP2A6 involved in 3'-hydroxylation of cotinine in human liver microsomes. J Pharmacol Exp Ther 277:1010–1015

Nemeth-Coslett R, Henningfield JE, O'Keeffe MK, Griffiths RR 1987 Nicotine gum: dose-related effects on cigarette smoking and subjective ratings. Psychopharmacology (Berl) 92:424–430

Patten CJ, Smith TJ, Friesen MJ, Tynes RE, Yang CS, Murphy SE 1997 Evidence for cytochrome P450 2A6 and 3A4 as major catalysts for N'-nitrosonornicotine alpha-hydroxylation by human liver microsomes. Carcinogenesis 18:1623–1630

Rao Y, Hoffmann E, Zia M et al 2000 Duplications and defects in the CYP2A6 gene: identification, genotyping, and in vivo effects on smoking. Mol Pharmacol 58:747–755

Schoedel KA, Hoffmann EB, Rao Y, Sellers EM, Tyndale RF 2004 Ethnic variation in CYP2A6 and association of genetically slow nicotine metabolism and smoking in adult Caucasians. Pharmacogenetics 14:615–626

Sellers EM, Kaplan HL, Tyndale RF 2000 Inhibition of cytochrome P450 2A6 increases nicotine's oral bioavailability and decreases smoking. Clin Pharmacol Ther 68:35–43

Sellers EM, Tyndale RF, Fernandes LC 2003a Decreasing smoking behaviour and risk through CYP2A6 inhibition. Drug Discov Today 8:487–493

Sellers EM, Ramamoorthy Y, Zeman MV, Djordjevic MV, Tyndale RF 2003b The effect of methoxsalen on nicotine and 4-(methylnitrosamino)-1-(3-pyridyl)-1-butanone (NNK) metabolism in vivo. Nicotine Tob Res 5:891–899

Silagy C, Mant D, Fowler G, Lancaster T 2000 Nicotine replacement therapy for smoking cessation. Cochrane Database Syst Rev, CD000146

Smith GB, Bend JR, Bedard LL, Reid KR, Petsikas D, Massey TE 2003 Biotransformation of 4-(methylnitrosamino)-1-(3-pyridyl)-1-butanone (NNK) in peripheral human lung microsomes. Drug Metab Dispos 31:1134–1141

Takeuchi H, Saoo K, Yokohira M et al 2003 Pretreatment with 8-methoxypsoralen, a potent human CYP2A6 inhibitor, strongly inhibits lung tumorigenesis induced by 4-(methylnitrosamino)-1-(3-pyridyl)-1-butanone in female A/J mice. Cancer Res 63:7581–7583

Tan W, Chen GF, Xing DY, Song CY, Kadlubar FF, Lin DX 2001 Frequency of CYP2A6 gene deletion and its relation to risk of lung and esophageal cancer in the Chinese population. Int J Cancer 95:96–101

Tyndale RF 2003 Genetics of alcohol and tobacco use in humans. Ann Med 35:94–121

Xu C, Goodz S, Sellers EM, Tyndale RF 2002 CYP2A6 genetic variation and potential consequences. Adv Drug Deliv Rev 54:1245–1256

Yamazaki H, Inui Y, Yun CH, Guengerich FP, Shimada T 1992 Cytochrome P450 2E1 and 2A6 enzymes as major catalysts for metabolic activation of N-nitrosodialkylamines and tobacco-related nitrosamines in human liver microsomes. Carcinogenesis. 13:1789–1794

Zhang W, Kilicarslan T, Tyndale RF, Sellers EM 2001 Evaluation of methoxsalen, tranylcypromine, and tryptamine as specific and selective CYP2A6 inhibitors in vitro. Drug Metab Dispos 29:897–902

DISCUSSION

Caggiula: You were talking about the CYP2A6 enzyme: did you say that nicotine is metabolized by CYP2A6 to carcinogens?

Tyndale: No. Nicotine is metabolized to cotinine, which is essentially pharmacologically inactive and non-carcinogenic. The nitrosamines are metabolized to hydroxyl-nitrosamines by the same enzyme, CYP2A6, but using different substrates in this case procarcinogen nitrosamines.

Gasparini: I have a question related to a potential liability because of drug–drug interaction using a blocker of CYP2A6. There is probably very little endogenous use of CYP2A6 except as detoxifying enzymes. Wouldn't this require that you preselect patients in the absence of any ongoing metabolism through 2A6?

Tyndale: That's a good question. If we give inhibitors, how much will we affect drug metabolism of other therapies? We have screened about 400 clinical drugs so far and have found only a very few, one antineoplastic and coumarin (which is off the market throughout most of the world). Protoxins present in the environment are frequently activated to toxins by this enzyme, so blockade of CYP2A6 seems to be a good thing.

Gasparini: What about food components and other drugs of abuse?

Tyndale: To be affected drugs have to be going through this enzymatic pathway fairly exclusively, because there are other very large capacity enzymes in the system. There are some drugs that have 5–10% of their metabolism by CYP2A6, but are primarily metabolized by these other large capacity enzymes such as members of the CYP3A family. We think it is unlikely that we will run into this problem. Also, there is a very large population, 5–10% of Japanese, who don't have any functional CYP2A6 at all. If it is important in terms of food we think we would have seen a problem in them.

Shiffman: Why did God put this enzyme here?

Tyndale: These are families of enzymes that have multiple subfamilies with massive diversity of substrate specificity. They appear to have been selected over time depending on dietary constituents; we believe that this may be one reason why populations from different parts of the world, with different dietary and environmental influences, have large differences in the function of these enzymes.

Perkins: In your study in which you videotaped patient smoking behaviour, did you collect self-reported ratings of smoking pleasure?

Tyndale: We did afterwards, but not during that 90 min. We have data on that component. There was some reduction.

Perkins: I wondered whether it might be the other way round: with sustained nicotine increases with each cigarette, subsequent cigarettes might be rated more desirable.

Tyndale: The key question there was whether they had increased nicotine. There was fairly modest amounts of nicotine being given to these people. It was 4 mg, which is equivalent to a cigarette. We tested for a short period so this may not be the best study to look at this issue of altered desirability.

Perkins: I was referring to the nicotine from the smoking, not from the nicotine gum.

Tyndale: It's an interesting question but I don't have the answer.

Hajek: Do they feel sick? Does this limit their smoking?

Tyndale: We see no indication of adverse responses. In kinetic studies where we altered nicotine levels we measured a large number of variables, for example related to cardiovascular concerns and nausea, without any sign of adverse response. In the smoking study, when they are smoking they are free to titrate their own nicotine levels and seem to do so quite well with no sign of adverse events.

Hajek: Could the reason they smoke less be that they would feel sick if they smoked at their usual intensity?

Tyndale: We don't have the data to answer that. In the study where we ask them to maintain their smoking while on an inhibitor they clearly didn't smoke at the same levels. They wanted to smoke less. It's something we need to look at more carefully. In terms of topography we are seeing changes in intensity of smoking as well as amount smoked.

Hajek: One analogy that might be relevant here could be obese people who have stomach banding surgery. They lose lots of weight, and there is evidence that they are not as hungry as you would expect them to be. The fact that eating makes them uncomfortable seems to reduce their appetite.

Tyndale: We see no indication of nausea in our subjects. They are able to titrate their nicotine by reducing their smoking.

Shiffman: I am interested in exploring the studies you showed us in the context of avoiding the activation of NNK. This helps us address the question of whether nicotine is carcinogenic, because here's a population that has much higher exposure to nicotine but lower cancer rates.

Tyndale: They have consistent exposure to nicotine with fewer cigarettes. There is also the confound of reduced activation of carcinogens by slow metabolizers so it is hard to make this conclusion about nicotine. To get at some of the kinetic questions there are ways we could use within individual study designs to look at what the descending plasma nicotine curves are doing to smoking ratings. We have induced this enzyme with phenobarbital and we can increase smoking. We think we can move individuals through a range of rates of metabolism from slow to fast and look at some of the impacts.

Picciotto: If you are decreasing smoking but keeping nicotine levels the same, you could ask across the variants whether there is a decreased cardiovascular risk among slow metabolizers.

Tyndale: We are going into both the chronic obstructive pulmonary disease (COPD) and myocardial infarction groups to see whether slow metabolizers with similar nicotine levels have lower risk. This might be answered in the Japanese population because we get a lot more power if we go down to zero metabolism by CYP2A6 as is seen in fully inactive individuals.

Perkins: Heart disease risk isn't a dose-dependent effect of smoking, unlike cancer.

Jarvis: I am wondering whether this will help throw light on just what aspect of nicotine intake people are regulating. You have shown that it relates to cotinine. Have you measured the immediate post-smoking nicotine peak? Is this invariant across the different rates of metabolism?

Tyndale: No, people are adjusting differently. As we go down the rates of metabolism we tend to get an adjustment by numbers of cigarettes per day. There is also some indication of smaller puff volumes. As we go up to the faster metabolizers we see this effect primarily in intensity. There are different styles of adjusting for variable metabolic rates.

Shiffman: We have talked a lot about bolus effects. How do we know that this enzyme is even relevant for a bolus effect? You are sending nicotine from the lung to the brain and this should have no chance to act on that initial dose.

Tyndale: Absolutely. This is where the route of administration makes a huge difference to how much influence CYP2A6 will have. It doesn't make any difference to the peak nicotine levels from the first cigarette, but it does for subsequent ones because of differences in the baseline level of nicotine in slow and normal metabolizers; this will either alter the interval between cigarettes or suggests that at a

similar interval the slow metabolizers have much higher peaks on the second cigarette due to the higher resting levels.

Balfour: Is CYP2A6 only found in the liver?

Tyndale: It is not well characterized elsewhere. We have looked in a number of
tissues. There are a pair of sibling CYPs in the brain but we don't know what influence they have on nicotine metabolism *in situ*. It doesn't appear to have any impact
on the plasma levels of nicotine, but in small environments in the brain it may alter
the levels.

Picciotto: Is there end product inhibition of 2A6 by cotinine?

Tyndale: Neal Benowitz has done elegant studies looking at why smokers have
lower rates of nicotine metabolism than non-smokers. He looked at CO, cotinine
and a number of other different variables as potential inhibitors, but he wasn't able
to show that these were causing the reduction. We did a study in monkeys where
we gave nicotine chronically and saw similar reductions in the rates of nicotine
metabolism as were seen in human smokers. We think nicotine is causing a down-
regulation of the enzyme, although it could be a form of mechanism-based inhibition as well. We can see this decrease in rates of nicotine metabolism in mice
treated chronically, too. We can't rule out a cotinine interaction because once you
give nicotine, cotinine is present, however Neal's data suggests this isn't the case.

Picciotto: There have been a few papers looking at the effects of cotinine on nicotinic receptors. In some of your non-metabolizers, or those treated with the antagonists, the levels of cotinine should be significantly higher than they would be in a
normal smoker.

Tyndale: It's a bit more complicated than that because we are blocking the routing
of nicotine to cotinine, so the levels of cotinine are reduced. But we are also blocking much more readily the subsequent metabolism of cotinine to 3-hydroxycotinine
because of the relative affinities of CYP2A6 for nicotine (higher) and cotinine
(lower).

Picciotto: In the high metabolizers, is there any evidence for an effect of the elevated cotinine, rather than simply the nicotine?

Tyndale: Where higher levels of cotinine are seen these are paralleled by dramatically higher levels of 3-hydroxycotinine as well. Neal Benowitz has done some nice
studies of taking cotinine up to high concentrations without seeing any pharmacological effects.

Stolerman: There have been a number of behavioural studies of cotinine in
animals. There has been some variation between species, but generally there is
extremely low pharmacological activity in the procedures that have been used.

Clarke: Isn't nicotine-N′-oxide another metabolite?

Tyndale: Yes, people make the N-oxide. Humans actually make lots of different
metabolites, but this hasn't been something that we have focused on. CYP2A6 is
responsible for about 90% of the metabolism of nicotine to cotinine; this pathway

represents about 70–80% of nicotine's removal from the body which is why we have focused on this major pathway. Manipulating the CYP2A6 pathway doesn't change the flow of nicotine to the other metabolites substantially.

Clarke: Do you think the levels of nornicotine in human smokers are sufficient to contribute at all to nicotine dependence?

Tyndale: What levels do you need? There is some interesting work being done in some of the animal models, but I'm concerned about these because the metabolism of those other pathways is really different in rat. Even the proportion of nicotine that goes to cotinine and the enzyme used are quite different in rat.

Challenges in discovery and development of pharmacotherapies for tobacco addiction

William A. Corrigall

Corrigall Consulting, 48 Highland Park Boulevard, Thornhill, ON L3T 1B3, Canada and Minneapolis Medical Research Foundation, 914 South Eighth Street, Minneapolis, MN 55404, USA

Abstract. This paper describes several tactical issues that would advance discovery science and the translation to development. There is a need to broaden target discovery with respect to the disease mechanisms of tobacco addiction. Secondly, discovery and target validation needs to be done in a more integrated fashion; there is a need to apply existing models in concerted fashion, recognizing that tobacco addiction is a complex, multifaceted disease. Discovery research would benefit immediately from the increased availability of molecular tools, both molecular probes for various receptor systems and compounds that can be used in human experimental laboratory studies to validate observations from cell, tissue and animal experiments. Fourth, tobacco addiction/dependence would benefit from broad agreement on its definition, its core elements and treatment targets for the disease. Finally, research with human subjects could make a greater contribution to target validation and to development, and improved networking of clinical trials sites could provide an appealing platform to augment development. The paper argues that advances in pharmacotherapies will be helped by collaborative activities, translational activities built upon existing knowledge, and partnership between publicly funded discovery researchers and the pharmaceutical industry.

2005 Understanding nicotine and tobacco addiction. Wiley, Chichester (Novartis Foundation Symposium 275) p 249–261

Three elements would improve our ability to respond to the health needs of the vast numbers of individuals who are addicted to tobacco through the pharmacological action of nicotine in the central nervous system; the development of pharmacotherapies or medications to treat nicotine addiction, an increased capacity to test tobacco addiction medications in real world settings with real world populations where their effectiveness and cost-effectiveness can be evaluated, and an enhanced delivery of tobacco addiction medications to relevant populations. This paper focuses on challenges that exist within the first of these elements. However, these three elements should function as a system. As such, activities in the latter two areas can lead to the listing and coverage of medications by health care providers, and to the delivery of medications to underserved populations such as individuals with co-occurring mental disorders or alcohol abuse problems, groups that contribute heavily to the real burden of tobacco disease. Indeed there is benefit in translating existing treatments more effectively for the very reason that it establishes an effective delivery system to support better medications as they are developed, in turn presumably a stimulus to development by enhancing the overall market for them. Thus it is important not to lose sight of the broader context that can influence development *per se*.

With respect to medication development for tobacco addiction, this paper describes several strategic issues and concludes with some tactical efforts that have been or could be used to advance them. One cautionary note: the points made here are personal opinions. They are factually based, but they reflect views formed over a career as a researcher in the field of behavioural neuroscience, as a scientist involved with program development at the National Institutes of Health (NIH), and currently as an independent consultant with a significant interest in the translation of science to practice.

There is a need to broaden target discovery with respect to the disease mechanisms of tobacco addiction

Logically following a direction established by research on psychomotor stimulants and opioids, the initial focus in the neuroscience of nicotine with respect to reward and reinforced behaviour was the midbrain dopamine system (Corrigall et al 1992, 1994). There has since been a real growth in understanding the role of the mesolimbic dopamine system at a multiplicity of levels of analysis (Balfour 2005, this volume, Di Chiara 2000). However, there has been limited success in translating this extensive knowledge to practice in terms of the development of dopamine-based medications for tobacco dependence. Contemporary discovery research, such as that focused on furthering the details of dopamine signalling that may be particularly relevant in nicotine addiction, for example the D_3 system (Heidbreder 2005, this volume, Le Foll et al 2005) may afford critical insights to allow medication development; similarly contemporary treatment research such as the investigation of monoamine oxidase (MAOB) manipulations may change the perspective on translation to pharmacotherapies (George et al 2003).

There are reasons to be concerned about the future for dopamine-based interventions as a sole approach, including the relatively small response exhibited by tobacco users to dopamine challenge in laboratory settings (e.g. Caskey et al 2002), the effort–outcome balance for dopamine-based medications that we have seen in the psychomotor stimulant field to date, and the involvement of the mesolimbic dopamine system in reward signalling generally (Tobler et al 2005). Clearly dopamine is a target for nicotine, but probably not a selective one, perhaps not a sufficient one, nor perhaps a drug-able one for tobacco (and, yes, this same criticism could be raised for other single-neurotransmitter approaches). Hence, while it is reasonable to capitalize on the solid base of knowledge regarding the effects of nicotine on the dopamine system, there is a very real need to understand the broader mechanisms of nicotine addiction (Wonnacott et al 2005), from nAChR mechanisms that control neurotransmitter release (e.g. Salminen et al 2005), to potentiation of synaptic responses (e.g. Mansvelder et al 2003). To build a base for pharmacotherapeutic approaches requires an expanded target discovery agenda (Cryan et al 2003, Heidbreder & Hagan 2005), and this has already begun. In our own research, for example, we chose to approach the problem by looking for other systems, both anatomical and neurochemical that might modulate the mesolimbic reward pathway. This allowed us to unmask the involvement of a brainstem pontine nucleus in nicotine reinforcement (Lança et al 2000a), a locus of projections to the dopamine cells in the ventral tegmental area (VTA) that have cholinergic, GABAergic and glu-tamatergic elements, and are influenced by opioid mechanisms (Corrigall et al 1999, 2001, 2002, Lança et al 2000b). Within the vicinity of the dopamine cells of the VTA we found that opioid and GABA mechanisms are also operative in reinforcement (Corrigall et al 2000). Others have advanced this field substantially, implicating other neurochemical systems and other pathways, some not synaptically intimate with the mesolimbic dopamine system (Markou 2005, this volume). This diversity of effects is not surprising given the wide distribution of high-affinity and other nicotinic recep-tors (nAChRs) throughout the CNS (Maskos et al 2005, this volume).

It is logical from an anatomical perspective to search for other brain loci given, as already noted, the diverse distribution of nicotinic acetylcholine receptors (nAChRs) within the CNS, and it is logical functionally to look for targets that might underlie the wide range of nicotine effects on human behaviour, asking about mechanisms underlying the explicit components of nicotine addiction, about the potential involvement of CNS systems that regulate food as a common target, about what we can learn from the mechanisms of executive functioning, task focusing and attention, and of course memory. In addition, a more reductionist approach would support looking within neuronal and synaptic processes for drug-able sub-strates for nicotine addiction—signal transduction processes (Picciotto 2005, this volume) or micro-structural changes seen after drug exposure that confer lasting functional changes (Robinson & Kolb 2004), along with ongoing efforts to iden-tify nAChR subtypes that play unique roles and confirming those roles *in vivo*.

Discovery and target validation needs to be done in a more integrated fashion

While the above issue concerns implementation, integration of research is also required. A variety of models and approaches have been used to discover nicotine's biological mechanisms of action at different levels of analysis, as exemplified by the presentations in this symposium. However, in the absence of successful pharmacotherapies for tobacco addiction, it has not been possible to establish the predictive validity of any of these model systems vis-à-vis medication development. Given that it has often fallen to behavioural paradigms such as operant self-administration to be used *de facto* as the tools of translation of basic neuroscience to potential application, it is worth noting that we are still learning what these behavioural models measure, and that parameters of the self-administration model influence the nature of the data acquired (W. A. Corrigall et al unpublished work 2003, Donny et al 2003, Stolerman 2005, this volume). This is not intended as an indictment of the solid research done with these models. Nor should it be construed as a statement that new models are required. In fact an explicit search for new models would be compromised by lack of knowing exactly what we need. Rather, nicotine addiction is a complex, multi-component disease, and tactically it will be necessary to approach the disease with the assumption that we can make progress by using a combination of approaches in a coordinated fashion. To do this, we need to use existing models differently, integrating the data and conclusions from a reasonable aggregate to reach overall conclusions about the validity of targets for medication development. In its simplest version, this could take the form of integrating information from experiments conducted with simple biological model systems, with animal behavioural pharmacological research, with human laboratory behavioural studies that can provide information on choice preferences, subjective effects and relapse cues, and human neuroscience data gained from approaches such as neuroimaging (Brody 2005, this volume). More creative approaches than this can be developed. Conceptually, an integrative approach such as this recasts discovery as a search for targets acting in concert. Operationally, it could move discovery to consider other targets elucidated by related fields such as mental health/behaviour-in-excess disorders or consumption disorders such as obesity. The value of an approach such as this is the potential identification of a 'fingerprint' or profile for the disease that will subsequently be useful in identifying candidates for development. It would be valuable if this integrative approach, which does happen, could be encouraged more widely.

Discovery research would benefit immediately from the increased availability of molecular tools

There are two aspects to this issue. First, there is quite simply a shortage of selective molecular probes for various receptor systems which presents a critical challenge to discovery of mechanisms in nicotine addiction for *in vitro* studies and animal research. This is well exemplified by the nAChR field in which there is a need for ligands with selectivity for the range of receptor subtypes that occur naturally *in vivo* as well as those that can be expressed *in vitro*. Although genetically manipulated mouse strains collectively are valuable tools to advance understanding of the function of various receptor systems, these models, too, would benefit from validation with selective probes.

Secondly, there is a lack of compounds that can be used in discovery research with human subjects, for studies in human experimental paradigms to validate in tobacco users observations from cell, tissue and animal experiments, and for development as imaging ligands to extend neuroscience discovery to the human CNS.

Tobacco addiction/dependence would benefit from broad agreement on its definition, its core elements and treatment targets for the disease

Definitions in the field of addiction or dependence related to all drugs have evolved substantially over time as new research and clinical observations change our understanding. However, various measurement instruments exist in which different core elements are given primacy (e.g. American Psychiatric Association 1994, Heatherton et al 1991, Piper et al 2004, Shiffman et al 2004, West 2005, this volume). There are several implications. Presumably, in research in which genetic information is collected across treatment trials, a common phenotype would be beneficial. In basic discovery research it would be useful to have the elements of the disease well described. For example, the definition of relapse should shape basic research with animal models of reinstatement of drug-taking behaviour, and in a truly translational sense, the reverse should also occur. Thirdly, consistent definition of the phenotype would support the use of common language, and presumably would lead to a more consistent approach to the choice of clinical endpoints. Certainly in the process of medication development it would enhance communication with regulatory bodies.

An additional benefit would accrue from agreement on core elements and treatment targets. Tobacco addiction is frequently described as a chronically relapsing disorder, accompanied by the explicit statement or tacit assumption that this characteristic justifies, as a *sine qua non*, protracted treatment. In addition, certain chronic use medications in general medicine have recently been withdrawn from the market or placed under increasing regulatory scrutiny. Coupled with the fact that there is increasing regulatory pressure on medications, likely greater on ones intended for chronic use, it may be that there will be increasing inertia to medication development for tobacco addiction, when the intended use is long term. A context in which agreement on exactly what constitutes dependence/addiction and the core elements of the disease could allow a clearer articulation of treatment goals and timelines according to disease components. This in turn could allow improved collaboration with regulatory bodies in the process of medication development.

Research with human subjects could make a greater contribution to target validation and to development

Identified biological targets should be the focus of increased human experimental research and clinical trial activities. As noted earlier in this commentary, there have been advances in the identification of potential neurochemical targets for nicotine addiction. In some cases there are compounds that have reasonable fidelity for these neurochemical targets and that can be administered to human subjects. Some of these compounds exist within the public domain, others very likely within the pharmaceutical industry. It would be valuable if such compounds were explored in human experimental studies to permit at least a first-order assessment of the role of these neurochemical targets alone or in combination in tobacco smoking behaviour.

Secondly, medication development would be augmented by a clinical trials 'network' for tobacco addiction, envisioned as an affiliation of clinical sites with expertise in tobacco addiction permitting early stage controlled clinical studies to obtain preliminary data on a potential medication. Such an affiliation could provide a valuable preferred partnership platform for the pharmaceutical industry on which to conduct Phase 2 studies in tobacco addiction, or for treatment researchers who are so inclined to conduct similar studies when the pharmaceutical industry may not be prepared to pursue them. A network would function with a relatively standardized set of assessments, consistent behavioural therapy, and uniform clinical endpoints. The network could ensure that stratification in the clinical response would be taken into account in a consistent fashion, could work in a systematic fashion to develop surrogate markers for efficacy at various disease treatment endpoints, and would provide a more direct and cohesive link to genetic repositories while ensuring that standard phenotypic descriptors accompany the genetic data. Moreover, tobacco addiction does not occur in isolation, but co-occurs with other diseases—with mental illness, alcoholism and substance abuse aetiologically, and as a factor in the development of and recovery from a range of other diseases, such as cardiovascular and pulmonary disease, and cancers. A clinical trials network that afforded access to patient profiles in which tobacco cessation treatment could be tested as a viable intervention to improve another outcome would provide an additional attractive opportunity to test the utility of medications.

Implementation challenges and possibilities

For some of the issues identified as challenges in this paper, there do not appear to be obvious tactics that can be used to progress significantly more quickly and/or on a larger scale. Rather they will evolve as the research field itself moves. Groups of like-minded individuals certainly can address issues such as the definition of nicotine and tobacco addiction, the core elements and disease endpoints, and indeed are doing so. Groups of treatment researchers can form clinical trials networks, but may have to do so without initial access to grants to cover infrastructure costs. The need to broaden discovery science, activity squarely within the domain of public sector research funding, unfortunately comes at a time at which recent dramatic increases in funding for research, such as the 'budget doubling' at the US NIH, has reached a plateau, and major grant-giving bodies in general are not in an expansionist mode of operation. Nonetheless, discovery science in addiction has been increasing in breadth, and this will progressively move the research field. Perhaps counterintuitively, the current fiscal climate may actually help to drive breadth if it encourages preclinical researchers to collaborate across multidisciplinary domains.

There are however, three areas in which steps can be taken to make greater progress. The first continues the theme of collaboration. Integrated research approaches are being viewed with increasing favour in some quarters. One example is the convocation sponsored recently by the US National Academies on the topic of facilitating interdisciplinary research. The report identifies challenges and ways to address them. At the same time, the NIH has recognized the need to enhance interdisciplinary research concretely. As a result, awards have been made for planning grants to support team building, and the near future may see the opportunity to apply for funding for interdisciplinary research consortia. Although this initiative may afford an opportunity for tobacco researchers to build research on a much broader platform, the main point in noting it here is to underscore that some funding agencies are endorsing approaches of this kind. In fact the tobacco field has been a leader in thinking in this direction. More than five years ago, the National Cancer Institute (NCI) and the National Institute on Drug Abuse (NIDA) jointly funded the Transdisciplinary Tobacco Use Research Centers (TTURCs), another integrative approach which is now in its second five-year cycle with the added partnership of the National Institute on Alcohol Abuse and Alcoholism. This initiative supports grants that are integrative across a range of disciplines. Included in the scope of the work is research in the area of medication discovery and development, and the development of human experimental research models.

The second opportunity lies in acting on known targets with a translational objective. There are now a number of neurochemical targets that have been identified in nicotine addiction. Where appropriate compounds exist, they can be tested in relatively smaller scale human experimental studies or in larger Phase 2 type clinical trials. Several years ago at NIDA we issued a request for applications to do this very thing, with positive results. In the absence of explicit funding mechanisms, these kinds of efforts should be continued as best they can through regular funding streams. Obviously the proposed clinical trials network noted above would be an asset for larger scale studies.

The third area is exemplified by an approach we initiated at NIH to facilitate the interaction between publicly funded discovery research, primarily based in academia, and development activities based primarily in the pharmaceutical and biotechnology industries. These two streams of activity are interdependent with respect to medications—the publicly funded base is unlikely to develop a medication and hence relies on industry to take its knowledge to application, and the industry base relies heavily on publicly funded discovery research for the knowledge to advance. Yet the systems tend to function in parallel with limited interaction. NIH itself appears to have recognized the gap and the need for action with its Roadmap initiative in New Pathways to Discovery in which there is explicit resource allocation to, for example, development of a bioactive small-molecule library and screening centres, cheminformatics and imaging probes (Zerhouni 2003).

For nicotine addiction, we took an approach that we believed would both advance the translational agenda and at the same time provide an opportunity to build partnerships with the pharmaceutical industry. Called the National Cooperative Drug Discovery Groups (NCDDG), it is an ongoing effort designed to enhance discovery and the early translation to development. The NCDDG is fundamentally a ligand discovery/development program that encourages investigators with a multidisciplinary range of appropriate expertise to form research groups to advance a molecule towards medication development over a portion of the translational spectrum. That is, the award can support studies over any portion of the range from molecular design to clinical trials. The range of activity across the five groups currently supported in the area of nicotine addiction includes:

- molecular modelling for nAChR ligands and positive modulators of the $GABA_B$ receptor
- synthesis of molecular probes for these receptors
- *in vitro* screening using nAChRs expressed in oocytes and in human cell lines
- screening *in vitro* for effects in neurotransmitter release and on monoamine transporters
- evaluation of brain bioavailability and pharmacokinetics
- evaluation in animal behavioural pharmacology models
- using industry-provided lead compounds in clinical trials for smoking cessation
- developing batteries based on neurophysiology and behaviour that are predictive of clinical outcome
- using neuroimaging to develop correlates and predictors of relapse

The rationale for the NCDDG was the recognition of several realities, including the need for mechanism-of-action-based medications in nicotine addiction, for molecular tools for discovery research, and to facilitate partnerships between academic and industry groups. The awards are not grants in aid of research, but rather cooperative mechanisms in which NIH retains a substantial partnership role by working with the awardees to help overall planning and to look for opportunities to enhance collaboration between the funded groups and thereby build infrastructure. That this should be possible is evident from the impressive range of activities across discovery and development in the funded groups. Although the pharmaceutical partnership is not mandatory, clearly it plays a key role in many of the projects either as a future for the molecules that are developed or in the provision of tools themselves. This latter is a critical point, because it capitalizes on the opportunity for synergy between publicly supported discovery research and the needs of the pharmaceutical industries for target identification and validation in addiction. The NCDDG has the potential to accelerate the discovery of new therapeutics for nicotine addiction, and it also should increase the availability of new pharmacological research tools for both pre-clinical and clinical research. It provides a model of how to increase discovery, increase integration, and derive molecular tools and validate potential medications in a single initiative. In addition, it may be that the partnerships so established increase the comfort level for industry in dealing with granting agencies and tobacco addiction researchers. One benefit of this approach might see industry sharing tools with preclinical investigator teams which have a key set of interdisciplinary models and are focused on discovery and validation for nicotine addiction medications, much in the way that industry uses 'preferred partnerships' with clinical investigators on occasion for trials in which investigators have clinical populations with special characteristics.

References

American Psychiatric Association 1994 Diagnostic and Statistical Manual of Mental Disorders (DSM-IV), 4th edn. American Psychiatric Association, Washington, DC

Balfour D 2005 Complementary roles for the accumbal shell and core in nicotine dependence. In: Understanding nicotine and tobacco addiction. Wiley, Chichester (Novartis Found Symp 275) p 96–115

Brody AL 2005 Localizing tobacco dependence pathways with functional brain imaging. In: Understanding nicotine and tobacco addiction. Wiley, Chichester (Novartis Found Symp 275) p 153–170

Caskey NH, Jarvik ME, Wirshing WC et al 2002 Modulating tobacco smoking rates by dopaminergic stimulation and blockade. Nicotine Tob Res 4:259–266

Corrigall WA, Franklin KB, Coen KM, Clarke PB 1992 The mesolimbic dopaminergic system is implicated in the reinforcing effects of nicotine. Psychopharmacology (Berl) 107:285–289

Corrigall WA, Coen KM, Adamson KL 1994 Self-administered nicotine activates the mesolimbic dopamine system through the ventral tegmental area. Brain Res 8:278–284

Corrigall WA, Coen KM, Adamson KL, Chow BL 1999 Manipulations of mu-opioid and nicotinic cholinergic receptors in the pontine tegmental region alter cocaine self-administration in rats. Psychopharmacology (Berl) 145:412–417

Corrigall WA, Coen KM, Adamson KL, Chow BL, Zhang J 2000 Response of nicotine self-administration in the rat to manipulations of mu-opioid and gamma-aminobutyric acid receptors in the ventral tegmental area. Psychopharmacology (Berl) 149:107–114

Corrigall WA, Coen KM, Zhang J, Adamson KL 2001 GABA mechanisms in the pedunculopontine tegmental nucleus influence particular aspects of nicotine self-administration selectively in the rat. Psychopharmacology (Berl) 158:190–197

Corrigall WA, Coen KM, Zhang J, Adamson L 2002 Pharmacological manipulations of the pedunculopontine tegmental nucleus in the rat reduce self-administration of both nicotine and cocaine. Psychopharmacology (Berl) 160:198–205

Cryan JF, Gasparini F, van Heeke G, Markou A 2003 Non-nicotinic neuropharmacological strategies for nicotine dependence: beyond bupropion. Drug Discov Today 8:1025–1034

Di Chiara G 2000 Behavioural pharmacology and neurobiology of nicotine reward and dependence. In: Clementi F, Fornasari D, Gotti C (eds) Handbook of experimental pharmacology. Springer, Berlin p 603–750

Donny EC, Chaudhri N, Caggiula AR et al 2003 Operant responding for a visual reinforcer in rats is enhanced by noncontingent nicotine: implications for nicotine self-administration and reinforcement. Psychopharmacology (Berl) 169:68–76

George TP, Vessicchio JC, Termine A, Jatlow PI, Kosten TR, O'Malley SS 2003 A preliminary placebo-controlled trial of selegiline hydrochloride for smoking cessation. Biol Psychiatry 53:136–143

Heatherton TF, Kozlowski LT, Frecker RC, Fagerstrom KO 1991 The fagerstrom test for nicotine dependence: a revision of the fagerstrom tolerance questionnaire. Br J Addict 86:1119–1127

Heidbreder C The dopamine D3 system: new opportunities for dopamine-based reward. In: Understanding nicotine and tobacco addiction. Wiley, Chichester (Novartis Found Symp 275) p 116–131

Heidbreder CA, Hagan JJ 2005 Novel pharmacotherapeutic approaches for the treatment of drug addiction and craving. Curr Opin Pharmacol 5:107–118

Lança AJ, Adamson KL, Coen KM, Chow BL, Corrigall WA 2000a The pedunculopontine tegmental nucleus and the role of cholinergic neurons in nicotine self-administration in the rat: a correlative neuroanatomical and behavioral study. Neuroscience 96:735–742

Lança AJ, Sanelli TR, Corrigall WA 2000b Nicotine-induced fos expression in the pedunculopontine mesencephalic tegmentum in the rat. Neuropharmacology 39:2808–2817

Le Foll B, Sokoloff P, Stark H, Goldberg SR 2005 Dopamine D3 receptor ligands block nicotine-induced conditioned place preferences through a mechanism that does not involve discriminative-stimulus or antidepressant-like effects. Neuropsychopharmacology 30:720–730

Mansvelder HD, De Rover M, McGehee DS, Brussaard AB 2003 Cholinergic modulation of dopaminergic reward areas: upstream and downstream targets of nicotine addiction. Eur J Pharmacol 480:117–123

Markou A 2005 Pathways and systems involved in nicotine dependence. In: Understanding nicotine and tobacco addiction. Wiley, Chichester (Novartis Found Symp 275) p 132–152

Maskos U, Granon S, Faure P, Changeux J-P 2005 Nicotinic acetylcholine receptor functions in the central nervous system investigated with a novel method of stereotaxic gene re-expression in knockout mice. In: Understanding nicotine and tobacco addiction. Wiley, Chichester (Novartis Found Symp 275) p 64–82

Picciotto M 2005 Nicotine-mediated activation of signal transduction pathways. In: Understanding nicotine and tobacco addiction. Wiley, Chichester (Novartis Found Symp 275) p 83–95

Piper ME, Piasecki TM, Federman EB et al 2004 A multiple motives approach to tobacco dependence: the Wisconsin Inventory of Smoking Dependence Motives (WISDM-68). J Consult Clin Psychol 72:139–154

Robinson TE, Kolb B 2004 Structural plasticity associated with exposure to drugs of abuse. Neuropharmacology 47 (suppl 1):33–46

Salminen O, Whiteaker P, Grady SR, Collins AC, McIntosh JM, Marks MJ 2005 The subunit composition and pharmacology of alpha-Conotoxin MII-binding nicotinic acetylcholine receptors studied by a novel membrane-binding assay. Neuropharmacology 48:696–705

Shiffman S, Waters A, Hickcox M 2004 The nicotine dependence syndrome scale: a multidimensional measure of nicotine dependence. Nicotine Tob Res 6:327–348

Stolerman I 2005 Animal models for nicotine dependence. In: Understanding nicotine and tobacco addiction. Wiley, Chichester (Novartis Found Symp 275) p 17–35

Tobler PN, Fiorillo CD, Schultz W 2005 Adaptive coding of reward value by dopamine neurons. Science 307:1642–1645

West R 2005 Defining and assessing nicotine dependence in humans. In: Understanding nicotine and tobacco addiction. Wiley, Chichester (Novartis Found Symp 275) p 36–58

Wonnacott S, Sidhpura N, Balfour DJK 2005 Nicotine: from molecular mechanisms to behaviour. Curr Opin Pharmacol 5:53–59

Zerhouni E 2003 The NIH roadmap. Science 302:63–72

DISCUSSION

Balfour: I am going to start with a prejudice. This is that granting bodies in Britain feel that in preclinical research tobacco dependence is solved. People are given nicotine replacement therapy or bupropion-containing medications such as Zyban®. There is no value in researching this further. What we know is that this doesn't work well, but this is a difficult concept to communicate.

Stolerman: I think you'll find that GPs, who should be encouraging their patients to use nicotine replacements or bupropion, are not particularly supportive of these approaches because of their low success rate.

Corrigall: Is the issue that you can't get the funding for the research?

Stolerman: I don't think there is a bias against funding research on nicotine or tobacco. It is driven by the perceptions of review boards on the quality of proposals.

Bertrand: I don't agree. Michele Zoli coordinated an EU project, Tobacogen, that was rated highly and still we couldn't get funding. I know that in Switzerland people feel that nicotine dependence isn't an important challenge.

Corrigall: In the current funding climate, we should remember to build networks and work collaboratively. If there is an issue with funding in the UK or Europe, I would encourage building bridges through the Society for Research on Nicotine and Tobacco (SRNT) or meetings like the present one, and forming partnerships with like-minded investigators based internationally.

Shiffman: We have a different sort of problem. If one puts in a basic science proposal that talks too much about drug development, it is going to be seen as too applied. We have encouraged in this way a style of research that generates basic knowledge but doesn't result in drug development. Conversely in human research if you don't say how this is going to produce a solution or treatment the year after next, it is seen as irrelevant. We are driving human population research in a too-applied direction, and animal research not applied enough.

Corrigall: The first part of your comment is one of the reasons why we put the cooperative group on drug development in place.

Shiffman: I think this meeting has been productive, but I am struck at how little we talk to each other, and the degree to which some of the animal research proceeds without an acute awareness about what we think we know about human nicotine use and tobacco smoking. The human clinical research also proceeds without a lot of knowledge of what is going on in the lab. We almost need to force the situation where a human researcher has to say to an animal researcher, 'Here's the study I want you to do', and vice versa.

Corrigall: I agree, but this is also a two-way street. I think that researchers who work with animal models should be aware of the clinical situation. For example, I was struck in your presentation that people who do reinstatement studies with animal models could benefit from an appreciation of the nature of relapse to tobacco smoking in various human populations, both clinical trial based as well as in real-world populations.

Markou: Part of the NIH roadmap is the emphasis on translational science. Perhaps there should be funding that forces clinical and basic science people to get together so they can do parallel studies in experimental animals and humans to address the same questions. Currently there is no incentive for us to spend our time doing this.

Shiffman: There is actually disincentive, because we each have a different constituency of colleagues who appreciate our work and we respond more to them.

Corrigall: Clearly one issue is that we should talk more frequently. How do we accomplish this?

Shiffman: It takes more than talk; it may take incentives.

West: I think it needs structures. The SRNT potentially has a role to play here, and it turns out that they have a bit of money to spend.

Balfour: There are two issues that strike me. The first is the integration of pre-clinical and clinical research. It does not integrate as well as it should. The second relates to funding. In theory we can do this perfectly well. But in practice it is sometimes more difficult. In the USA, SRNT has access to people who have influence. SRNT does not have access to the right sort of people in Europe. How would you want to spend the money?

Shiffman: The role SRNT could play is not to try to do something on its own, but to help coordinate the efforts to influence the funding.

Corrigall: Could SRNT have an influence on European funding?

West: Probably not. Europe doesn't have the same kind of coherence as the USA does. In the USA an NGO that would be relevant would be SRNT; in Europe there isn't such a thing. But within countries there are potential influential bodies. ASH

UK has a lot of influence, and retains strong links with the academic and political communities.

Chiamulera: Let's try to think of something practical that we can do. You mentioned, in terms of experimental strategies, the 'fingerprinting' of a target. We could also fingerprint a behavioural phenomenon relevant to tobacco addiction from molecular to clinical analysis. From a scientific point of view it is fundamental to have cross-validation across the different levels of investigation. But more resources are needed and it is difficult to do this because we don't have the money: we need sponsors.

Bertrand: What is frustrating is that the tobacco industry has given important amounts of money to European countries on the basis of special agreements, but none of this money has found its way to basic research.

Balfour: Through our local member of the European Parliament, I had some correspondence with the relevant European Commissioner and was told specifically that the money taken from tobacco companies could not be used for research.

Bertrand: I can see a fruitful interaction that could begin any day. I am sure that it would be profitable for us to share more data and influence each others' research. However, I am confident that if we show this and go to politicians they will say that we have been able to do this without supplementary support, so why would they provide further grants?

Shiffman: That is the approach of the politicians. I don't understand European funding mechanisms, but in the USA this would likely ease the way for grant proposals to be regarded more favourably.

Caggiula: Last year at the COGDOP meeting, which is a gathering of chairs of Psychology Departments at research universities in the USA, two people from the American Psychological Association who were liaisons between APA and NSF and NIH, briefed us on projected future trends at those funding agencies. They said that the explicit policy trend at both agencies is big science. It's the physics science model: moving away from funding individual investigators towards a more transdisciplinary, cross-investigator, cross-lab or even cross-campus approach.

Corrigall: You can see this approach in NIH with things like the roadmap. An example is the molecular libraries imaging effort: millions of dollars are being invested to generate new molecules for research purposes, to develop imaging probes, and as starting points for potential new therapeutics.

Final discussion

Nicotine comorbidity

Markou: I wanted us to discuss nicotine comorbidity. This is a topic that hasn't really figured in the presentations. There is a high comorbidity of smoking with psychiatric disorders. Perhaps if better mental health treatment was provided to these populations, then it would be easier for these people to quit smoking. These people are probably self-medicating part of their psychiatric symptoms with nicotine and other components in tobacco. This self-medication provides some clues to basic science as to how aspects of psychiatric disorders can be treated with nicotine receptor agonists.

Jarvis: There are widespread views that nicotine is in some way self medication, either as an anxiolytic to improve mood or counter stress, or as a cognitive enhancer. At the moment we have discrepant views on this. People working in the human area remain unconvinced. The apparent relationships can all be explained in terms of withdrawal relief and so on. Yet we have heard from people on the animal side that nicotine is indeed an anxiolytic and a cognitive enhancer.

Stolerman: I am not among those who argue that the animal data suggest nicotine to be an anxiolytic. Findings are conflicting and other interpretations are possible.

Picciotto: I think there are specific human data out there which are very telling, and explain some of the animal data. For example, Tony George has done nice studies on the effect of quitting smoking on cognitive function in the relatively normal population and in schizophrenic subjects (reviewed in Sacco et al 2004). In his task he has shown that quitting smoking makes the normal subjects get better at his particular cognitive tasks and it makes the schizophrenics get worse. There is a clear dichotomy in the effect of stopping the self-medication on people who started at different baseline. This goes along extremely well with the animal literature. The best effects on cognitive enhancing properties of nicotine come in models of impaired cognition. In normal animals there is some cognitive improvement with nicotine but it isn't that impressive. However, the improvements in impaired animals are greater. The idea that nicotine has very different effects not just on cognition but also on mood depending on the baseline state is supported in many animal and human studies.

Perkins: There is a critical distinction that needs to be made here. When you say 'cognitive enhancer' people assume that it makes you better than normal, but in the human literature no improvement is seen in optimally functioning adults.

Stolerman: We have just spent five years studying improvements in performance induced by nicotine in an attentional task that parallel improvements in attention that are seen in humans; such effects may be the most reproducible form of cognitive enhancement in humans. The effects are small and require a certain amount of pressure on the animals' attentional ability to be seen. It is an oversimplification to say that such effects just don't matter. We need to know more about their importance in relation to self-administration.

Chiamulera: It partly is a matter of definition and nomenclature. What is important is the category of the subject that we study in animal research versus what is studied clinically in humans.

Perkins: Perhaps we should substitute the term cognitive 'restorer' for cognitive enhancer. The former refers to improvement from a suboptimal level.

Shiffman: We tend to take the wrong lesson from the data on comorbidity. Not long ago 80% of British males smoked. This makes it very hard to explain nicotine use as matter of psychopathology. What it suggests is heterogeneity: there may be very different reasons for smoking. Even in the human work we do very little segmentation. The animal research goes so far in the other direction: everything is done with the purest, most homogeneous conditions possible that it becomes completely impossible to address heterogeneity. When we see a result we don't know how much it is due to the homogeneity in that strain and condition. Obviously, you can do a different study in another animal. But it seems that in both camps we are trying too much for universal homogeneity.

Stolerman: The point that you make about animal research is its main strength, not weakness. Conditions are better controlled so that effects of relevant variables can be identified one by one, in the absence of noise due to uncontrolled factors. Heterogeneity is studied all the time, but not on the basis of single individuals for whom results cannot be reproduced, but by comparing between groups of subjects with different previous histories, or by examining how current environmental conditions influence behavioural effects of nicotine, or by working with groups of animals with differing but defined genetic compositions. These are sources of heterogeneity that have been examined in innumerable published studies.

Caggiula: There is a rather large literature in the animal addictions field that specifically addresses individual differences. These studies range from work in rodents showing that behavioural and physiological characteristics of individual animals can predict their response to drugs like amphetamine and nicotine all the way to non-human primate studies demonstrating how polymorphisms in genes controlling neurotransmitter function interact with rearing conditions to determine individual differences in response to alcohol. So the animal research arm of the addictions field is not as 'homogeneous' as you might think.

Hajek: The human data suggest the opposite of what a lot of people believe: that smoking contributes to anxiety and stress.

Picciotto: We see the same in animals. It depends on the condition.

Tyndale: The suggestion from the genetic literature is that there are very different genetic influences on why people start smoking and why they maintain smoking. These genetic influences don't necessarily overlap with how people quit. You can start smoking for all sorts of heterogeneous reasons. Whether you then maintain smoking for those same reasons is not clear. The literature from heritability suggests that there is not a lot of overlap between these stages. There may be something to take from this in terms of how we model the issues that alter who starts smoking from those that then keep them smoking in these different subpopulations.

Animal models

Bertrand: I have one question about animal models. How much of a fluctuation in the blood nicotine level is there when the animal presses the lever? This must be important if nicotine is the determining factor.

Shiffman: Especially the local effects on the brain: because of the disposition in smoking humans from lung directly to brain without passing the liver, the levels seen in before first-pass metabolism are much higher. There has been speculation that this is an important effect, which may not be modelled in the animal studies.

Picciotto: There are certainly differences in pharmacokinetics. But in terms of first-pass metabolism, the confound is not there during jugular self administration. The models aren't bad.

Shiffman: This raises a basic question. There are at least two human studies that purport to show the pharmacokinetics in arterial blood on its way up to the brain. Have such data been published for different methods of administration in the animal literature? There may be an effect for an acute reinforcement that needs a certain level of quick change. This is not to preclude that there is an effect from non-contingent nicotine in the manner that Tony Caggiula's group has proposed.

Balfour: When a rat or human takes a bolus of nicotine, increased dopamine overflow in the nucleus accumbens is quickly established and persists for an hour or more. Thereafter, very little probably happens to dopamine overflow even if the individual takes more drug. We now take the view that this persistent increase in extracellular dopamine plays a central role in the attribution of reinforcing properties to stimuli paired with delivery of the drug. Persistent exposure to nicotine also desensitizes the receptors that mediate its effects on dopamine overflow and during the periods when these receptors are desensitized, as Tony's studies have implied, a rat in an intravenous self-administration paradigm is responding primarily for the conditioned stimuli rather than nicotine itself. Thus, the effects of nicotine are rapid and, when given to abstinent animals, fairly persistent. Importantly, however, once the nicotine has exerted its effect, probably within the first few minutes of the trial, subsequent nicotine injections have little or no further effects. Nevertheless, the rat learns to press for nicotine because the behaviour continues to be reinforced over the period that extracellular dopamine in the nucleus accumbens remains elevated. The hypothesis predicts that, similarly, when people smoke, the first two or three puffs produce increased dopamine release in the accumbens; thereafter they continue to smoke primarily for the reinforcing properties of the habit *per se* and the conditioned stimuli present in the smoke.

Stolerman: There never will be a complete model. The real situation is too complex. What we try to do is to hypothesize about the importance of specific mechanisms and then try to isolate them so that they can be studied.

Bizarro: I would like to remind people that a lot of research in psychology progressed studying self administration of food in rats that pressed levers to get the food. No one really cares that the food is completely different, or the amount of food ingested is different from human feeding.

Shiffman: Everyone is saying that it doesn't matter, but we don't know that it doesn't.

Bizarro: I'm not saying that. The problem is with the model itself or the acceptance of the data derived from the animal models. I have one foot in clinical work and one in basic science. Basic science can bring important hypotheses to the clinic and vice versa. However, it is necessary to accept the imperfections of models. Models are not complete or perfect. This is not what models are for. Models are for providing straight answers to specific questions. In the clinical field we don't have this, but we do have the validity and relevance of the subject. Unfortunately, due to limitations of the scientific method, if you control too much you may be sure of your results but these can't be transposed directly. This bridge has to be built by both clinicians and basic scientists. I would also add that all science is 'basic science': the moment one uses scientific method, this is one approach of the subject one would like to study, it is not the subject itself. Scientists have to accept and understand the limitations of scientific method

Reference

Sacco KA, Bannon KL, George TP 2004 Nicotinic receptor mechanisms and cognition in normal states and neuropsychiatric disorders. J Psychopharmacol 18:457–474

Contributor Index

Subject Index

A

α-bungarotoxin (α-BgT) 66, 85, 92
α-calcitonin gene-related peptide (α-CGRP)
    111
α-conotoxin MII 66
α7 antagonists 91–92
abstinence *see* cessation of smoking
acamprosate 128
ACC *see* anterior cingulate cortex
accumbal shell and core *see* nucleus
    accumbens
acetaldehyde 23, 106, 206
acetylcholine *see* nicotinic receptors
acquired drive 36
adrenal chromaffin cells, signal transduction
    84, 86
alcohol 233, 263
    dependence criteria 37, 39, 53, 57
    dopamine system 116–117, 125, 126,
        128–129
    pharmacogenomics 184
Alzheimer's disease 168
American Psychiatric Association 19, 36–48,
    50, 52–54
ammonia 206
amphetamine 263
    functional brain imaging 158
    nucleus accumbens 97, 98–100, 105, 109
amusias 110
amygdala 118–119, 127, 134, 140
anhedonia 132, 138, 148–150
animal models 17–35, 264–265
    advantages 20–22
    cessation of smoking 17–18, 24–26
    chronic conditions 19–20
    conditioned place preference 21
    defining addiction 1

drug discrimination methods 21–22
extinction behaviour 33–34
hedonic effects 30, 31
limitations 20–22
measurement issues 22–23
motivation to quit 24–26, 30, 33
punishment 24–26
reinforcement 20–21, 25–26, 28–30,
    32–34, 264
stereotaxic gene re-expression 64–82
target definition 18–19
tobacco versus nicotine 23, 29
withdrawal syndromes 19, 21, 34
see also reinforcement; self-administration
ANKK1 gene 180, 184, 186, 191, 195
anterior cingulate cortex (ACC) 118–120,
    124, 126, 154–155, 162–163, 191–192
anterior temporal lobe 154–155
antidepressants 18, 148–150, 185, 198, 239
antineoplastics 239, 244
antipsychotics 123–124
anxiety 168–169, 262, 263
aortic aneurysm 5, 6
ASH 260–261
associations 168
autocrine action 202
autoradiography 153
aversion levels 61–62

B

β2 nicotinic receptor subunits 22
baclofen 18, 128, 136–137, 152
basolateral subregion of the amygdala (BLA)
    118–119, 127
Bayesian approaches 197
BDNF *see* brain-derived neurotrophic factor
behavioural factors 2